Instructor's Manual to Accompany
Radiographic Imaging

Instructor's Manual to Accompany
Radiographic Imaging

Mosby's Radiographic Instructional Series

Mosby

St. Louis Baltimore Boston Carlsbad Chicago Minneapolis New York Philadelphia Portland
London Milan Sydney Tokyo Toronto

Mosby
Dedicated to Publishing Excellence

A Times Mirror Company

Publisher: Don Ladig
Executive Editor: Jeanne Rowland
Developmental Editor: Carole Glauser
Project Manager: Gayle May Morris
Associate Production Editor: Lisa M. Kearney
Manufacturing Manager: Betty Mueller

Photographic assistance generously provided by the Radiology Department staffs at Missouri Baptist Medical Center, St. Louis, Missouri and Ana Jaques Hospital, Newburyport, Massachusetts.

Scripting and editorial services provided by Tom Lochhaas.

Audio production by Smith/Lee Productions, Inc.

Multimedia program development by Monotype Composition Company, Inc.

Printed in the United States of America
Composition by Black Dot

Mosby
11830 Westline Industrial Drive
St. Louis, MO 63146

www.mosby.com

ISBN 0-8151-5409-7

99 00 01 02 03 / 9 8 7 6 5 4 3 2 1

REVIEWERS

Kathleen P. Euganeo, MS, RT(R)
Instructor, Radiologic Technology Program
Delaware Technical Community College
Christiana Care Health System
Wilmington, Delaware

Jon Hartwein, BA, RT(R)
Faculty, Radiologic Technology
St. Louis Community College at Forest Park
St. Louis, Missouri

Kevin C. Seisler, BA, RT(R)
Assistant Director, Mayo Radiographic Program
Mayo Clinic
Rochester, Minnesota

Dwayne TerMaat, MEd, RT(R)
Professor, Radiologic Technology
St. Louis Community College at Forest Park
St. Louis, Missouri

Introduction

This instructor's manual is designed to accompany *Mosby's Radiographic Instructional Series: Radiographic Imaging*. This manual will be a valuable resource for use with both the slide/audiotape and the CD-ROM versions of the program. Another resource that will enhance teaching and learning from the multimedia program is the *Radiographic Imaging Study Guide*, which your students may purchase for their own use. Details on the study guide and how to use it appear at the end of this introductory section.

THE MULTIMEDIA PROGRAM

The slide/audiotape and the CD-ROM versions of the program are similar in many respects, although the CD-ROM version contains additional material, including images and audio, not included in the slide/audiotape version. The slide/audiotape version of *Radiographic Imaging* covers the topics typically taught in the imaging component of the radiography curriculum, organized to follow the ASRT curriculum outline. Each of the eight modules is approximately 1 hour in duration, if presented without interruptions.

Instructor Mode

The CD-ROM version functions in two different ways, depending on how you chose to use it with your students. In the "instructor" mode, you run the program on the computer in the same way as a slide/audiotape program. Students view the program on one or more monitors, or you may project the images if you have the equipment capability. In the instructor mode, students do not interact with the program from a computer keyboard. Even in the instructor mode, however, the CD-ROM program offers options such as running only selected portions or selecting individual image/sound segments. Another feature is the use of animation in certain subject areas—a functionality obviously not possible in the slide version. The content of the program in the instructor mode is, however, essentially the same as in the slide/audiotape program.

Student Mode

In the "student" mode, the other way of using the CD-ROM, the student interacts individually with the program using the computer's keyboard and mouse. The student may select topic areas within each of the eight modules or view the module in a linear manner from start to finish. Along the way the student has options, such as asking for more information or repeating particular segments for review. The program interacts with the student by asking questions at intervals and then providing feedback on the individual student's responses. Because of the additional material available in the student mode, the time required to work through a given module will generally be longer than the slide/audiotape program or instructor mode CD-ROM presentation. Some students may complete the material in an hour; others may need or want more time. In any case, students control the pace and can quit at most points along the way.

Testing Options

Both the slide/audiotape and CD-ROM versions include a self-assessment quiz followed by an examination at the end of each module. The self-assessment is intended as just that: a series of questions followed by a discussion of the correct and incorrect answers to help students assess how well they understand the material after working through the program. As the instructor, if you are using the slide/audio or CD-ROM instructor mode program, you can ask students to write their answers on a sheet of paper and score these themselves. The examination, on the other hand, is more like formal testing. All the questions are multiple choice, and students are not given the answers afterward. (The answers to the examination for each module are in the corresponding modules of this manual.) In the CD-ROM version functioning in the student mode, the student's answers are scored and saved on the computer's hard drive and can be accessed by the instructor. Documentation provided with the CD-ROM version describes this process.

INSTRUCTOR'S MANUAL ORGANIZATION

The eight modules in this instructor's manual have the following parts:

Overview

This section begins with a brief outline of the multimedia module's content and then describes the key concepts and information. This is intended to help you review, in a brief format, the material your students have experienced or are about to experience.

Learning Objectives

Learning objectives are stated in the behavioral terms, listing the expectations one can have for student learning for each module.

Key Terms

Key terms used in each module are listed alphabetically; these are terms that may be new to students. The study guide provides full definitions of these terms for students.

Instructional Outline

This section is a more detailed presentation of the content in the multimedia program.

Teaching Tips

Specifically designed for instructors who may be new to the teaching of radiographic imaging, this section presents ways of looking at the material in the module and tips for how to explain it to students. In general, you may choose to have students experience the multimedia program first or after reading a textbook chapter, and then follow up this experience with study guide assignments and/or your own instruction. The tips in these sections of the instructor's manual are directed to this last stage of teaching.

Study Guide Posttest Answers

Answers are provided along with brief rationales for the correct answer.

Testbank Questions

A group of 20 multiple-choice questions are provided for your use for further teaching or evaluation of students.

Audiovisual Script

This is a listing of the images and narration used in the slide/audiotape and CD-ROM program. With this listing you may customize your use of the multimedia program by selecting or reordering images or by showing them individually with your presentations.

Answers to the Multimedia Examinations

At the end of each of the modules is a multiple-choice examination, the answers to which are not included in the multimedia program. The correct answers appear at the end of each module in this instructor's manual.

THE STUDY GUIDE

This multimedia instructional program, along with the accompanying study guide, will provide students with a solid foundation in the principles of radiographic imaging such as equipment components, factors affecting recorded detail, technique, and film processing, and how these principles can be applied in the clinical setting. This program may be used for both initial instruction and review. It is intended to supplement, not replace,the use of a textbook in the radiographic imaging curriculum.

The accompanying study guide was developed to enhance the teaching value of the multimedia presentation. The eight modules in the study guide correspond to the eight modules of the multimedia program. Students should experience the multimedia program first, and then read and work thorough the accompanying module in the study guide. The different parts of each module encourage students to review and apply what they learn from the corresponding multimedia module.

Self-Assessment Pretest

The Self-Assessment Pretest is a group of 10 multiple-choice questions designed to help students determine how much of the material they have already mastered from the multimedia program before beginning to review this material in the study guide. The correct answers are presented afterward. Students who incorrectly answer some questions are encouraged to pay more attention to those subjects as they proceed through the other part of the study guide module.

Key Terms

Key Terms is a brief glossary section that defines important terms introduced in the multimedia program. A clear understanding of these terms—and the concepts represented by the terms—is important for students before they proceed. These terms are used in following parts of the module, helping students become more familiar with them and their importance in radiography.

Topical Outline

The Topical Outline presents in a brief format the primary information and knowledge covered by the multimedia module. As when reading the definitions of key terms, students should pay particular attention to areas they do not understand as well.

Review

The Review asks students to interact with the material that has been briefly introduced through the Key Terms and Outline sections. They are encouraged to write in the terms and phrases indicated by the blank lines in these descriptive and explanatory statements. It is important in this exercise that students become more familiar with the terminology and concepts related to the module's content. Some artwork is included in this section, usually a variation of illustrations used in the multimedia program, to enhance the learning and retention of important concepts or processes.

Learning Quiz

The Learning Quiz is unique among the various parts in that it is not intended to be used by students who have worked through the CD-ROM version of the multimedia program in what is called the "student mode" (a student at the computer working through the learning program). In other words, this section is intended only for those students who have seen the slide/audiotape version or the CD-ROM program presented to them in instructor mode, without experiencing the program individually at the computer. If your students have already worked through the full interactive program at the computer, they can, if they choose, skip over this section, which includes exercises they will already have experienced in the computer tutorial. On the other hand, repeating these exercises in the study guide format may be valuable as additional review. These exercises are designed to increase mastery of the material by answering questions that require knowledge and understanding of key information that has been presented so far.

Applications

Applications addresses the module's concepts and information at a higher level by asking questions that require students to apply what they have learned in different situations or examples. Working these programs necessitates a fuller understanding of the material—how the principles of imaging apply to the specific topic. These questions are in some ways the most difficult in the module because they involve more than just defining terms or repeating information. Ask students to take their time with these. If they have difficulty with certain topics, they should return to the Key Terms and Outline sections to review them. Students who do well in answering these questions usually have a good grasp of the material in this module.

Posttest

The Posttest is the final section in each module. It consists of an average of 20 multiple-choice questions designed to assess student understanding and retention of the information in the unit. The answers to this section, unlike other sections, are not included in the study guide, but are printed here in the instructor's manual at the end of each module. This allows you to use the posttest for more formal evaluation of your students if desired.

Note that the study guide is not intended for use without the multimedia program. The study guide presentation is effective as a review, but does not convey the wealth of information given by the multimedia program. The study guide does not attempt, therefore, to replace a textbook in radiographic imaging. It is intended to make the learning experience more satisfying, while at the same time helping students learn, master, and remember what may be new or difficult material.

As always, Mosby welcomes your comments on this and all our publications for students and practitioners in the imaging technologies.

Contents

Radiographic Equipment 1

Overview

X-ray discovery
- Dr. Roentgen and Crookes tube
- Early hazards discovery
- Current medical and dental uses

Types of equipment and exams
- Radiography and fluoroscopy
- Tubes, tables, consoles
- CT

Suspension systems
- Radiation protection

This module introduces students to the basics of radiographic equipment, forming the basis for future use of this equipment for a variety of examinations.

The module begins with an overview of radiography's history, starting with Dr. Roentgen's experiments with a Crookes tube and progressing to modern uses of radiography, fluoroscopy, and CT scanning. Radiation burns and the earliest interest in protection are included.

Modern equipment that is briefly introduced and described includes multipurpose radiographic units, dedicated units such as head units and mammographic units, mobile units, and fluoroscopic units. The basic elements of the tube, table, and console are described.

The tube housing and various kinds of tube suspension systems are included also to introduce students to the wide variety of equipment in use today.

Finally, many types of radiation protection equipment and barriers are described, to complete the student's understanding of the design of a radiographic suite.

Learning Objectives

Upon completion of this module, the student should be able to do the following:

1. Define all the key terms in the module.
2. Give a brief history of radiography from Dr. Roentgen's experiments to the present.
3. Explain why radiation protection is important.
4. Describe the differences between radiography and fluoroscopy and give examples of how each is used.
5. Describe several different types of general purpose and dedicated radiographic units.
6. Describe at least four types of tube suspension systems.
7. Explain the difference between primary and secondary radiation protection.
8. Successfully complete the activities and posttest in the Study Guide.

Key Terms

Bucky assembly
C-arm unit
Cathode ray
Contrast medium
Computed tomography
Control console
Crookes tube
Floating table top
Fluoroscopy
Grid
Head unit
Housing
Linear tomography
Mammographic unit
Primary radiation
Radiation protection
Radiolucent
Scatter radiation
Secondary radiation
Suspension system
Upright unit

Instructional Outline

I. X-rays were discovered in the late nineteenth century and became the focus of much experimentation for decades.
   A. Dr. Roentgen, in 1895, discovered the unknown, invisible rays produced by a Crookes tube could pass through objects and make a fluorescent screen glow.
      1. Roentgen discovered that some objects are radiolucent and others radiopaque.
      2. By chance Roentgen discovered he could obtain an image of bones within the body by passing x-rays through his hand. A radiograph of his wife's hand was the first published radiograph.
   B. In 1896 the first medical use was made of radiography to view a broken wrist.

C. In 1898 Dr. Rollins first published warnings of the potential harmful effects of radiation after experiencing skin burns from his experiments with x-rays.
D. In the 1940s and 1950s the hazards of x-rays were examined more carefully, leading to an increasing interest in protective devices.
E. Now, some 200 million medical and 100 million dental radiographs are made every year in the United States.
F. In the middle and late twentieth century, imaging technology has continued to expand and now includes computed tomography, magnetic resonance imaging, and other diagnostic modalities for imaging body structures. Radiation is also used in the treatment of some conditions such as tumors.

II. Modern radiography has evolved into a wide spectrum of imaging procedures using a variety of types of equipment.
  A. Radiography and fluoroscopy are the two main types of radiologic examinations.
    1. Radiography uses x-rays to produce static images on film.
    2. Fluoroscopy uses x-rays to produce dynamic images on a monitor.
    3. Specialized examinations are used to image different structures and to observe changes within the body such as with the insertion of a catheter or the movement of a fluid through vessels.
  B. There are many types of radiographic equipment.
    1. Dedicated radiographic equipment is used only for specific functions, such as a head unit or mammography unit.
    2. Multipurpose radiographic equipment is used for many different types of examinations.
    3. Mobile radiographic or fluoroscopic units are used outside the radiology department, often in emergency rooms, intensive care units, or surgical suites.
  C. Examination tables, like the x-ray tube itself, can be angled and moved in various ways to allow very controlled exposure of the desired body area.
  D. In addition to the tube and the table, the third key element in all radiographic equipment is the image receptor device, such as the film cassette or the Bucky tray that holds the film and grid, usually mounted under the examining table.
  E. The fourth key element is the control, or operating, console, which contains the controls the radiologic technologist uses to set the tube current, voltage, exposure time, and other settings for an examination.
  F. Conventional tomography and computed tomography are additional modalities using x-ray exposure.
    1. Conventional, or linear, tomography uses special equipment that moves the film and x-ray tube to produce images that highlight structures in a certain focal plane.
    2. In computed tomography, also called CT scanning, a computer creates a cross-sectional image from exposures taken in a complete circle around the body.

III. In addition to the x-ray tube and image receptor, other parts of radiographic equipment are important.
  A. The tube housing absorbs x-rays that otherwise would "leak" out from the tube in directions other than in the useful beam.
  B. The x-ray tube and tube housing are structurally supported, or suspended, in different ways in different types of equipment.
    1. An overhead suspension system is mounted on the ceiling, with rails and adjustments to allow the tube to be directed in many different ways.
    2. A floor-to-ceiling suspension system mounts the tube on rails mounted to both ceiling and floor.
    3. A floor-mounted suspension system uses rails or support columns mounted on the floor or the table.

4. A variety of mobile systems have been developed in which the tube is suspended from a stand on a mobile base.
5. The C-arm suspension system holds the tube on one end of the arm and the image receptor on the other; these systems may be mobile or fixed.

IV. Modern radiology suites generally have permanently installed equipment in a design that also incorporates radiation protection devices.

A. Lead sheets are often built into the walls of examination rooms to prevent exposures by primary, scatter, or leakage radiation.

B. Secondary radiation protective barriers and shields include a variety of devices to absorb secondary radiation and protect both the radiographer and patient from unwanted exposure.

Teaching Tips

History

Students do not automatically find history interesting. However, because the historical roots of radiography do have relevance for modern radiographers, students can gain from an understanding of the early years of radiography, starting with Dr. Roentgen. As you talk with students, try to help them see the tremendous excitement of discovering how one can look inside the body, a capability we might take for granted now but that was such a great breakthrough for medicine. This helps provide a context for the meaning of the profession. Similarly, help them glimpse how it was that the hazards of x-ray beams were not fully appreciated by many at first; however, the dangers surfaced almost immediately in the form of skin burns experienced by the early experimenters. Point out that as they learn more and more about performing radiographic examinations, the focus on protection and safety concerns will never diminish; the hazards are still as real as they once were, although radiography may now seem much more routine than a century ago.

Radiography and Fluoroscopy

After ensuring that all students understand the similarities and differences in radiography and fluoroscopy, it may be helpful to briefly look ahead in their education to a discussion of image receptors. Some students may be tempted to oversimplify the difference between radiography and fluoroscopy and think only that the former is done with film, the latter with a television monitor. Explain that with both, the image can be preserved and analyzed on film, on a monitor, or in a computerized digital format. Make sure they see that the essential difference is static vs. moving images. Although this module does not discuss the higher patient exposures that result from fluoroscopy rather than radiography, you may choose to discuss this briefly so that they understand that fluoroscopy is used only when it is essential to be able to see movement within the body.

Radiographic Equipment

Obviously students can learn more about radiographic equipment by actually seeing it in person, moving it about, and working with it; however, the basic concepts behind the equipment and its various types are well suited for the classroom. This module introduces several basic types, urging students to understand the variety of types of equipment in practice today, although they may not see all types in their clinical student experience. To help students grasp the similarities and differences among different types of equipment, you might point out and comment upon details shown in the illustrations in this module. For example, it can be helpful to show students how the equipment they will soon work with is similar to or different from the equipment they are observing in this module. Always remind them that equipment is continually evolving with new technological advances, and help them understand the general principles behind the equipment so that they don't get lost in the details. For example, keep the focus on why the examination table top should be designed for flexibility in positioning the patient in different ways for different exams; this general principle is much more important than details of a floating vs. a fixed table top.

As students learn about other aspects of the equipment, such as the tube housing and the tube suspension system, keep the focus on the principles involved. It is not as important for students to describe the difference between an overhead suspension system and a floor-to-ceiling suspension system as it is to understand why the unit should allow movement of the tube in almost all directions and be capable of holding the tube perfectly motionless during the examination.

Understanding dedicated radiographic units also is important, both for the theoretical understanding of why such units have value and for introducing students to the world of practice awaiting them. Mammographic units are found in most larger departments everywhere, for example, and students should come to understand not only the technical reasons for the unique aspects of this equipment but also the larger context of how the equipment is used. You might even take a moment to explain the importance of mammographic screening at different ages in light of the current recommendations from the American Cancer Society. Such a context helps students understand not only a particular piece of equipment but also the value of their profession within the larger health community.

Finally, an effective way to help students grasp the uses of such a variety of equipment is to describe for them a "day in the life" of a radiographer in a busy hospital, using descriptions of real or fictional patients. Include special examinations such as arteriography for someone with a suspected renal blockage, and include applications for mobile equipment, such as a trauma patient in the emergency room who needs a cervical spine radiograph. You may also help students retain this material by providing them with a variety of patient scenarios and ask them what equipment might be used in different situations. Such discussions help students move away from the "dry facts"of equipment to a larger perspective involving the radiographer's daily practice.

Radiation Protection

Only the very basics of radiation protection are introduced in this module. It is important for students to understand from the beginning, as they learn about equipment in the radiographic suite, that protection is important and involves many different types of equipment and safeguards. This module introduces only the basics: lead lining in the walls, the tube housing, and barriers. In your teaching you can link the need for such protection to the historical roots at the beginning of this module; the radiation burns and the deaths suffered by so many of the first experimenters with x-rays. Particularly important is scatter radiation; students easily grasp that they need to be protected from exposure to the primary beam, but some students will not easily conceptualize how scatter can be produced virtually anywhere in the area of the x-ray equipment exposure and spread out in virtually all directions.

Workbook Posttest Answers and Rationales

1. What was the earliest tube used in the discovery of x-rays called?
   a. Roentgen tube
   b. Crookes tube—This early cathode tube was being used in experiments when Roentgen first discovered x-rays.
   c. Rollins tube
   d. Sodium vapor tube

2. About how many medical and dental radiographs are taken every year in the United States?
   a. 1 million
   b. 50 million
   c. 300 million—Of these, about 100 million are dental radiographs.
   d. 2 billion

3. Radiography, computed tomography, ultrasonography, and MRI are similar in that all involve which of the following?
   a. X-radiation passing through the body
   b. Electromagnetic energy passing through the body
   c. Imaging structures inside the body—Note that ultrasonography uses sound waves, not radiation of any sort.
   d. None of the above

4. Which of the following is a common use of fluoroscopy?
   a. To track the insertion of a catheter
   b. To observe a fluid moving through the gastrointestinal tact
   c. To see the movement of a contrast medium in blood vessels
   d. All of the above—All these gain from the dynamic imaging of fluoroscopy.
   e. None of the above

5. Dynamic fluoroscopic images are shown on which of the following?
   a. A monitor—Fluoroscopy does not normally use film, although images can be stored and printed out.
   b. Fluoroscopic film
   c. Both a monitor and fluoroscopic film
   d. Standard radiographic film

6. Which of the following is true of a floating radiographic table?
   a. It floats over a shallow pool of water.
   b. It moves laterally but not longitudinally.
   c. It moves longitudinally but not laterally.
   d. It moves both laterally and longitudinally—It is called "floating" because it can move in any direction.

7. The standard radiographic tabletop must always be which of the following?
   a. **Radiolucent**—It must let x-rays pass through because the film is positioned under the tabletop.
   b. Radiopaque
   c. Shielded from the primary beam
   d. All of the above

8. What is the source of most of the scatter radiation that grids are designed to absorb?
   a. The Bucky assembly
   b. The x-ray tube housing
   c. The radiographic film
   d. **The patient**—Scatter radiation may be produced in any substance through which x-rays pass, but most scatter radiation is produced as the primary beam passes into and through the patient.

9. Why is a barrier positioned between the patient area and the operating console?
   a. To prevent the patient from seeing the controls and settings
   b. **To prevent radiation from reaching the radiographer**—Scatter radiation from the patient and the entire area around the patient may be radiated toward the console area, which is therefore protected to shield the radiographer.
   c. To protect delicate electronic equipment from x-ray damage
   d. To prevent scatter radiation from the console from reaching the film

10. Upon which principle does linear tomography work?
   a. Alpha and gamma rays react in special ways to create a different image.
   b. Averaging multiple exposures produces a clearer image than any one exposure.
   c. **By moving the x-ray tube and film in opposite directions, only structures in a certain focal plane are in focus**—This is the basic process underlying linear tomography; other structures outside the focal plane are blurred and have less visibility in the image produced.
   d. The computer can assemble a cross-sectional image from multiple exposures.

11. In computed tomography, how does the x-ray tube move?
   a. **In a full circle around the patient**—The computer then assembles a cross-sectional image from the exposures from all sides of the patient
   b. Back and forth in a half-circle under and around the patient
   c. Side to side in a horizontal plane over the patient
   d. None of the above

12. Which of the following would occur without a housing around the x-ray tube?
   a. No x-rays could reach the patient.
   b. The x-ray tube would rapidly overheat.
   c. The x-ray tube would be easily broken when moved.
   d. **X-rays would emerge out in all directions from the tube**—The primary function of the housing is to absorb radiation exiting the tube in all directions expect for the primary beam out the tube window.

13. Which of the following is true of a tube suspension system?
    a. It supports the x-ray tube.
    b. It may be fixed or mobile.
    c. It allows movement of the x-ray tube.
    d. **All of the above are true**—These are different ways x-ray tubes are held suspended.
    e. None of the above

14. In a C-arm suspension system, you can adjust which of the following?
    a. The distance between the tube and the image receptor
    b. **The angle of the C-arm**—The distance between tube and receptor is fixed, but the arm's angle can be adjusted in different directions.
    c. Both of the above
    d. Neither of the above

15. Locks on an overhead tube suspension system prevent which of the following?
    a. Theft
    b. Electrical shock
    c. **Unwanted movement of the equipment**—Movement of the equipment during an exposure could lead to a less clear image.
    d. All of the above

16. A mobile radiographic unit may be used in which of the following?
    a. An emergency room
    b. An operating room
    c. An intensive care unit
    d. **All of the above**—These are all common uses of mobile units.
    e. None of the above

17. Which of the following is a challenge in using mobile radiographic equipment?
    a. **Positioning very ill patients**—Often these patients are too ill or injured to be moved to the radiology department, so the radiographer takes a mobile unit to them.
    b. Moving the heavy equipment
    c. Arranging for necessary electrical power levels outside the radiology department
    d. All of the above
    e. None of the above

18. Radiation protection built into the radiology department may include which of the following?
    a. Thick aluminum walls
    b. Flowing water absorption systems
    c. **Sheets of lead built into the walls**—Lead is the best material to absorb x-radiation.
    d. All of the above
    e. None of the above

19. Protection from scatter radiation includes which of the following?
   a. X-ray tube housing
   b. The radiographic tabletop
   c. **Barriers between the radiographer and the patient**—Because most scatter radiation is produced in the patient, barriers between the patient and the radiographer are important.
   d. All of the above
   e. None of the above

20. Materials that may be used in secondary radiation barriers include which of the following?
   a. Glass
   b. Lead acrylic
   c. Gypsum board
   d. **All of the above**—Although lead is used mostly for barriers to primary radiation, these other materials have lead equivalency for protection from secondary radiation.
   e. None of the above

Testbank Questions

1. The Crookes tube has all but which one of these parts in it?
   a. Anode
   b. Partial vacuum
   c. Focus cup
   d. Cathode

2. One of the earliest medical applications of x-rays was for imaging which of the following?
   a. Bone fractures
   b. The brain
   c. Cardiac arrhythmias
   d. All of the above

3. Which one of these imaging modalities does *not* use x-rays?
   a. Fluoroscopy
   b. CT scanning
   c. Ultrasonography
   d. Conventional tomography

4. Cardiac catheterization is a procedure usually accomplished with the help of which imaging modality?
   a. Fluoroscopy
   b. CT scanning
   c. Ultrasonography
   d. Conventional tomography

5. Which of the following statements is false?
   a. Fluoroscopy and radiography both use x-rays.
   b. Fluoroscopy and radiography both are used to make static images only.
   c. Fluoroscopy and radiography both involve patient exposure.
   d. Fluoroscopy and radiography can both be performed with some equipment.

6. Which of the following is considered a "dedicated unit"?
   a. A BRS (basic radiographic system)
   b. A CT scanner
   c. An R/F (radiographic/fluoroscopic) unit
   d. A mammographic unit

7. The best radiographic table top is made from which of the following?
   a. Lead
   b. Wood
   c. Plastic
   d. Any of the above

8. What is the purpose of a grid?
   a. To absorb scatter radiation
   b. To help hold the patient motionless during the exposure
   c. To focus the x-ray beam only on the part being examined
   d. To protect the radiographer from leakage radiation

9. Scatter radiation inside the examining room may move in what direction?
   a. From the patient outward in any direction
   b. From the table outward in any direction
   c. From the air between the tube and the patient, in any direction
   d. All of the above
   e. None of the above

10. In most examining rooms, where is the control console located?
    a. Immediately beneath the tube
    b. Attached to the front of the table
    c. Outside the room or behind a barrier
    d. Wherever the radiographer positions it

11. What moves during a conventional tomography exposure?
    a. The patient
    b. The tube only
    c. The film only
    d. Both the tube and the film

12. The image produced by CT scanning is which of the following?
    a. An anteroposterior view
    b. Dynamic (moving)
    c. A cross section
    d. All of the above

13. Which of the following is true of an overhead suspension system?
   a. Often mounts the tube from rails on the ceiling
   b. Is used for dedicated head units
   c. Holds the radiographic film in a special tray on the ceiling
   d. Is used only for large patients

14. What kind of equipment is most likely to be used in an intensive care unit?
   a. Mobile unit
   b. CT scanner
   c. R/F unit
   d. Linear tomographic unit

15. Who needs to be protected from radiation during the radiographic examination?
   a. The patient
   b. The radiographer
   c. Others in the building
   d. All of the above
   e. None of the above

16. Scatter radiation is what type of radiation?
   a. Leakage radiation
   b. Primary radiation
   c. Secondary radiation
   d. Gamma ray radiation

17. Which of the following types of radiographic units can ONLY make exposures with the patient standing?
   a. Floor-to-ceiling suspension systems
   b. Floor-mounted suspension systems
   c. Ceiling-mounted suspension systems
   d. All of the above
   e. None of the above

18. A cracked tube housing could result in what kind of problem?
   a. An underexposed image
   b. Leakage radiation
   c. Heat burns to the patient
   d. All of the above
   e. None of the above

19. A contrast medium is used to do which of the following?
   a. To immobilize a certain body area or part to prevent motion blur
   b. To mix the light and dark tones on a radiograph to a medium gray
   c. To make a certain body area or part more radiopaque
   d. To make a certain body area or part more radiolucent

20. The "C" in CT scanning stands for which of the following?
    a. Conventional
    b. Computed
    c. Coordinated
    d. Circular

Answers to Testbank Questions

1. c	6. d	11. d	16. c
2. a	7. c	12. c	17. e
3. c	8. a	13. a	18. b
4. a	9. d	14. a	19. c
5. b	10. c	15. d	20. b

Audiovisual Script

SLIDE 1-1/CD 1-i Welcome
Welcome to Mosby's Radiographic Instructional Series.

SLIDE 1-2/CD 1-ii Radiographic equipment
The module you are about to experience is the first of eight in the Radiographic Imaging program: Radiographic Equipment.

This module will introduce you to the many types of radiographic equipment and their components. You'll learn the purposes of different types of equipment and how the images they record are used in diagnosing the patient's condition. You'll also learn about equipment installed for permanent use, as well as mobile units, and how to use proper radiation protection when new units are installed.

SLIDE 1-3/CD 1-1 Introduction
Over the course of your studies in radiography, you'll come to understand a great deal about radiographic equipment and how it works. This will set the stage for what you will learn later about using radiographic equipment and performing radiographic examinations of patients.

We'll begin this module by looking at how the use of x-rays developed and how they are used to diagnose patients.

SLIDE 1-4/CD 1-2 Creation of x-rays

The idea behind the way radiographic equipment works is simple. Imagine many high-speed electrons bombarding a piece of metal. The kinetic energy from the electrons turns into electromagnetic energy. The energy from the electrons becomes x-rays.

The job of radiographic equipment is to convert the energy of electrons into electromagnetic energy and direct it in useful ways to help diagnose and treat illness. The equipment must produce and control electron flow so that the x-rays created are of a diagnostically useful quality.

SLIDE 1-5/CD 1-3 Roentgen

Amazingly, x-rays were discovered quite by accident. The first person to see the "unseeable," the inside of a living body, was an obscure German physicist, Dr. Wilhelm Conrad Roentgen.

In November of 1895, Dr. Roentgen was experimenting with a Crookes tube, the forerunner of fluorescent and neon lamps. At the time, researchers in physics departments of many European universities were studying the way cathode rays, or electrons, were conducted through glass tubes. Colorful flashes of energy were created by applying electricity to metal electrodes in the tubes.

There were several different types of Crookes tubes. Most of them could produce x-rays, although no one understood that yet. Several other physicists had seen the results of x-radiation, but they didn't recognize what it was or how important it would be. Dr. Roentgen did, however, and his discovery changed the world.

CD 1-3A Crookes tube

Sir William Crookes was a late nineteenth century English scientist after whom the Crookes tube was named. There were many different types of Crookes tubes capable of producing x-radiation.

The basic design of the tube was simple: it consisted of a positive and a negative electrode within a sealed glass tube. When air was removed from it with a vacuum pump, trace amounts of elemental gases (hydrogen, mercury, sodium, or neon vapor) could then be introduced into the tube so their electrical conductive properties could be studied. When a current, what we know today to be a flow of electrons, passed through the gas in the tube, the gas would glow with a distinctive color.

SLIDE 1-6/CD 1-4 Roentgen's discovery

While he was working in his lab on November 8, 1895, Dr. Roentgen wrapped his Crookes tube in black paper so he could get a better idea of the effects of the cathode rays in the tube without being distracted by the flashes inside it. Then he energized the cathode ray-producing tube.

As it happened, a screen coated with a fluorescent material, barium platinocyanide, was sitting on a table about a yard away. When Dr. Roentgen switched on the current, a faint glow came from the area near the screen. Dr. Roentgen lit a match and saw that the mysterious invisible light was illuminating the screen. He knew the screen was too far from the Crookes tube for that to have been the source of the light.

SLIDE 1-7/CD 1-5 Dr. Roentgen

Dr. Roentgen kept repeating the experiment with the same results. He discovered the rays could pass through a playing card, a book, and a thin sheet of aluminum and cause the screen to fluoresce, but a small lead disk blocked the path of the rays. When he held the lead disk with his thumb and finger in the path of the rays, he saw the outline of the bones of his hand on the screen behind the disk. The sight stunned him. No one had ever imagined that it would be possible to see inside the body.

Dr. Roentgen toiled constantly with his discovery, and within a few months, he'd learned just about everything we know today about x-radiation. He called the phenomenon "x-light." The "x" stood for unknown, and although we know what it is now, the name stuck. Dr. Roentgen didn't tell the world about this mysterious kind of invisible but penetrating light that passed through solid materials for a few months, until January of 1896.

In a time before televisions or fax machines, the news traveled quickly as soon as Dr. Roentgen disclosed it. Within a year, excited scientists had published 49 books or pamphlets and 1,044 papers on x-rays. In 1901, Dr. Roentgen won the Nobel Prize in physics for his work. A shy man, he didn't like the fanfare and attention that came with his discovery, and within 2 years he published his final observations on x-rays and turned to work on other projects.

CD 1-5A Roentgen demonstrating x-rays

Once Dr. Roentgen opened the door, the interest in x-rays exploded. Scientists experimented with them in all sorts of ways. They made pictures of lizards and frogs, took x-ray film of objects in boxes and pockets, and used x-rays on patients afflicted with pneumonia, skin conditions, cancer, and carbuncles.

In those days the use of x-rays, which were thought to be harmless, wasn't regulated. There were plenty of "x-ray martyrs to science" before people caught on to their harmful effects.

SLIDE 1-8/CD 1-6 Historical hand radiograph

Fortunately, Dr. Roentgen understood the medical value of his discovery very quickly. Because his wife Bertha had faith in him, she allowed him to radiograph her hand and publish the image, although the process terrified her. Bertha thought that this first radiograph ever produced was a premonition of death.

Today, about 200 million medical radiographs and 100 million dental radiographs are taken in the United States every year.

CD 1-6A Other uses of x-rays

Although their first use was in medicine, the impact of x-rays outside of medical fields was also remarkable. A byproduct of electron beams creates the picture in your television set. Security guards at the airport increase the odds of your safety when they use x-rays to examine luggage for bombs and weapons. Manufacturers use x-rays to find flawed metal parts. And scientific labs use them to analyze the crystal structure of molecules that might be the next miracle drug.

SLIDE 1-9/CD 1-7 First American radiograph

What is generally acknowledged to be the first radiograph taken in the United States was done at the physics laboratory at Dartmouth College in Hanover, New Hampshire in 1896. Eddie McCarthy, a young man who broke his wrist ice skating, agreed to have his wrist photographed by the new "x-light."

MORE INFO LEADS TO THIS AUDIO RESPONSE: It was another American, the Boston doctor and dentist William Herbert Rollins, who was one of the first to sound the alarm about the dangers of x-rays after experiencing radiation burns on his hand during experiments in 1898. Because there was no way to measure the intensity of x-rays in those early years, operators would hold one hand up to the beam while the machine warmed up until they could see on the imaging screen that there was enough energy for good pictures.

Rollins' pamphlet, "X-Light Kills," wasn't taken too seriously by his colleagues. However, that didn't stop him from inventing protective devices like boxes covered with lead paint to shield x-ray tubes and other gadgets that forced radiologists to keep the tube a certain distance away from patients.

SLIDE 1-10/CD 1-8 Medical uses of radiographs
Today, x-ray departments are vital components of any medical facility. Since Dr. Roentgen's discovery, they've been important in diagnosing diseases and medical disorders.

Originally, Dr. Roentgen and others found x-rays to be helpful in showing skeletal fractures. Over the years, increasingly sophisticated equipment has been invented that can image virtually every tissue and organ system in the body. Since the 1920s, many technological advances have helped radiography become safer, more accurate, and a very valuable diagnostic tool.

CD 1-8A Radiation burns
It wasn't until the 1940s and 50s that the hazards of radiology were really understood and dealt with, but there had been reports of many injuries before that. Those dealing with x-rays suffered radiation burns and skin ulcers, some so severe that hands and arms had to be amputated. By 1936, there were so many victims that a stone column was erected in the courtyard of a German hospital to honor 168 men and women who had died from overexposure. The list was to grow much longer when the latent effects of radiation were recognized.

SLIDE 1-11/CD 1-9 CT console
Dr. Roentgen would be amazed if he could see how his discovery has developed and how many ways it can be used in diagnosing illness. Although the basic principles of x-rays remain the same, new equipment continues to refine the imaging process. In the 1970s, computed tomography (CT) was developed. And in the 1980s, magnetic resonance imaging (MRI), was added to the examination arsenal, although it uses neither x-rays nor sound waves.

CT scanning, which began in 1973, allowed radiologists to visualize structures inside the skull, including the brain, for the first time. It is also valuable for diagnosing a variety of conditions, such as tumors, skeletal fractures, herniated vertebral discs, and congenital abnormalities.

SLIDE 1-12/CD 1-10 Radiation protection
The good German physicist probably would be further amazed to learn that now x-rays are also used to treat, not just identify, disease in patients. Research has shown that because x-rays cause biologic change in tissue, radiation therapy can help to shrink tumors.

But x-rays aren't wonder techniques that can be prescribed indiscriminately. Technologists and patients still must be protected from the dangers of excessive radiation, such as with the protective wear shown here. We'll talk more about protection at the end of this module and in a later module in this series.

CD 1-10A Historical foot radiograph

Let's take a moment to review. At the turn of the century, scientists and others had a field day with x-rays. For the first time in history, it was possible to see inside a living human being. Many x-ray exposures were taken with little regard for the safety of the people involved. The historic radiograph shown here of a foot inside a shoe was taken in 1896.

Yes or No: Were there signs that radiation was dangerous?

Click on your answer now.

PRESENT THIS AUDIO IF ANSWER WAS yes: Yes, of course you're right. Scientists and technologists were receiving radiation burns to their hands as they held them in front of the x-ray source while waiting for the machine to heat up. The American doctor William Rollins warned about the hazards in 1898. But people were so excited about the possibilities of x-rays that they ignored the dangers and didn't take the precautions they should have.

PRESENT THIS AUDIO IF ANSWER WAS no: No, you missed this one. The dangers existed all along, but people were so excited about the new technology they chose to ignore them. The American doctor William Rollins tried to warn people in 1898, but it wasn't until the 1940s and 50s that protection from x-rays was taken seriously.

SLIDE 1-13/CD 1-11 History of x-rays: conclusion

This concludes the section on the discovery of x-rays and their use in diagnosing illness. As you have seen, Dr. Roentgen's surprise discovery has had a huge impact on the world in the past 100 years.

The technology improves each year so that better images at lower doses of radiation are the norm these days in the United States. Radiology is more accurate and safer for radiographers and patients as long as safety precautions are followed.

SLIDE 1-14/CD 1-12 Radiographic procedures

You have begun the topic of radiographic procedures, the purposes of different machines, and their diagnostic and treatment uses. This subject builds on information covered in the preceding topic of the discovery of x-rays and their use in diagnosing illness. If you have not yet worked through that topic, you may want to quit this section now and return later after going through the earlier one.

There are two basic kinds of radiologic procedures. They are radiographic examinations and fluoroscopic examinations.

Although there are many variations in radiographic and fluoroscopic machines, the basic equipment is generally quite similar.

SLIDE 1-15/CD 1-13 Preparing for examination

A radiographic exam uses special radiographic film. In dedicated radiology suites, the equipment is often mounted on a track on the ceiling and can be moved in many directions. It produces radiographic images of many parts of the body.

MORE INFO LEADS TO THIS AUDIO RESPONSE: Despite differences in the size of radiographic suites, the general purpose x-ray unit is probably the most common type. It's used to take images of bones and joints, the skull, abdomen, chest, pelvis, spine, and extremities.

SLIDE 1-16/CD 1-14 Fluoroscopic examination
A fluoroscopic exam is usually done with an x-ray tube that's located under the examining table. In contrast to a radiographic exam, it shows moving, or dynamic, images on a fluoroscopic screen or a monitor.

This is a useful procedure when it's important to see the path of fluids such as barium moving through the gastrointestinal tract, or to monitor a contrast medium reaching the heart, or to track the positions of catheters being inserted into the body.

CD 1-14A Radiographic/fluoroscopic unit
A more versatile piece of equipment than the general purpose radiographic machine is the radiographic and fluoroscopic unit, called an R/F unit. It has an x-ray tube above the table to use in conventional radiography and another under the table for fluoroscopic studies. They can be used independently of one another.

SLIDE 1-17/CD 1-15 Many uses of radiography
Today, no medical facility could function without radiographic equipment. You'll find it everywhere, including hospitals, clinics, doctors' and dentists' offices, and outpatient diagnostic centers. This is no wonder, because as you learned earlier, 200 million medical x-rays and 100 million dental x-rays are taken in the United States every year!

Radiographic machines are classified by the energy of the x-radiation they produce or by the rays' purpose. Equipment comes in many different sizes and shapes. New technology is being developed all the time, so the equipment you'll come in contact with will vary depending on where you are. These days, the average life span of any radiographic machine is about 5 to 10 years, although well-maintained equipment can last 20 or more years.

SLIDE 1-18/CD 1-16 Tube voltage
X-ray machines that are used to diagnose illness usually operate at top voltages that range from 25 to 150 kVp (kilovolts peak). Their tube currents range from 25 to 1,200 mA (milliamperes).

Equipment known as therapeutic x-ray machines are used to treat disease and can operate at higher or lower voltages. But their tube currents can't go over 20 mA.

Just about all radiographic equipment operates from an incoming line of 210 to 220 volts.

SLIDE 1-19/CD 1-17 Chest radiograph
Some equipment, especially in large facilities, is designed to be installed in a dedicated radiographic room or a radiographic/fluoroscopic room. Patients come here to be radiographed with machines such as mammographic equipment, head units, and chest imaging equipment. In other units, the same equipment is used for a variety of different radiographs, such as the unit shown here being used for a chest radiograph.

MORE INFO LEADS TO THIS AUDIO RESPONSE: Hospitals have traditionally placed radiology departments on the ground floor, originally because that area could bear the weight of protective shielding. Many of them are still there because a ground floor location provides easy access to the emergency room, surgery, and the outpatient area.

SLIDE 1-20/CD 1-18 Mobile radiographic unit
Other x-ray equipment is designed to be mobile so that it can be used when a patient can't come to the radiography suite. Mobile equipment is ready to roll into an operating room or to a patient's bedside when needed. This kind of movable equipment includes radiographic and fluoroscopic units. You'll learn more about this equipment at the end of this module.

SLIDE 1-21/CD 1-19 X-ray tube
The fact that a piece of equipment is permanently installed doesn't mean that you can't move some of its parts around to make your work easier and to get better images.

As you've seen, basic x-ray equipment consists of a radiographic table with an x-ray tube above it. The x-ray tube is one essential part of the basic equipment. Because some parts move, you can position the x-ray tube so that the beam is either perpendicular or parallel to the table. And depending on how you position the tube, you can use the table top or a wall-mounted cassette holder to take a variety of radiographs.

SLIDE 1-22/CD 1-20 Positioning patient
The table where the patient lies is the other part of the basic equipment. Usually, it's in a horizontal position so the patient can lie down (although not very comfortably, if you ask the patients). Sometimes, you may be able to put a pillow under a person's head or knees to make the table feel a little less hard.

Tables are designed to be at a height to make it easy to position patients on them with a minimum of bending and lifting for you. But what makes your work easier can make climbing on and off them awkward for patients. Some new table designs can be raised and lowered: lower to make it easier for patients to climb on and off, higher to be at a comfortable height for the technologist to perform the study.

SLIDE 1-23/CD 1-21 Tilting radiographic table
Radiographic tables are often designed to move, too, so that you can more easily perform the radiographic procedure. Design features such as the floating table top enable you to more easily move the patient to achieve the most accurate centering and obtain the best possible images. Tables can also be tilted. Most equipment has this capacity.

Surfaces made of synthetic resins and plastics are common on tables because they allow the x-rays to pass through with minimal loss of x-ray intensity. The table top has to be uniformly radiolucent, easy to clean and hard to scratch. It has to be smooth, without crevices where contrast media could accumulate.

SLIDE 1-24/CD 1-22 Patient on tilted table
Many tables can be tilted to place the patient at different angles. You can move them to an upright position or to the Trendelenburg position, which means the patient's head is lower than the patient's feet.

Sometimes tilting tables are described by their ability to tilt. For example, 90-15 means a table could tilt at 90 degrees in one direction and 15 degrees in another.

CD 1-22A Radiographic suite

Here's a good point to stop and review x-ray equipment that's permanently installed in a radiology suite.

True or false: Even though this equipment isn't mobile, there are still some parts of it you can manipulate to get better images.

Click on your answer now.

PRESENT THIS AUDIO IF ANSWER WAS true: You're right, you do have some leeway in using this equipment. You can change the direction of the tube to alter the direction of the x-ray beam. And you can either move or tilt the table to get views of the patient from different directions.

PRESENT THIS AUDIO IF ANSWER WAS false: No, you aren't as restricted in using this equipment as you think. You can change the direction of the tube to alter the direction of the x-ray beam. And you can either move or tilt the table to get views of the patient from different directions.

SLIDE 1-25/CD 1-23 Grid

One part of most radiographic tables is a device called a "Bucky assembly," or tray, invented by the radiologist Gustav Bucky in 1913. This device is suspended directly under the x-ray table and consists of a grid and a tray in which to place a cassette loaded with film.

The grid is made up of many thin lead strips separated by a material that lets some x-rays pass through but absorbs scatter and secondary radiation before they hit the film. This results in a better quality image. Shown here is an early Bucky grid.

MORE INFO LEADS TO THIS AUDIO RESPONSE: Dr. Bucky's first grid was rather crude. He designed it so that two wide strips of lead were crisscrossed on the film. That meant viewing the patient through a checkerboard pattern.

In 1920, a Chicago radiologist, Hollis Potter, reworked Dr. Bucky's design and had the lead strips going in just one direction. He made the strips thinner and then designed a grid that could move during the exposure. As it moved, the strips blurred and couldn't be seen on the film, which made for a clearer image.

SLIDE 1-26/CD 1-24 Grid use

Scatter radiation is produced when a primary x-ray photon interacts with an outer-shell electron in an atom in the patient's body. This x-ray photon loses energy, changes direction, and becomes what is known as a scattered photon. Scattered photons aren't part of the useful beam, so the number of them reaching the film must be kept to a minimum. That's best done by using a grid and by restricting the size of the x-ray beam. The two radiographs shown here illustrate how using a grid improves the contrast.

MORE INFO LEADS TO THIS AUDIO RESPONSE: Almost all the scatter radiation in diagnostic radiology comes from what is called Compton scattering. It happens when a portion of the energy of a higher-energy photon ejects an outer shell electron from an atom of the medium it's moving through. The result is that the incident photon is scattered in a different direction and has less energy than when it entered the atom.

SLIDE 1-27/CD 1-25 Positioning patient

Not all x-ray equipment has the two basics: a tube and a table. A head unit, for example, which is used to get precise images of the bones in the head and face, has an x-ray tube and a Bucky tray but no table. Patients either stand up or sit in a chair to be examined. The unit has a floor-to-ceiling tube mount with either a C-shaped or a U-shaped arm attachment on the pivoting collar.

A dedicated head unit can obtain better skull and facial images because of the ways the tube and film holder can be angled. The patient remains in one position while the equipment moves around him or her.

SLIDE 1-28/CD 1-26 Positioned for radiograph

You'll see many upright units in radiographic rooms. They're also called upright film cassette holders and Bucky units. Radiographic examinations of the chest are usually done when the patient is standing upright. Other procedures, such as acromioclavicular joints, abdomen, and cervical spine imaging, provide the best results when the patient is standing.

SLIDE 1-29/CD 1-27 Radiographic equipment

No matter what kind of radiographic equipment you're likely to see, it will have three main parts. Those are the tube and table, as you've already seen, or the tube and a Bucky tray, plus the control console, or control panel (sometimes called the operating console). A high-voltage generator powers the equipment.

You may sometimes see all of these parts housed together, as in dental or mobile machines, for example. But most have the tube and table in one room, the control console in another, and a protective barrier separating the two. There's a lead glass window in the barrier that lets you see the patient during the exam.

SLIDE 1-30/CD 1-28 Photograph: generator

The generator will be either in a cabinet against the wall in one corner of the examining room or in a false ceiling.

SLIDE 1-31/CD 1-29 Control panel

One component of x-ray equipment that you're going to become very familiar with is the control, or operating, console. Just as it sounds, this is the part of the equipment that lets you control the tube current and voltage so you'll get a good quality image. Voltmeters and ammeters on the console monitor kVp and mA levels. Some machines might emit a beep to let you know when the beam is on.

MORE INFO LEADS TO THIS AUDIO RESPONSE: Although you're dealing with high voltage levels, the meters and controls within the console are at a low voltage to keep the chance of hazardous shock to a minimum. You'll learn more about how control panels operate in a later module.

SLIDE 1-32/CD 1-30 Cardio-cath exam

As we mentioned before, there are times when getting an accurate diagnosis involves seeing motion within the patient's body. For example, seeing the path of a contrast medium can show what's going on in the gastrointestinal tract. Some surgical procedures involve inserting a device in the body, such as a catheter to the heart. It's important to be able to guide the catheter's route.

When producing images that require motion like this, the radiographic unit swings out of position and is replaced by the fluoroscopic unit. X-rays that emerge from the patient are converted to images you can see on a monitor and can be put on videotape to be studied more at a later time. In contrast, conventional radiographs are static (nonmotion) images.

SLIDE 1-33/CD 1-31 Mammography unit
There are other, more specialized types of x-ray equipment. The mammography machine is one. Because of the emphasis on the importance of early detection of breast cancer and the high incidence of this disease in the United States, mammography has become a common imaging tool.

Mammography units are used only in breast imaging, which is why they're called dedicated units, or machines used for a specific purpose only. You'll find them in hospitals, women's health care clinics, and other health care facilities.

SLIDE 1-34/CD 1-32 Mammographic exam
Mammography units are designed to take detailed images of the soft tissue in the breast. It's important to position the patient to get the best images that show structural and pathological changes.

Because the female breast is cone-shaped, thicker at the chest wall than at the nipple, it has to be compressed to try to get all the tissue at an even thickness and bring it as close to the image detector as possible. Many women find this very uncomfortable, so it's important to tell them why compression is necessary.

SLIDE 1-35/CD 1-33 Tomography
There are times when the area of the body to be radiographed is hidden by the images of tissues and organs lying above or below it. That's when tomography is likely to be used. Tomography produces a radiograph of a selected body plane at a specific thickness and level in the body.

SLIDE 1-36/CD 1-34 Conventional tomography
In conventional or linear tomography, the x-ray tube and the film can be moved in opposite directions at the same time so that only the structures in the chosen focal plane stay in focus. Other tissues and organs are blurred, leaving a sharper image of the area of interest. This technique is most commonly used for imaging kidney abnormalities.

SLIDE 1-37/CD 1-35 Computed tomography
Computed tomography is a more sophisticated way of getting images of organs or structures that are masked because of where they lie in the body. A computed tomography, or CT, unit looks quite different from traditional x-ray equipment. It's square and has a circular opening.

The patient lies in the center of the unit, and a thin beam of x-rays makes exposures from many angles as it rotates around the patient. A computer program puts all the views into an image that looks like a slice through the head or body, showing details of structures deep inside.

MORE INFO LEADS TO THIS AUDIO RESPONSE: To put it another way, in a CT scan, an x-ray tube rotates around the patient on a mechanized track and produces tomographic images. A series of detectors opposite the tube records how many x-rays pass through the patient's body at different angles. This information is fed into a computer, which generates an image.

CT imaging is complex and exposes the patient to higher doses of radiation. It's used when more detailed images are needed for a diagnosis.

SLIDE 1-38/CD 1-36 Contrast medium

There are other types of radiological exams that involve giving the patient contrast medium through an injection or a catheter. Sometimes the patient drinks the contrast medium. Some of these special procedures are performed by a doctor or radiologist under sterile conditions, generally in a restricted access area in the department. They usually involve complicated radiologic and fluoroscopic equipment.

SLIDE 1-39/CD 1-37 Angiography

Here are some of the special procedures and the reasons they're done:
Cardiac catheterization is used to show blockages in coronary arteries.
Renal arteriography is used to view the renal arterial system.
Cerebral arteriography is used to show blood vessels that support the brain.
And therapeutic catheterization techniques are used to diagnose and alleviate blood vessel diseases.
Shown here is the special equipment used in one angiography suite for special imaging of blood vessels.

SLIDE 1-40/CD 1-38 Tube housing

As you've seen, there's quite a variety of radiographic equipment that can be used in many different situations. Although many of the diagnostic outcomes are specialized, you can recognize the basic design of much radiography equipment.

For example, all machines contain an x-ray tube that produces x-rays. The rays are emitted in all directions, which is why the tube is placed inside a heavy housing lined with lead. This housing absorbs the x-rays that are not part of the primary beam and prevents technologists and patients from being exposed to leakage radiation.

SLIDE 1-41/CD 1-39 Functions of tube housing

The housing has several openings for electrical connections. It also has a port, or window, through which the x-rays pass to expose the patient and produce radiographs.

The housing is important in other ways. For one thing, it protects the x-ray tube from all the handling it gets and from the damage that can come with frequent use.

It also supports the tube. The housing can hold the tube immobile during exposure. And because it's easy to move around, it can be manipulated into different positions to get the best images.

SLIDE 1-42/CD 1-40 Overhead suspension system

There are five ways to support tubes in place. They're called the tube support, or suspension, systems.

When a support system is located above a table, it's called an overhead suspension system or ceiling suspension. It has locks to keep it in place so that the radiographic images won't be affected by unwanted movement. Those same locks allow you to raise and lower the tube, release it, and use it somewhere else in the room.

SLIDE 1-43/CD 1-41 Telescoping column

An overhead suspension system has three main parts that make it easy to move the tube when you want to take images of patients in different positions. One is a telescoping column that controls the vertical, or up-and-down, distance. You can also angle the tube up to a 300 degree arc toward the head or the foot of the table. It can rotate 360 degrees and roll up to 60 degrees from side to side.

SLIDE 1-44/CD 1-42 Rails of overhead system

The other parts of the over-head suspension system are two sets of rails. One regulates the longitudinal position, or the lengthwise adjustment, of the tube. The other regulates the transverse, or side-to-side, position of the tube. You control all of these possible movements of the equipment.

SLIDE 1-45/CD 1-43 Floor-to-ceiling suspension

The second kind of suspension system, floor-to-ceiling, is also used for longitudinal, or lengthwise, positioning of the tube. It has a pair of rails, one on the ceiling and one on the floor. Sometimes a room will have such high ceilings that the ceiling rails will have to be suspended from a wall.

This kind of system is quite versatile. It can do more than take images of a person lying flat on a table. It has a telescoping arm for side-to-side movement. It also has a main column collar that slides up and down for vertical positioning. Although you can angle the x-ray tube, you can't rotate it in this kind of system.

SLIDE 1-46/CD 1-44 Floor-mounted suspension

Just as it sounds, the floor suspension system is mounted on the floor. Stationary tube-support columns are attached to the table. Movable columns run on either one or two rails that are also mounted on the floor. You operate this system much like the floor-to-ceiling one.

Because this kind of system can tip over rather easily, it must be anchored by a counterweight at the back of the telescoping tube arm. It also means that the tube system and the table must be installed farther from the back wall than other systems so there is room for the counterweight. This system does not have the flexibility to be moved around the room.

SLIDE 1-47/CD 1-45 Mobile suspension system

There are many kinds of mobile tube suspension systems. They're all different, but just remember that most of them are based on the floor suspension model.

They consist of a very simple piece of equipment with a tube attached to a mobile stand and can be used for special procedures such as angiography.

SLIDE 1-48/CD 1-46 Basic radiography system

There are other, even more simple systems that you might encounter if you find yourself working in an area with few medical resources. The basic radiography system, or BRS, was designed to provide access to radiology in developing countries. It's very portable and can be mounted on a tripod or a patient lift system.

SLIDE 1-49/CD 1-47 C-arm suspension system

The C-arm tube suspension system isn't hard to imagine. It contains an arm shaped like the letter C that holds the tube and image receptor. These two parts are anchored to opposite ends of the C-arm. When you release the clamp or lock that holds the tube in place, the tube and receptor can be moved to a new position.

C-arms are commonly used in head units, mobile fluoroscopy units, and ceiling-suspended angiography and surgical units.

SLIDE 1-50/CD 1-48 Procedures and equipment

This concludes the section on radiologic procedures, the purposes of different radiographic equipment, and their diagnostic and treatment uses. With this basic understanding of x-ray equipment and its capabilities, you should be ready to learn more about radiography.

SLIDE 1-51/CD 1-49 Radiation protection

You have begun the topic of radiation protection methods for radiography equipment. This subject builds on information covered in the preceding topics of the different kinds of radiographic equipment and their diagnostic uses. If you have not yet worked through those topics, you may want to quit this section now and return later after going through the earlier topics.

At this point, you have an idea of the range of x-ray equipment that's permanently installed in medical facilities. Now, let's take a look at mobile equipment, the kind that can be moved around from place to place as needed.

There are two major types of mobile equipment: portable, light-duty units and full-power, institutional units.

SLIDE 1-52/CD 1-50 Mobile unit

Most often mobile radiographic equipment is used when the patient is too ill to be taken to the radiology suite. The emergency room, operating room, or intensive care unit are typically the places where you'll find patients who need to be radiographed but who are physically incapable of being moved.

MORE INFO LEADS TO THIS AUDIO RESPONSE: Madame Curie was probably the first person to see the value of mobile equipment. Curie, who co-discovered radium in 1898, was upset by the number of wounded soldiers who were misdiagnosed by doctors in World War I. She convinced the French military leaders to let her outfit 18 cars as mobile x-ray units. These cars, called "little Curies," went right to the front lines, where they were used to diagnose an estimated 10,000 soldiers.

SLIDE 1-53/CD 1-51 Mobile exam

Another common use of mobile equipment is follow up chest x-ray screening at bedside to monitor potential complications from surgery and to assess how the patient is doing.

Using mobile equipment is one of the biggest challenges you'll face, because positioning seriously ill patients and manipulating the equipment to get the best results possible is difficult. Sometimes patients may not be able to communicate with you. Once you use mobile equipment, you'll realize that it's relatively easy to use stationary equipment in rooms especially designed for it.

SLIDE 1-54/CD 1-52 Mobile fluoroscopic unit
Do you remember learning about fluoroscopy at the beginning of this module? It involves taking dynamic images with an x-ray tube located under the examining table. These images are then shown on a fluoroscopic screen or a monitor.

There are mobile fluoroscopy machines with C-arm units that can produce the same dynamic and static images when they're connected to a video recording system.

SLIDE 1-55/CD 1-53 Protective barrier
In this module, we've briefly discussed a variety of radiographic equipment. Along the way in your studies, you'll learn much more about exactly how different machines work and your role in operating them.

One consistent factor, and an area that you'll also study in greater detail, is the need to protect radiographers, radiologists, and patients from radiation. That's a concern that's always in the minds of people in the field and one that's planned for and taken seriously.

SLIDE 1-56/CD 1-54 Lead in walls
People who design radiology departments or x-ray rooms know how important radiation protection is, both for the radiographer and the patient. Usually they incorporate sheets of lead into the walls of examining rooms to act as protective barriers.

MORE INFO LEADS TO THIS AUDIO RESPONSE: Although most hospital radiology departments are located on the ground floor, it's possible to locate them anywhere in the building. And it can be practical too, because you don't need thick protective barriers up on the thirtieth floor, where it's unlikely anyone's walking around outside!

SLIDE 1-57/CD 1-55 Scatter and leakage radiation
When architects and medical physicists design x-ray facilities, they consider three types of radiation. They are primary radiation (the useful beam) and two kinds of secondary radiation (scatter radiation and leakage radiation).

SLIDE 1-58/CD 1-56 Cassette holder
Designers consider an extra protective barrier anytime an x-ray unit can be positioned against a wall. An upright cassette holder, which intercepts many x-ray photons in the course of a day, is a good example. Often extra protective shielding, such as lead or concrete block, is installed directly behind it.

SLIDE 1-59/CD1-57 Barriers for scatter radiation
Secondary radiation requires some thinking in advance about the need for protective barriers, too. For example, when a useful beam is intercepted by matter, such as the human body, it can cause some of the x-ray photons to scatter in many different directions. Protective barriers help to absorb that scattered radiation.

Leakage radiation can come from the x-ray tube housing assembly and leak in directions other than the direction of the useful beam. That's why it's very important for the tube housing to be designed and installed properly. When it is, even with the machine operating at its maximum output, the level of this kind of radiation will never go above the regulated limits.

SLIDE 1-60/CD 1-58 Secondary radiation barriers
Most new suites contain additional radiation barriers to protect against both scatter and leakage radiation. They're thinner than primary protective barriers and can be made from materials other than lead, such as gypsum board, glass, or lead acrylic. Most control booth barriers are secondary protective barriers.

SLIDE 1-61/CD 1-59 Quiz instructions
THIS AUDIO FOR SLIDE/TAPE ONLY: This concludes the presentation section of this module. If you are not going to work through the self-assessment quiz that follows, you may stop the program at this point and turn off the equipment.

If your instructor has asked you to take this self-assessment quiz on the material you have learned in this module, you should have a piece of paper ready. There will be 10 questions with multiple-choice or short answers. After this self-assessment we will go back through these questions and briefly talk about the reasons for the correct answers. Ready?

THIS AUDIO IN CD ROM LECTURE MODE ONLY: You have reached the self-assessment quiz for this module. Here you will be asked 10 questions to help you assess how well you understand what you have learned in this module. The questions are multiple choice or have short answers. After this self-assessment we will go back through these questions and briefly talk about your answers and the reasons for the correct answers. Ready?

THIS AUDIO IN CD ROM STUDENT MODE ONLY: You have reached the self-assessment quiz for this module. Here you will be asked 10 questions to help you assess how well you understand what you have learned in this module. The questions are multiple choice or have short answers. For multiple-choice questions, click on the box next to your answer choice. For those questions that require a short answer, type in your answer at the keyboard and press enter. After this self-assessment we will go back through these questions and briefly talk about your answers and the reasons for the correct answers.

SLIDE 1-62/CD 1-60 Quiz question 1

1. What is the main purpose for the use of x-rays?
   a. Therapeutic
   b. Diagnostic
   c. Preventive
   d. Holistic

SLIDE 1-63/CD 1-61 Quiz question 2

2. What are the two main types of radiographic exams?
   a. Radiography and fluoroscopy
   b. Radiography and tomography
   c. Electromagnetic imaging and fluoroscopy
   d. Fluoroscopy and mammography

SLIDE 1-64/CD 1-62 Quiz question 3

3. The primary purpose of a fluoroscopic exam, compared with a radiographic exam, is to show which of the following images?
   a. Static
   b. Longitudinal
   c. Dynamic
   d. Cross-sectional

SLIDE 1-65/CD 1-63 Quiz question 4

4. What unit of measurement is used for x-ray tube voltages?
   a. Volts
   b. Millivolts
   c. Voltmeters
   d. Kilovolts

SLIDE 1-66/CD 1-64 Quiz question 5

5. Radiographic equipment can be permanently installed in a medical facility or it can be mobile. When and where is mobile equipment most likely to be used?
   a. In the emergency room
   b. At the patient's bedside
   c. In the operating room
   d. All of the above

SLIDE 1-67/CD 1-65 Quiz question 6

6. What is a Bucky assembly?
   a. A device to hold a grid and a loaded cassette tray
   b. A part of a mobile chest x-ray unit
   c. A unit that controls movement on an x-ray table
   d. A part of the control panel

SLIDE 1-68/CD 1-66 Quiz question 7

7. What are the main components of basic radiographic equipment?
   a. Grid, operating console, and table
   b. Operating console, x-ray tube, and suspension system
   c. Radiographic table, operating console, and x-ray tube
   d. X-ray tube, table, and film

SLIDE 1-69/CD 1-67 Quiz question 8

8. Mammography is used a great deal now in the United States. Which of these reasons would you choose to explain this?
   a. It is inexpensive.
   b. It is easy to use.
   c. The radiation dose is low.
   d. There is a high incidence of breast cancer now in this country, and when properly done, mammography can detect tumors early.

SLIDE 1-70/CD 1-68 Quiz question 9

9. Conventional tomography is used to obtain clear images of parts of the body that are otherwise hidden by other organs or tissues. It blurs other body parts so only the area of interest is shown. It is often used to diagnose which of the following?
   a. Heart problems
   b. Renal problems
   c. Brain tumors
   d. Breast masses

SLIDE 1-71/CD 1-69 Quiz question 10

10. All radiography equipment contains an x-ray tube that produces x-rays. Why is the tube placed inside a lead-lined housing?
    a. To absorb x-rays that are not in the primary beam
    b. To prevent x-rays from leaking from the tube
    c. To protect radiologic technologists and patients from radiation
    d. All of the above

SLIDE 1-72/CD 1-70 Quiz review

That concludes the self-assessment quiz for Module 1: Radiographic Equipment. Let's quickly go back through the questions and see how you did.

SLIDE 1-73/CD 1-71 Review question 1

Question 1 asked you about the main purpose of radiographing patients. It's a basic question but one for you to keep in mind as you work in this field.

The correct answer is b, diagnostic. Congratulate yourself if you got it right! The images a radiologist sees on a film or on a screen can indicate what's going on inside the patient's body. Without x-rays, doctors might have to perform surgical procedures to get at the root of illness.

CD 1-71A Review question 1

Question 1 asked you about the main purpose of radiographing patients. It's a basic question but one for you to keep in mind as you work in this field.

PRESENT THIS AUDIO IF ANSWER WAS b: Yes, you're right. The correct answer is b, diagnostic.

PRESENT THIS AUDIO IF ANSWER WAS a, c, or d: Sorry, you missed it. The correct answer is b, diagnostic. The images a radiologist sees on a film or a screen can indicate what's going on inside the patient's body. Without x-rays, doctors might have to perform surgical procedures to get at the root of illness.

SLIDE 1-74/CD 1-72 Review question 2

Question 2 asked you to name the two basic kinds of radiographic exams. This was probably easy for you.

The correct answer is a, radiography and fluoroscopy. Basic radiography provides static images of body tissue and organs. Fluoroscopy provides moving images that are projected on screen or monitor. They can be stored for future study.

CD 1-72A Review question 2
Question 2 asked you to name the two basic kinds of radiographic examinations.

PRESENT THIS AUDIO IF ANSWER WAS a, radiography and fluoroscopy: Yes, you correctly answered this question.

PRESENT THIS AUDIO IF ANSWER WAS b, c, d: You incorrectly answered. The right answer is a, radiography and fluoroscopy.

SLIDE 1-75/CD 1-73 Review question 3
Question 3 asked you the main reason for performing a fluoroscopic exam. The correct answer is c, to provide dynamic, or moving, images to help in diagnosis.

CD 1-73A Review question 3
Question 3 asked you the main reason for performing a fluoroscopic exam.

PRESENT THIS AUDIO IF ANSWER WAS c: Yes, you're correct in answering c, to provide dynamic, or moving, images to help in diagnosis.

PRESENT THIS AUDIO IF ANSWER WAS a, b, or d: Sorry, you missed this one. The correct answer is c, to provide dynamic, or moving, images to help in diagnosis.

SLIDE 1-76/CD 1-74 Review question 4
Question 4 asked how x-ray tube voltages are measured.

The correct answer is d, in kilovolts.

CD 1-74A Review question 4
Question 4 asked how x-ray tubes voltages are measured.

PRESENT THIS AUDIO IF ANSWER WAS d: You're right! They're measured in kilovolts.

PRESENT THIS AUDIO IF ANSWER WAS a, b, or c: Sorry, your answer is wrong. The correct answer is d, kilovolts.

SLIDE 1-77/CD 1-75 Review question 5
Question 5 asked when mobile radiographic equipment is most likely to be used.

The correct answer is d, in all the situations mentioned: in emergency rooms, at bedside, and in the operating room.

CD 1-75A Review question 5
Question 5 asked when mobile radiographic equipment is most likely to be used.

PRESENT THIS AUDIO IF ANSWER WAS d: You're right! The correct answer is d, in all three situations mentioned: in emergency rooms, at bedside, and in the operating room.

PRESENT THIS AUDIO IF ANSWER WAS a, b, or c: Sorry, you missed this one. The correct answer is d, in all three situations mentioned: in emergency rooms, at bedside, and in the operating room.

SLIDE 1-78/CD 1-76 Review question 6
Question 6 asked what a Bucky assembly is.

The correct answer is a, the device that holds the grid and a tray in which to place a loaded cassette. It's usually located under the x-ray table.

CD 1-76A Review question 6
Question 6 asked what a Bucky assembly is.

PRESENT THIS AUDIO IF ANSWER WAS a: You got the correct answer a, a device to hold a grid and a loaded cassette tray.

PRESENT THIS AUDIO IF ANSWER WAS b, c, or d: No, you missed it. The correct answer is a, a device to hold a grid and a loaded cassette tray.

SLIDE 1-79/CD 1-77 Review question 7
Question 7 asked you to identify the main components of basic radiographic equipment.

The correct answer is c, the x-ray tube, the table, and the operating console.

CD 1-77A Review question 7
Question 7 asked you to identify the main components of basic radiographic equipment.

PRESENT THIS AUDIO IF ANSWER WAS c: Yes, you are right, the answer is c, the x-ray tube, the table, and the operating console.

PRESENT THIS AUDIO IF ANSWER WAS a, b, or d: No, you missed it. The correct answer is c, the x-ray tube, the table, and the operating console.

SLIDE 1-80/CD 1-78 Review question 8
Question 8 asked about the reason for the increase in the use of mammography in the past several years.

The correct answer is d, because there's a high incidence of breast cancer now in this country and, properly done, mammography can detect tumors early.

CD 1-78A Review question 8
Question 8 asked about the increase in the use of mammography in the past several years.

PRESENT THIS AUDIO FOR ANSWER d: Congratulate yourself, you got it right. The high incidence of breast cancer in the United States has caused more and more women to seek early detection through one of the few tools we have, mammography.

PRESENT THIS AUDIO IF ANSWER WAS a, b, or c: No, you missed this one. The answer is d. The high incidence of breast cancer in the United States has caused more and more women to seek early detection through one of the few tools we have, mammography.

SLIDE 1-81/CD 1-79 Review question 9
Question 9 asked what is conventional tomography often used to diagnose.

The correct answer is b. Renal organs can easily be masked by other tissues and organs, and the tomogram can blur them so the organs in question stand out clearly. The patient is given a contrast medium that also helps the organs to stand out clearly.

CD 1-79A Review question 9
Question 9 asked what is conventional tomography often used to diagnose.

PRESENT THIS AUDIO IF ANSWER WAS b: Yes, you're right. The correct answer is b, renal problems. They can easily be masked by other tissues and organs, and the tomogram can blur them so the organs in question stand out clearly. The patient is given a contrast medium that also helps the organs to stand out clearly.

PRESENT THIS AUDIO IF ANSWER WAS a, c, or d: Sorry, but you missed it. The correct answer is b, renal problems. They can easily be masked by other tissues and organs, and the tomogram can blur them so the organs in question stand out clearly. The patient is given a contrast medium that also helps the organs to stand out clearly.

SLIDE 1-82/CD 1-80 Review question 10
Question 10 asked why x-ray tubes are placed inside a lead-lined housing.

The answer is d. The lead housing absorbs the x-rays that are not in the primary beam, prevents them from leaking from the tube, and protects people from radiation.

CD 1-80A Review question 10
Question 10 asked why x-ray tubes are placed inside a lead-lined housing.

PRESENT THIS AUDIO IF ANSWER WAS d: Well, you're right. The lead housing absorbs the x-rays that are not in the primary beam, prevents them from leaking from the tube, and protects people from radiation.

PRESENT THIS AUDIO IF ANSWER WAS a, b, or c: Sorry, you missed it. The correct answer is d. The lead housing absorbs the x-rays that are not in the primary beam, prevents them from leaking from the tube, and protects people from radiation.

SLIDE 1-83/CD 1-81 Quiz conclusion

This concludes the self-assessment quiz. This was not intended as a test, so don't feel bad if you missed some. All that means is that you probably need to review this module or study your textbook more carefully.

CD 1-81A Quiz feedback
FOR SCORE OF 10, THIS AUDIO: You've done an excellent job here with a difficult subject. Clearly you are studying well, and you seem to have worked through the tutorial carefully.

FOR SCORE OF 9, THIS AUDIO: You've done well with a difficult subject. Clearly you are studying and paying attention to the subject. Maybe next time you'll get the perfect score!

FOR SCORE OF 7-8, THIS AUDIO: Your score is about average. I'd suggest you review this material in your textbook. You may also find it helpful, next time, to read the material in your book before coming to the computer to take the tutorial. And don't hesitate to talk to your instructor if you have trouble after both reading the textbook and working through the multimedia tutorial.

FOR SCORE OF 5-6, THIS AUDIO: Your score is below average. You need to review this material in your textbook, and perhaps you should come back and take this tutorial again afterwards. You may have just been unprepared this time, or if you are having trouble after both reading the textbook and working through the multimedia tutorial, be sure to talk to your instructor.

FOR SCORE OF 0-4, THIS AUDIO: Your score is rather low. Don't feel too bad; these are, after all, difficult concepts to grasp. If you tried your best here but are having this much difficulty with the material, you should first go to your textbook and see if you can understand the material there. If it still seems difficult, please ask your instructor for additional study aids.

SLIDE 1-84/CD 1-82 Exam instructions
In the next 7 or 8 minutes you will be presented with 15 multiple-choice questions. Select the one best answer choice. Get ready a blank sheet of paper numbered 1 to 15 down the left side. As you take the examination, write the letter corresponding to your answer choice next to the number for each question.

Ready? You will not be asked to perform any complicated calculations.

CD 1-82A More exam instructions
In the next 7 or 8 minutes you will be presented with 15 multiple-choice questions. Select the one best answer choice. This examination covers the material you've been learning about in this tutorial over the last hour or so. It is designed to help you and your instructor determine how well you now grasp this material. You can use scratch paper during the exam if you want, but it shouldn't be necessary for any complicated calculations.

SLIDE 1-85/CD 1-83 Exam question 1

1. Basically, radiographic equipment produces images when high-speed electrons bombard a piece of metal. The energy from the electrons turns into which of the following?
   a. Mechanical energy
   b. Electromagnetic energy
   c. Kinetic energy
   d. Human energy

SLIDE 1-86/CD 1-84 Exam question 2

2. What is the name of the German physicist who first recognized "X-ray light" in 1895?
   a. William Crookes
   b. Wilhelm Conrad Roentgen
   c. Madame Curie
   d. E. B. Frost

SLIDE 1-87/CD 1-85 Exam question 3

3. There have been many advancements since Dr. Roentgen first discovered x-rays. Which of the following was made in the past 3 decades alone?
   a. Mammography
   b. X-ray computed tomography
   c. Magnetic resonance imaging (MRI)
   d. All of the above

SLIDE 1-88/CD 1-86 Exam question 4

4. How are radiographic machines classified?
   a. By how clear the images are
   b. By how low a dose of radiation they expose the patient to
   c. By the energy of the x-radiation they produce or by the purpose those x-rays are used for
   d. By how inexpensive they are

SLIDE 1-89/CD 1-87 Exam question 5

5. Radiographic machines used to diagnose illness usually operate at top voltages measured in kVp, or kilovolts peak. What is their range?
   a. 25 to 200 kVp
   b. 50 to 100 kVp
   c. 25 to 125 kVp
   d. 25 to 150 kVp

SLIDE 1-90/CD 1-88 Exam question 6

6. X-ray tube currents are measured in mA, or milliamperes. What is the currents' range?
   a. 500 to 1,000 mA
   b. 25 to 1,200 mA
   c. 50 to 1,500 mA
   d. 25 to 750 mA

SLIDE 1-91/CD 1-89 Exam question 7

7. Most facilities have radiology rooms with the basics: a radiographic unit and a fluoroscopic unit. These allow them to handle just about every kind of radiographic and fluoroscopic exam they need. With a radiographic exam, the x-ray tube is generally positioned over the examining table. Where is the fluoroscopic x-ray tube usually placed?
   a. Over the table
   b. Under the table
   c. In the Bucky assembly
   d. On the floor

SLIDE 1-92/CD 1-90 Exam question 8

8. Basic x-ray equipment consists of a radiographic table with an x-ray tube above it. The tube, an essential part of the equipment, can be moved so that the beam is in which of the following positions?
   a. Either perpendicular or parallel to the table
   b. Under the table
   c. It can't be moved; it must stay in position over the table
   d. Focused on the wall

SLIDE 1-93/CD 1-91 Exam question 9

9. Radiographic tables can also be moved so you can center patients at different locations and get good images. Many tables can be tilted in which of the following positions?
   a. To an upright position
   b. To the Trendelenburg position
   c. To place the patient at other angles
   d. All of the above

SLIDE 1-94/CD 1-92 Exam question 10

10. Some equipment, like a head unit, is used to get precise images of the bones in the head and face. Which of the following is true of a head unit?
   a. The unit has a floor-to-ceiling tube mount.
   b. Better images can be obtained because of the ways the tube and film holder can be angled.
   c. Patients either stand up or sit in a chair to be examined.
   d. The patient remains in position while the equipment moves around him or her.
   e. All of the above are true.

SLIDE 1-95/CD 1-93 Exam question 11

11. Why is the control, or operating, console important?
   a. It lets you control tube current and voltage.
   b. It lets you position the patient.
   c. It lets you talk to the patient.
   d. It lets you decrease the time the patient is being radiographed.

SLIDE 1-96/CD 1-94 Exam question 12

12. Fluoroscopic studies are usually done for which of the following?
   a. Hands
   b. Hips
   c. Gastrointestinal tract
   d. Head

SLIDE 1-97/CD 1-95 Exam question 13

13. All radiography equipment contains a tube that produces the x-rays. To prevent the rays from being emitted in all directions, which is what they do naturally, they're enclosed in a heavy housing. This protects technologists and patients. Which of the following is true of the housing?
   a. It is lined with lead.
   b. It has a port, or window, through which the x-rays pass.
   c. It protects the x-ray tube from handling and frequent use.
   d. All of the above are true.

SLIDE 1-98/CD 1-96 Exam question 14

14. Mobile equipment is used to take bedside radiographs, to assess how a patient is doing after an operation, or when a patient is too ill to come to the radiology department. Why is using mobile equipment a challenge?
    a. Because it's heavy to move around
    b. Because positioning seriously ill patients and manipulating the equipment to get good images is difficult
    c. Because doctors and nurses in the emergency room, intensive care unit, or operating room think mobile equipment gets in their way
    d. Because it's hard to find the right electrical outlets

SLIDE 1-99/CD 1-97 Exam question 15

15. When designers are creating new radiologic facilities, they consider several different types of radiation and build protective barriers in the walls. What are the three kinds of radiation?
    a. Secondary, scatter, leakage
    b. Primary, secondary, scatter
    c. Primary, scatter, leakage
    d. Leakage, secondary, primary

SLIDE 1-100/CD 1-98 Conclusion

INSTRUCTOR CD/SLIDE AUDIO: This concludes the examination section of Module 1 of Radiographic Imaging. Please follow your instructor's directions for your answer sheet to the questions.

STUDENT CD AUDIO: This concludes the examination section of Module 1 of Radiographic Imaging. Your score has been saved on the computer. Your instructor will report it to you later.

Answers to the Multimedia Examination

1. b	6. b	11. a
2. b	7. b	12. c
3. d	8. a	13. d
4. c	9. d	14. b
5. d	10. e	15. c

Radiographic Density and Contrast

2

Overview

- Density
  - Film exposure and development
  - mA and kVp
  - SID
  - Intensifying screens, grids
  - Beam-restricting devices
  - Filtration
  - Film processing
- Contrast
  - Subject contrast and film contrast
  - Scatter, fog
  - Film-screen combinations
  - Contrast media

This module introduces students to visual characteristics of radiographs, density and contrast, and their importance in making a diagnostic image. The focus throughout the module is on factors within the radiographer's control, so that students understand what they can do in practice to help ensure the highest quality images. In addition, factors beyond their control are discussed to widen their perspective of the many variables involved in imaging.

The module begins with a review of what happens when a film is exposed. This helps students recall that density in the image is a result of exposed silver halide crystals being converted to black metallic silver in the development process. With this understanding of density, students are led through the effects of exposure variables on density, with emphasis on the relationship of mAs and kVp to density. Other factors affecting density are then discussed, including SID, intensifying screens, grids, the anode-heel effect, beam restriction, patient size, and film processing.

From density the module moves to contrast, reviewing how many of the same factors also affect contrast. Students learn that achieving the best density and contrast is not simply a matter of getting "the right" selection of variables but a fluid interplay of factors, balancing the need for the best diagnostic image with the desire to keep patient exposure low. This discussion includes devices to reduce scatter radiation, the use of film-screen combinations, other factors that cause fog, and contrast media.

Learning Objectives

Upon completion of this module, the student should be able to do the following:

1. Define all the key terms in the module.
2. Explain why density and contrast are important in creating a diagnostic image.
3. Describe how density is formed on the film in the exposure and development processes.
4. Explain the effects of each of the following factors on both density and contrast:
   - mAs
   - kVp
   - SID
   - Intensifying screens
   - Grids
   - Collimators, aperture diaphragms, cones, and cylinders
   - Filtration
   - Patient size, thickness of body part
   - Film processing and chemicals
   - Film contrast
5. Explain how the radiographer may adjust exposure variables to improve density and contrast.
6. Successfully complete the activities and posttest in the Study Guide.

Key Terms

Added filtration
Anode heel effect
Aperture diaphragm
Attenuation
Automatic processor
Black metallic silver
Characteristic curve
Collimator
Compensating filter
Cone
Contrast
Contrast medium
Densitometer
Density
Development fog
15% rule
Filter
Film contrast
Focus-film distance (FFD)
Grid
High-energy x-rays
Inherent filtration
Intensifying screen
mA
mAs
Pathology, pathological condition
Phosphor
Scatter radiation
Source-to-image receptor distance (SID)
Subject contrast
Trough filter
Wedge filter

Instructional Outline

I. Density and contrast are two important characteristics of radiographs.
   A. Both density and contrast are important for diagnostic quality.
   B. Both density and contrast are affected by a number of variables within the radiographer's control.

II. Density, also called optical density or radiographic density, is the overall amount of blackening on the film. Many factors affect the density of an image.
   A. Density results when silver halide crystals in the film emulsion are exposed by x-ray photons and then converted into black metallic silver by the development process.
      1. Density varies from total black to nearly clear (unexposed).
      2. A radiograph can be overexposed (too dark) or underexposed (too light).
      3. Contrast refers to the difference between adjacent areas of darkness and lightness in the radiograph.
      4. A densitometer measures density.
   B. Exposure is a key factor determining density.
      1. The characteristic curve measures the relationship between exposure and density.
      2. mAs is the primary factor affecting density, the product of the tube current and the exposure time.
      3. The x-ray exposure rate is directly proportional to the mAs.
   C. kVp also affects density.
      1. Increasing the kVp by 15% doubles the exposure and thus the density.
      2. Higher kVp may cause more scatter, which increases the density caused by fog.
      3. Because of other factors related to kVp (such as penetration, patient dose, scatter, and contrast) usually mAs rather than kVp is manipulated if a radiograph must be repeated because it is too light or too dark.
   D. Source-to-image receptor distance (SID) also affects density.
      1. Because of the inverse square law, the intensity of the x-ray beam decreases as the SID increases.
      2. Even slight differences in SID affect density.
   E. Intensifying screens help increase density without increasing the exposure.
      1. The phosphor layer in the intensifying screen emits light when struck by x-ray photons.
      2. The light photons produced by the screen increase the film exposure without the patient having to be exposed to as much radiation.
   F. The anode-heel effect, which causes the beam to be more intense on the cathode side than on the anode side, can be used to advantage to produce more even density when imaging certain body areas.
   G. Grids also improve density by absorbing much of the scatter radiation produced inside the patient's body.
   H. Collimators, aperture diaphragms, and cones also help reduce scatter radiation, and thereby improve diagnostic density, by restricting the size of the beam penetrating the patient.
   I. Filtration provides additional control over density.
      1. Filters absorb low-energy (long wavelength) x-rays and thereby increase the average energy of the beam.
      2. Added filtration, such as aluminum filters, adds to the inherent filtration of the tube glass port.
      3. Compensating filters, such as wedge filters and trough filters, provide more filtering in one area than in another and are used to even out densities that would otherwise vary too much because of differences in body structures.

J. The patient's size and body thickness, as well as certain pathological conditions, also affect density, with larger patients and body areas requiring greater exposures to produce adequate density in the image.

K. Film processing affects density.
   1. In the developing stage, density is affected by the developer time and temperature, the chemical concentration, and the size of the film crystals.
   2. The fixing stage prevents the image from fading, the density from decreasing.
   3. The washing and drying stages complete the process.

III. Contrast, defined as the density differences on adjacent areas of the radiograph, is important for diagnostic images.

A. Subject contrast refers to the different densities in the image resulting from attenuation differences in the body.

B. Film contrast is the inherent ability of a particular film to record a range of densities.
   1. High-contrast films, also called short scale films, show sharp differences in density, but with relatively few steps in the gray scale from light to dark.
   2. Low-contrast films, called long scale films, show more subtle differences with slight tissue variations, with more shades of gray.

C. Other factors within the radiographer's control also affect contrast.
   1. Scatter radiation causes fog, which reduces the contrast in a radiograph.
      a. Grids, collimators, and other beam-restricting devices reduce the amount of scatter radiation.
   2. Film-screen combinations have been developed that produce the best density and contrast for different types of examinations.
   3. Fog, which uniformly increases density and reduces contrast, may result from poor film storage or development conditions.
   4. The use of standardized SIDs prevents density and contrast deviations that could result from inconsistent SIDs.
   5. Contrast media are used to increase contrast in body areas into which the medium is injected, ingested, or otherwise inserted.
      a. Positive contrast agents (such as barium ingested into the stomach) attenuate x-rays and decrease the density in that area of the radiograph.
      b. Negative contrast agents (such as air injected into an organ) help let x-rays pass through the area and increase the density in that area of the radiograph.
   6. Problems with the film processing solutions can cause chemical fog that reduces contrast.

Teaching Tips

The Radiographic Image

This module covers such a wide variety of variables that influence density and contrast that some students may feel a bit overwhelmed at first trying to keep it all straight. Reassure students that although the quality of the radiographic image can be affected by a dozen different factors, in practice they are generally concerned with only two or three. In fact, with the use of technique charts and automated systems, they usually will not have to make decisions about even these few selections. Yet it is important that they understand how density and contrast are controlled and the various factors that affect diagnostic quality. First, they need this knowledge to help complete their theoretical understanding of the entire imaging process. They may be asked questions by patients, for example, about why an examination is being done in a certain way. Secondly, if a problem occurs that results in an image having poor contrast or density, they may need to know how to change exposure variables if the radiograph must be retaken, or they may need to inform others in the department about a possible problem with the equipment, the developer, or other factors. Finally, there will be examination circumstances in which automated or standardized examinations using technique charts just won't work, and they will have to adjust their technique to get the best images. Talk about these factors with your students, and share your own experiences with density and contrast problems, so that they have a wider perspective on how all this information matters.

Density

It may be effective to begin your class discussions of density with a quick review of the whole process of what happens when x-ray photons strike the film to make an exposure through to the development process that leads to the final image of black metallic silver on the film. Once students clearly understand this process, virtually all variables affecting contrast and density can be related back to these fundamental concepts. For example, it is relatively easy to understand how doubling the mA will double the density, because twice as many x-ray photons penetrate the body to have twice as much effect on the silver halide crystals and so on, resulting in twice as much black metallic silver being deposited on the film.

The same underlying explanations can be given for the effects of other variables too. For example, as the SID is increased by the inverse square law, the beam is more dispersed, such that fewer x-ray photons penetrate the body to reach the film to interact with the silver halide crystals and so on. Fog can be understood in terms of density and contrast as a generalized darkening of the film when x-ray photons scattered in all directions within the patient reach the film to expose and darken the film all over, including areas of dense tissue where the primary x-ray beam was mostly attenuated inside the patient—so that "white" areas of bones, for example, become darker. Even postexposure variables such as unacceptable variations in developer solution strength or temperature can be better understood through the same consistent explanation: although the correct amount of film crystals were exposed to result in good density and contrast, if the chemical processes in the developer fail to properly convert just the right amount of these crystals into black metallic silver, then the image density will suffer. For example, overdevelopment will turn even some unexposed crystals into black metallic silver, resulting in an image that is too dark.

Again, using this perspective throughout your discussions of density and contrast will help students gain a unified understanding of how so many different factors can affect density and contrast. If class time permits, you may call upon students to explain, for each factor affecting density, what is happening at the level of the crystals in the film.

Although it is easier to refer to "film" through this discussion to help students understand, always remind students that most of the same principles hold true for other types of image receptors as well.

mAs, kVp, and Density

The effect of mAs on density was mentioned above. This is fairly easy for most students to grasp because it is a direct proportion: doubling the mAs doubles the number of x-ray photons, thereby doubling the metallic silver produced, which doubles the density. Understanding the 15% rule with kVp is more difficult for some students to understand, however, because it does not seem intuitive. To clarify this, you may have to lead students back through a review of how x-ray photons at different energy levels are more likely to interact with matter in different ways: absorption, scatter, or transmission.

Because this material is usually covered along with other principles of radiographic physics, this module only briefly describes the effects leading to the 15% rule. Most importantly, students need to understand why kVp is a more complex variable to manipulate when it comes to density and contrast. Increasing kVp, within limits, does increase density, but higher kVp may also increase scatter radiation that diminishes the contrast. The penetrating quality of the x-ray beam is also affected by changes in kVp, as is patient dose. In many situations, then, changing the mAs may be the preferred way to increase or decrease the density.

Throughout your discussions about density and contrast, use as many radiographs as practical to illustrate these concepts. Actually looking at a dark image has much more impact on students than saying "too much density." This module contains a number of radiographs showing desirable and undesirable levels of density and contrast, and you can supplement these with radiographs printed in textbooks. Most effective for teaching purposes are the same views or examinations with different exposure variables, so that students can see effective and ineffective images side by side.

Other Variables and Density

In addition to mAs and kVp, this module describes many other factors that influence density, including all the following: SID, intensifying screens, anode-heel effect, grids, collimators, aperture diaphragms, cones and cylinders, filters, patient size, and film processing. As noted earlier, it is important for students to understand the interplay of all these variables with the final image, however, students also need to know that most of these are devices or factors used for other reasons, not principally to change density or contrast. For example, a radiographer should understand how a change in SID affects density, but altering SID is not a normal way to control density. Collimators reduce fog and thereby improve contrast, but the main reason for using a collimator is not to improve contrast but to reduce patient exposure. Intensifying screens improve density, but the main reason for using them is to reduce patient dose; if the dose did not matter, then it would be easier just to increase the exposure variables to get the best density and not use an intensifying screen at all.

The exceptions here are the use of grids to reduce fog caused by scatter—to improve contrast—and the use of compensating filters to even out density in specific circumstances. Both of these are discussed in this module to help students understand how these devices work and the reasons for using them. But because only a limited amount of time could be spent on these subjects in this module, you may want to supplement this discussion by talking with students about practical circumstances for using them. Additional specific examples of when different kinds of compensating filters are used to improve contrast in specific examinations would help students better grasp the functions of this equipment.

Contrast Media

The effects of most variables on contrast have already been mentioned above. The use of contrast agents, however, is often of interest to students, in part because the effects often make for such dramatic and interesting images. Although this module gives only a few examples of the use of contrast media to improve contrast—to clarify the general principles—you may choose to bring in additional radiographs or texts showing the wide variety of uses of contrast media to image different organs and body areas. Showing students these images while discussing this way to manipulate contrast also makes an interesting conclusion for your class time spent on contrast, as it helps bridge from the understanding of theory into what students often find more exciting: the world of practice.

Workbook Posttest Answers and Rationales

1. The visible blackness on a finished radiograph is composed of which of the following?
   a. Silver halide crystals
   b. Metallic silver—The developer turns the exposed silver halide crystals into black metallic silver.
   c. Unexposed film emulsion
   d. Fixer

2. Contrast is defined as which of the following?
   a. The difference between adjacent areas of density in a radiograph—This is the basic definition, the difference between the light areas and the dark areas of the radiograph.
   b. The overall amount of blackness in a radiograph
   c. The characteristic ability of a grid to reduce scatter
   d. None of the above

3. The characteristic curve has to do with which of the following?
   a. mA and kVp
   b. mA and mAs
   c. Exposure and contrast
   d. Exposure and density—The curve shows this relationship, for example, how increasing the exposure increases the density.

4. If a radiograph was made at 100 kVp, and you wanted to double the amount of density to make a second radiograph (with all other factors remaining unchanged), what kVp would you use?
   a. 50 kVp
   b. 85 kVp
   c. 115 kVp—This is known as the 15% rule: to double the density, increase the kVp by 15%.
   d. 200 kVp

5. What is the result of scatter radiation reaching the film?
   a. Fog
   b. More density
   c. Less contrast
   d. All of the above—All these occur because the scatter radiation darkens the film overall (fog), which is an increase in density overall, which also lowers the contrast as the lighter areas become darker.
   e. None of the above

6. Which factor is most often manipulated if a radiograph must be repeated because it is too light or too dark?
   a. mAs—Changing the mAs is usually the preferred way to change density; changing kVp involves too many other factors (penetration, patient dose, contrast); SID is usually standardized, and OID is almost always as short as possible.
   b. kVp
   c. SID
   d. OID

7. If all other factors remained the same, increasing the SID would have what effect on density of the radiograph?
   a. Less density—Because of the inverse square law, a greater SID means a decreased intensity of the beam, which would result in decreased density.
   b. More density
   c. Same density
   d. Depends on patient size

8. Where is the intensifying screen usually positioned?
   a. Next to the filter
   b. Just inside the collimator
   c. On top of the patient
   d. Next to the film—The screen is usually in contact with the film, because the goal is to minimize any spreading out of the light photons produced in the screen before they reach the film.

9. What is the main reason for using an intensifying screen?
   a. To reduce scatter
   b. To reduce patient exposure—The screen works to expose the film mostly by light produced by x-rays penetrating the patient; so less x-ray exposure of the patient is required.
   c. To decrease density
   d. To make up for decreased penetration with large patients

10. Reasons to use a collimator or other beam-restricting devices include which of the following?
    a. Less scatter radiation
    b. Lower patient exposure
    c. Improved contrast
    d. All of the above—Reducing the beam's field size exposes the patient to less radiation, which also produces less scatter; with less fog from scatter, the contrast is improved.
    e. None of the above

11. What do compensating filters compensate for?
    a. Differences in body structures—Compensating filters even out the density in the radiograph when imaging body areas with very different levels of attenuation.
    b. Differences in kVp settings
    c. Variations in the cross section of the x-ray beam
    d. Variations in SID

12. Irregularities with the film developer can cause which of the following?
    a. Poor density
    b. Poor contrast
    c. Both poor density and poor contrast— Too much developer (from too strong a solution or too high a temperature) causes too much density, and other chemical problems can cause fog, which diminishes contrast.
    d. Neither poor density nor poor contrast

13. Film contrast is defined as which of the following?
    a. The variations in metallic silver resulting from how much of the beam is attenuated within the patient
    b. The color range of the film
    c. The film speed multiplied by the exposure time
    d. The inherent ability of a film to record a range of densities—This is the basic definition of film contrast, which is a characteristic of the film itself, not an exposure factor.

14. What can cause fog?
    a. Scatter radiation
    b. Improper film storage conditions
    c. Incorrect film developer temperatures
    d. All of the above—Fog, which is a uniform increase in density over the radiograph (thereby reducing contrast), may result from all these factors.
    e. None of the above

15. Which of the following is true of contrast media?
    a. They always increase the density in certain areas of the radiograph
    b. They always decrease the density in certain areas of the radiograph
    c. They affect the density in different ways depending on the media. Positive contrast agents attenuate x-rays and decrease the density in that area; negative contrast agents increase the density.
    d. None of the above is true.

Testbank Questions

1. What can happen when an x-ray photon from the primary beam enters a patient's body?
    a. The photon can be transmitted through the body to the film.
    b. The photon can be absorbed.
    c. The photon can be scattered.
    d. All of the above are true.
    e. None of the above is true.

2. What happens to exposed silver halide crystals in the film when they are developed?
    a. They turn into sensitivity specks.
    b. They turn into black metallic silver.
    c. They are washed off the film.
    d. None of the above is true.

3. A radiograph that is too dark has likely been which of the following?
    a. Overexposed
    b. Underexposed
    c. Underdeveloped
    d. Exposed at an unusually long SID

4. The amount of overall blackening on a radiograph is which of the following?
   a. Emulsion
   b. Exposure
   c. Contrast
   d. Density

5. The difference in density of adjacent areas on a radiograph is which of the following?
   a. Contrast
   b. Exposure
   c. Penumbra
   d. Characteristic curve

6. When might it be useful to use a densitometer?
   a. When checking the solution strength in the developer tank
   b. When measuring a patient for an examination
   c. When creating technique charts to get the best images
   d. None of the above

7. What does the characteristic curve shows us?
   a. Small exposure changes at low-range exposure levels cause larger density changes.
   b. Small exposure changes at mid-range exposure levels cause larger density changes.
   c. Small exposure changes at high-range exposure levels cause larger density changes.
   d. All of the above are true.

8. How is mAs calculated?
   a. mA in milliamps divided by time in seconds
   b. mA in milliamps minus time in seconds
   c. mA in milliamps multiplied by time in seconds
   d. mA in milliamps added to time in seconds

9. The density on a radiograph is doubled if you do which of the following?
   a. Double the mAs
   b. Reduce the mAs by half
   c. Increase the mAs by 15%
   d. Decrease the mAs by 15%

10. kVp controls which of the following?
    a. The number of x-ray photons in the beam
    b. The speed of x-ray photons in the beam
    c. The energy level of x-ray photons in the beam
    d. The size of x-ray photons in the beam

11. What percentage increase in kVp causes a doubling in the density?
    a. 100%
    b. 50%
    c. 25%
    d. 15%

12. Typically mAs selection is changed to improve density rather than the kVp. Why?
   a. Changing the kVp may produce scatter, too much patient exposure, poor contrast or problems in penetrating the body area.
   b. The amount of density is directly proportional to the mAs.
   c. Changing SID does affect density but is not the most practical way to adjust density.
   d. All of the above are true.
   e. None of the above is true.

13. The term "focus-film distance," seldom used anymore, refers to which of the following?
   a. Source-to-image receptor distance
   b. Source-to-object distance
   c. Object-to-image receptor distance
   d. Tube-to-focal point distance

14. What is the most common type of film-screen combination?
   a. Single-emulsion film next to one intensifying screen
   b. Double-emulsion film next to one intensifying screen
   c. Single-emulsion film between two intensifying screens
   d. Double-emulsion film between two intensifying screens

15. Why are grids able to absorb scatter radiation?
   a. Lead absorbs x-ray photons.
   b. Scatter radiation is produced at an angle to the beam.
   c. The primary beam travels in a straight line from the tube to the image receptor.
   d. All of the above are true.
   e. None of the above is true.

16. How does a cone function?
   a. By focusing the beam into a narrow, more concentrated conelike shape
   b. By absorbing x-rays except those in the part of the beam desired to reach the patient and image receptor
   c. By bending the beam in the desired direction
   d. All of the above
   e. None of the above

17. What is the primary reason for using a compensating filter?
   a. To even out density
   b. To reduce the exposure to the patient
   c. To reduce the exposure when a short SID must be used
   d. All of the above
   e. None of the above

18. When selecting exposure variables for a heavy and a thin patient, what is the best way to ensure the best density for each?
   a. Use double the mA for the heavier patient
   b. Use 15% higher kVp for the heavier patient
   c. Consult the technique chart for the examination
   d. Use a shorter SID for the heavier patient

19. Using a positive contrast medium can make the density of a soft tissue area do which of the following?
    a. Look closer to the density of bone on a radiograph than without the contrast
    b. Look even more different from the density of bone on a radiograph than without the contrast
    c. Look blacker in the radiograph than without the contrast
    d. None of the above

20. Intensifying screens do which of the following?
    a. Increase contrast
    b. Decrease patient exposure
    c. Have different speeds, which are paired with the appropriate films
    d. All of the above
    e. None of the above

Answers to Testbank Questions

1. d	6. c	11. d	16. b
2. b	7. b	12. d	17. a
3. a	8. c	13. a	18. c
4. d	9. a	14. d	19. a
5. a	10. c	15. d	20. d

Audiovisual Script

SLIDE 2-1/CD 3-i Welcome
Welcome to Mosby's Radiographic Instructional Series.

SLIDE 3-2/CD 3-ii Density and contrast
The module you are about to experience is the second of eight in the Radiographic Imaging program: Radiographic Density and Contrast.

This module will help you understand density and contrast, identify the acceptable range of density, differentiate between subject and film contrast, and analyze the relationships of factors that affect density and contrast.

SLIDE 2-3/CD 2-1 Introduction
There's a great deal of skill involved in producing a radiograph that will give good information the human eye can readily see. And a good image is very important: radiologists can only make accurate diagnoses from radiographic films that clearly show the parts of the body under examination.

Like the photographs you take yourself at home, the best radiographic images are the ones that are sharply recorded and distinctly show overall darkening with differences between adjacent densities. With your own photos, you know yourself that subjects are either washed out or lost in shadows (which makes them difficult to see) if you haven't taken film speed and light conditions into account. Those are the ones that don't make it into your album.

The same principles hold true with radiographic images. But in radiography, exposure involves the proper combination of kVp, milliamperes, and the exposure time used to produce the image. Here, the two terms to remember are density and contrast. The amount of radiographic density and its variations, what we call contrast, are what we'll study in detail in this module.

SLIDE 2-4/CD 2-2 Radiographs comparing density
Let's talk about density first. The amount of overall blackening on a radiograph, or of a certain part of the image, is referred to as optical density, radiographic density, or just plain density, which is what we'll call it. Density depends on two things: the amount of radiation that reaches a particular area of the film, and the mass of black metallic silver deposited when the film is developed. The radiograph on the left has excellent density and the one on the right has a density level that is too light.

When a radiologist looks at a radiograph, she or he looks for any anatomic or pathologic change that causes a change in the normal density. That could be, for example, a solid mass in the lung that stops x-rays from reaching the detector and decreases the amount of film darkening in that area.

CD 2-2A Absorption and transmission
When x-rays pass through a patient's body, three things can happen: (1) the x-ray photon is transmitted, it passes through the body, interacts with the film, and produces a dark area on the film; (2) the x-ray photon is absorbed, and because fewer x-rays penetrate bone than soft tissue, those areas appear light on the film; and (3) the x-ray photons are scattered, which darkens areas that would have been light if the direction of the rays hadn't changed.

SLIDE 2-5/CD 2-3 Black metallic silver
What the radiographer sees on the finished radiograph are the variations in the amount of black metallic silver (the silver bromide crystals) that stay on the film after film processing. The exposed silver emulsion is converted into black metallic silver as it's developed. The tiny particles look black because they're so finely divided. How black a radiograph is depends on the amount of exposure that reaches the emulsion of the film.

There can be a range of densities on the film, from total black (where there is no light transmitted) to nearly clear. Problems occur when the density of the image is too light or too dark. A radiograph that is too dark has been overexposed (too much radiation reached the image receptor). A radiograph that hasn't been exposed to enough radiation is underexposed. Both may be difficult to interpret.

CD 2-3A Density variations
Occasionally difficulty is encountered in attempting to get high-quality films. When deciding whether a repeat film is needed, you may be able to use a film that is slightly overexposed. A film that has absorbed too many photons has recorded more information than it needs.

The solution: Either a computerized optical scanner or a bright light can eliminate some of that extra information and salvage the film enough so it can be seen by the human eye; however, a repeat is typically done.

A film that's too light because it hasn't absorbed enough photons, however, can't be saved because it hasn't recorded enough information in the first place.

SLIDE 2-6/CD 2-4 Types of contrast
We'll get back to density and the factors that influence it in just a few minutes. But first, let's talk about radiographic contrast so you'll have an idea of how it relates to density.

A radiograph consists of light and dark areas. That means it shows variations in density. The range of that variation between light and dark is called the radiographic contrast. Another definition of contrast is the difference in density of adjacent areas on a radiograph.

As you've seen, density represents the amount of silver deposited in an area during film processing. Contrast, on the other hand, represents how that silver is distributed in various areas. Contrast is what enables us to see anatomical detail.

There are really three kinds of contrast, but two of them come under the general umbrella of radiographic contrast. They are subject contrast and film contrast. We'll talk in more detail about contrast a little later.

SLIDE 2-7/CD 2-5 Densitometer
But for now, let's consider the acceptable ranges of radiographic densities. You can figure that out with an instrument called a densitometer, which measures film blackness. Film blackness is the relationship of the intensity of the light that hits the film from the view box to the intensity of the light transmitted through the film. You can plot the measurements on a graph called a characteristic curve.

Here's the algebraic equation for density:

$$\text{Density} = \text{Log}\,\frac{\text{Io (Incident intensity)}}{\text{It (Transmitted intensity)}}$$

The limitations of the human eye affect the useful density range for diagnostic radiography. In numbers, the diagnostically useful range of densities is 0.25 to 2.5. You'll learn more about this in detail in the module on exposure calculation.

CD 2-5A Characteristic curve
The characteristic curve measures the relationship between density and exposure. When exposure is low or high, small exposure changes cause small changes in density. (Toe and shoulder refer to these ends of the curve.) At mid-range exposure levels, small exposure changes cause bigger changes in density. This area is the straight-line part of the curve, and it's where well-exposed films lie.

CD 2-5B Density and contrast
Let's pause for a moment for a quick review. Density and contrast are basic concepts in radiography and you should be sure you know what they are.

As you've seen, density refers to the amount of blackening on a radiograph. You see a lot of density on one of the radiographs shown here. How would you define contrast, as shown in the other?

Variations in light and dark areas OR

The relationship between incident and transmitted intensity

Click on your answer now.

PRESENT THIS AUDIO IF ANSWER WAS variations in light and dark areas: Yes, you're right. Density represents the amount of silver halide crystals deposited in an area of a radiograph during processing. Contrast represents the variation of those crystals spread out over various areas or the range of density levels shown.

PRESENT THIS AUDIO IF ANSWER WAS the relationship between incident and transmitted intensity: Actually, the correct answer is that while density represents the amount of silver halide crystals deposited in an area of a radiograph during processing, contrast represents the variation of those crystals spread out over various areas or the range of density levels shown.

SLIDE 2-8/CD 2-6 Ranges of density

You have begun the topic of acceptable ranges of density. This topic builds on the preceding topic of density and contrast. If you haven't yet worked through the earlier topic, you may want to quit this section now and return later after going through it.

Now let's talk about the acceptable ranges of density and the factors that affect it.

Many factors affect the density of a radiographic image. The primary controlling factors are milliamperage (mA) and exposure time, but kilovoltage (kVp), distance from the source, and the thickness and nature of the part of the body being radiographed, and other factors all influence density. We'll discuss them one-by-one.

SLIDE 2-9/CD 2-7 mA and density

Let's consider mA first. X-ray currents are measured in milliamperes; A stands for ampere, a measure of current, and m stands for the prefix milli, 1/1000 (0.001). Normal household current is a few amperes.

mA controls the number of x-ray photons produced in the tube and determines the exposure rate only, not the penetrating ability of an x-ray beam. The mA control on the operating console adjusts the current flowing through the filament in the cathode.

In other words, mA is a measure of the flow of electrons per second from the cathode to the anode of the x-ray tube. As the flow increases, more x-ray photons per second are produced at the target.

SLIDE 2-10/CD 2-8 High and low mA effect

The exposure rate, what's referred to as R/sec, is directly proportional to the mA. If x-rays have penetrated a part of the body being studied but the density is such that you can't see the part very well, you can adjust the mA level to compensate. When you double the mA, the x-ray exposure rate doubles, when you triple the mA, the rate triples, and so on. But the energy of the x-ray photons themselves isn't affected.

As shown here, a high mA produces more x-rays than a low mA.

MORE INFO LEADS TO THIS AUDIO RESPONSE: The R in R/sec stands for Roentgen, the German scientist who, you remember, discovered x-rays.

In 1928, the Second International Congress of Radiology designated the R as the international exposure unit. It's based on ionization in air. Ionization, which you studied in the Radiologic Physics module, is the process of changing atoms to ions.

SLIDE 2-11/CD 2-9 Milliampere-seconds

The combination of mA and the exposure time (measured in seconds) determines how many x-rays are produced during an exposure. mAs, milliampere-seconds, are the product of mA and time and control the number of electrons flowing from cathode to anode during the exposure. When you increase or decrease either mA or exposure time, the density is changed accordingly.

You can vary mA and time and still maintain the mAs you've selected without changing the density. For example, you can achieve 10 mAs if you use 10 mA and 1 second. Or 100 mA and 1/10 second. Or 300 mA and 1/30 second. Or 400 mA and 1/40 second. And so on. Each combination that leads to the same mAs produces an equal number of electrons to produce x-rays, and you end up with the same density.

In order to make a change in density that's visible to the human eye, you have to change the mA setting by at least 30%.

Or, you can change the mA and time (along with kVp) to either maintain or vary density and contrast.

SLIDE 2-12/CD 2-10 Review: effect of mA

Let's pause for a quick review.

How many and at what rate x-ray photons come from an x-ray tube depends on many things. But of all the factors that govern the exposure of radiation and the density that results (and which you as a radiographer can control) mA is the most influential.

The reason is that mA measures the x-ray tube current (how many electrons cross the tube from cathode to anode per second). So here's the question: As mA increases, what happens to the current?

It increases OR It decreases

Click on your answer now.

The correct answer is the current increases. As the mA level increases, so does the number of electrons that cross the tube. And as the flow increases, so does the number of x-ray photons per second produced at the target. Remember, when you double the mA, the current increases, but it's the x-ray exposure rate that doubles.

PRESENT THIS AUDIO IF ANSWER WAS increases: Good. As the mA level increases, so does the number of electrons that cross the tube. And as the flow increases, so does the number of x-ray photons per second produced at the target.

PRESENT THIS AUDIO IF ANSWER WAS decreases: No, it doesn't decrease. What happens is that as mA increases, so does the number of electrons that cross the tube. And as the flow increases, so does the number of x-ray photons per second produced at the target. Remember, when you double the mA, the current increases, but it's the x-ray exposure rate that doubles.

SLIDE 2-13/CD 2-11 Effect of kVp

Now let's take a look at kilovoltage (kVp). The kVp range determines two things: (1) the ability of the x-ray beam to penetrate the subject and (2) the quality of the beam itself. That means kVp affects density because it can produce higher-energy photons that will pass more easily through the body.

As kVp increases, the number of primary photons does too, because the tube current's kinetic energy is more efficiently converted into x-rays. These more penetrating photons aren't as easily absorbed, so a larger percentage of the primary radiation reaches the intensifying screens. (You'll learn more about screens later in this module.) The result is an increase in kVp that increases the exposure of the film and the resulting density.

MORE INFO LEADS TO THIS AUDIO RESPONSE: Here's a reminder of what voltage means. It's the difference in electrical potential that's needed in conventional circuits to move an electric charge from point to point. Kilovoltage is the potential difference placed across an x-ray tube's electrodes. Higher-energy x-rays are produced as the kVp increases.

SLIDE 2-14/CD 2-12 kVp 15% rule

An increase of 15% in kVp just about doubles the exposure. This principle is referred to as the "15% Rule." For example, you can double the exposure at 80 kVp by adding 12 kVp. But bear this in mind: While density increases as kVp does, this isn't a strictly proportional relationship.

Usually, with grids having a ratio of 8:1 or less (we'll talk more about grids a little later on), it's best not to exceed 85 kVp because increasing kVp will increase the amount of scatter radiation exiting the patient. Scatter radiation causes film fog and lowers the contrast.

CD 2-12A Scatter radiation

Scatter radiation is something to avoid because it reduces the contrast and visibility of a radiograph. X-rays are scattered when the direction they're traveling in changes and they lose energy. That causes unnecessary darkening on the film.

SLIDE 2-15/CD 2-13 Effect of exposure time

Exposure time has a role to play in the degree of density, too. Keep this general principle in mind: The longer the exposure time, the more x-ray photons emitted by the x-ray tube. And the same holds true when considering mA: Doubling the exposure time doubles the exposure, tripling the exposure time triples the exposure, and so on.

The longer the time the film is exposed to radiation, the more silver halide crystals in the film emulsion are affected. That increases density.

SLIDE 2-16/CD 2-14 Variations in contrast

Although it's true that increasing kVp will show a corresponding increase in density, altering kVp is complex. Changing the setting affects a lot of other properties, like penetration, patient dose, scatter, and contrast. As you gain more experience in radiography, you'll come to know whether the radiographic image can best be improved by a change in density or by changing the contrast.

SLIDE 2-17/CD 2-15 Radiographer control

All of this calculation may seem a bit complicated now, but as you learn more about radiography and actually begin to work in the field, you'll be more comfortable with this part of it.

As a general rule, keep this in mind: If a radiograph needs to be repeated because of improper density, you need to either double the original mAs, if it was too light, or cut the original mAs in half, if it was too dark. For example, if the resulting image was too light with an original mAs of 10, then you need to adjust it to 20. With more experience, you'll be able to make these adjustments with ease.

CD 2-15A Automatic control systems

As a radiographer, your job is to produce images with proper density. The mA setting is usually made by following the technique chart for that particular equipment.

Exposure time for any particular examination may be selected by the technologist based upon body part and thickness, or it may be controlled by an automatic exposure control system that shuts the exposure off when a proper density has been achieved.

SLIDE 2-18/CD 2-16 Effect of SID

Now we come to distance, referred to as focus-film distance (FFD) or source-to-image receptor distance (SID) in radiography. The terms mean the distance between the source of x-rays and the film, which affects the intensity of the exposure. We'll use the term most commonly accepted these days: SID.

A good way to understand the effect of distance on x-rays is to think about the way a flashlight works. When you shine it out into the dark, you can see things that are close because the source of light focuses directly on them. As you shine the light out over a wider arc, however, its impact becomes weaker and objects are less clearly visible. That's because the same amount of light is spreading out over a much larger area. You should remember from your study of Radiologic Physics that this is called the inverse-square law.

CD 2-16A Beam intensity and SID

Most people in radiography now use the term source-to-image receptor distance (SID), rather than focus-film distance, (FFD), which has become outdated.

Distance doesn't have any effect on the quality of radiation. But the SID you use to make an exposure is what determines a beam's intensity when it strikes the image receptor.

Note that most SIDs in radiography are standardized. Many radiographs are made using an SID of 40 inches. Chest radiographs routinely use an SID of 72 inches.

SLIDE 2-19/CD 2-17 Beam spread over distance

X-rays spread from a focal spot on the x-ray tube in a conelike shape in all directions. (The beam becomes wider as the distance from the target increases, so usually a beam limiting device called a collimator is used to modify it.) In other words, the same amount of radiation spreads out over a larger area the farther that area is from the tube focus.

When the area is larger, the amount of radiation thins itself out to cover it. That means the density at a farther distance is less for a given exposure because the area is getting less radiation than an area closer to the x-ray tube would get. You can compensate for this by increasing the mAs.

MORE INFO LEADS TO THIS AUDIO RESPONSE: A collimator has dials or levers you can adjust to change the radiation field size. It's mounted permanently on the tube housing.

SLIDE 2-20/CD 2-18 Inverse square law

Even slight variations in SID make a significant difference in density. That's because of the inverse-square law, which says that the intensity of x-rays, (and the film density), is inversely proportional to the square of the distance between the point at which the radiation is received and its source.

In other words, if you reduce the SID to half of the original distance, intensity and density will increase by a factor of 4.

SLIDE 2-21/CD 2-19 Intensifying screens

Now let's turn to different kinds of factors that affect radiographic density. As we mentioned earlier, one of these is the intensifying screen. An intensifying screen is a device inside the film cassette that converts some of the energy of the x-ray beam to visible light. The light interacts with the film in the cassette to create a latent image and greatly reduces the time a patient is exposed to radiation.

Only about one third of the x-rays that strike a screen interact with it. But each one emits many visible light photons. A screen amplifies the x-ray beam, meaning that fewer x-ray photons need to pass through the body in order to produce an image. That, in turn, allows a lower dose of radiation to the patient. Most radiographic exams use intensifying screens, even though they tend to cause a slight degree of image unsharpness.

In the early days of radiography, glass plates with a layer of photographic emulsion coated on one side were used, not film. It could take as long as a half hour to complete an exposure. Film with double-emulsion greatly reduced the exposure time and patient dose. It reached the market by World War I and was used with an intensifying screen.

MORE INFO LEADS TO THIS AUDIO RESPONSE: Before World War I, much of the glass used in radiography came from Belgium and other European countries. But with a war waging on, glass was difficult to get. At the same time, battlefield injuries increased the demand for radiography. A substitute base for the photographic emulsion used in radiography was clearly necessary. The one that was developed was cellulose nitrate, and it turned out to be more efficient than glass plates.

SLIDE 2-22/CD 2-20 Composition of screens

Intensifying screens usually look like sheets of plastic and usually have four layers. The base is made of plastic and supports the other layers.

The second layer is the reflective layer. It helps to redirect light, which is emitted in all directions, back toward the film. This helps increase screen speed, but it reduces detail in the image.

The third layer, the phosphor, is the active part of the intensifying screen. The phosphor crystals emit the light that exposes the x-ray film.

The fourth layer, the protective one, protects the phosphor layer and helps prevent static electricity.

CD 2-20A Review of screen function
Okay, let's pause for a minute to review intensifying screens, which were invented by the light bulb inventor, Thomas Edison, in 1896. You've seen that their function is to turn x-ray energy into visible light. Is it true that by doing so, screens cut down on the time a patient is exposed to x-rays during an exam?

Yes or No?
Click on your answer now.

PRESENT THIS AUDIO IF ANSWER IS yes: Yes, the reason is that intensifying screens produce a lot of light photons when they're struck by the x-rays, even though only about one third of them will interact with the screen. This light forms almost all of the latent image (99%); x-ray photons do the rest. That means much less radiation is needed to produce a good quality radiograph, so the patient receives much less exposure than he or she would have if there had been no screen.

PRESENT THIS AUDIO OF ANSWER IS no: No, screens do cut down on patient dose, which is why they're used so much in radiography. The reason is that intensifying screens produce a lot of light photons when they're struck by the x-rays, even though only about one third of them will interact with the screen. This light forms almost all of the latent image (99%); x-ray photons do the rest. That means much less radiation is needed to produce a good quality radiograph, so the patient receives much less exposure than he or she would have if there had been no screen.

SLIDE 2-23/CD 2-21 Comparison of radiographs
Radiographic film is sandwiched between two intensifying screens in a cassette, and the screens convert the energy of the x-ray beam into visible light. The light interacts with the film and forms the latent image. The image on the left was made using a screen and the one on the right without a screen.

Most radiographic procedures use film holders, called cassettes, that have a set of two screens and use double-emulsion film. Some, like mammography, use only one screen with single-emulsion film.

SLIDE 2-24/CD 2-22 Anode heel effect
One way to improve a radiographic image is to take advantage of the anode heel effect. This is a variation in the intensity of the x-ray beam along the anode-cathode axis. The part of the beam nearer the anode is less intense than the part of the beam nearer the cathode side.

The heel effect is something to think about when you radiograph body parts that vary in thickness. As a general rule, you'll get more uniform density on the film by positioning the cathode side of the x-ray tube over the thicker part of the body. You'll see cathode and anode directions indicated on the protective housing.

SLIDE 2-25/CD 2-23 Grids
There are other ways to improve the quality of radiographs. One way is to use a grid, which absorbs much of the radiation that is scattered in the patient by the moderate-energy x-rays used for diagnosis, before it reaches the film. Scatter radiation adds unwanted density to an image and also reduces contrast.

A grid is made of thin lead strips separated by a radiolucent material. It works this way: primary radiation passes through the material, and the lead strips absorb the scatter. Grids have a profound impact on contrast, so we'll discuss them in more detail when we get to contrast.

MORE INFO LEADS TO THIS AUDIO RESPONSE: Gustav Bucky, inventor of the grid, first experimented with grids in 1913. His design has been streamlined as technology has advanced, but the basic principle hasn't changed.

SLIDE 2-26/CD 2-24 Collimation

Another way to limit scatter radiation is to restrict the primary x-ray beam. A major factor contributing to the production of scatter radiation is a large primary beam field size. The more patient tissue that is exposed to the primary beam, the more scatter is produced. Beam restriction means reducing the beam to either the size of the film, or better yet, to the area of the body under study.

A collimator, the most common beam restrictor, can help to reduce the amount of scatter radiation produced in the patient but doesn't eliminate it. You control collimation by adjusting a double set of lead shutters that sit directly under the x-ray tube port, using two controls as shown here.

SLIDE 2-27/CD 2-25 Aperture diaphragms and cones

A less common way of controlling the size of the x-ray beam includes using aperture diaphragms and cones. They do limit the beam, but not to the extent of collimation.

Let's talk about aperture diaphragms first. They're sheets of metal placed below the tube port with a hole in the center of the sheet that corresponds to the desired field size. The opening lets part of the primary x-ray beam pass through to the patient.

The aperture can be any shape. You may use apertures that are commercially manufactured or ones that someone in the department has made. If they're used in all exams, you have to have a large supply on hand, and go through the inconvenience of changing them frequently.

Aperture diaphragms don't offer much flexibility because they're designed for a fixed film size and SID. You'll most often see them these days with dedicated chest units and some tomography units.

MORE INFO LEADS TO THIS AUDIO RESPONSE: An aperture diaphragm may not be the most efficient beam-limiting device, but it is the simplest, and one of the first to be used. One that is designed well projects an image 1 centimeter smaller than the film on all sides. You should see an unexposed border on the radiograph.

SLIDE 2-28/CD 2-26 Cones and cylinders

Cones are metal extension devices attached below the tube port that can be either flared or cylinder-shaped. Cylindrical cones produce a sharper image because they restrict the beam better than flared ones. You'll see them in mammography and in some head and spine radiography.

Cones were the next beam-limiting devices that came into use after aperture diaphragms, and they proved to be better at limiting the size of x-ray beams than their predecessors. They have metal plates with a round opening that attaches them to the tube housing. A metal sheet forms a ring and extends from the metal plate to the tube.

Cones eliminate most of the secondary radiation that's produced at the edge of the opening, as well as part of the radiation that comes from the tube.

SLIDE 2-29/CD 2-27 Filtration

Now let's discuss filtration. X-rays have mixed wavelengths. Some of the x-ray photons in the beam have a short wavelength and are highly penetrating, although others have a long wavelength and can be absorbed by the patient's tissues. The purpose of a filter is to absorb the long wavelengths before they reach the patient. That increases the average energy of the beam and reduces the dose to the patient by as much as 80%.

Just about any material (copper or leather, for example) could serve as a filter, but aluminum is the standard because it efficiently removes low-energy x-rays and because it's easy to shape into filters.

CD 2-27A Dr. William Rollins

Dr. William Rollins was a Boston physician/dentist who was the first to use collimation and filtration in the late 1800s. After receiving radiation burns to his hand in x-ray experiments in 1898, he used leather and aluminum filters when he made x-ray exposures of his patients' teeth.

He was concerned about the dangers of x-rays (in contrast to most other scientists of the time, many of whom suffered severe radiation burns and illnesses because of their indiscriminate use of the new technology). He experimented with guinea pigs and proved x-rays could be harmful. He published an article, "X-ray Light Kills," that was one of the first to warn about the dangers of this exciting new diagnostic tool.

SLIDE 2-30/CD 2-28 Inherent and added filtration

There are two types of filtration: inherent and added filtration. When they're added together they become total filtration.

Inherent filtration consists of the tube elements that act to filter the x-ray beam. This includes the tube's glass envelope, the insulating oil that surrounds the envelope, and the tube housing window. As the x-ray beam exits the tube, the inherent filtration removes the lower-energy, longer wavelengths.

Added filtration consists of thin sheets of aluminum placed between the protective tube housing and the collimator. The aluminum is similar to inherent filtration in that it removes low-energy x-ray photons that would otherwise contribute to an increased patient dose. Filters help produce an x-ray beam with higher effective energy and therefore greater penetrability.

SLIDE 2-31/CD 2-29 Compensating filters

Compensating filters are another common type of filter used in radiography. They come in many shapes. The most common are the wedge filter and the trough filter. They are often mounted on the collimator, as shown here.

Compensating filters even out variations due to patient thickness or pathology. For example, a chest radiograph could show very different densities if the left side has fluid or a mass and the right side is normal. The left would show low density and the right would show higher density.

In this situation a compensating filter is placed so that the thinner part is positioned over the left side. With a compensating filter used in this situation, the differences in anatomy are evened out.

You'll sometimes see trough filters in chest radiography, where they're usually used with dedicated x-ray machines. The thin part of the trough covers the mediastinum, and the thick parts filter the lungs. The result is a radiograph with more uniform density.

CD 2-29A Filtration standards

There are ways to measure filtration. Inherent filtration is about the same as a 1-mm aluminum equivalent (Al eq). That means it filters as much as 1-mm thickness of aluminum.

SLIDE 2-32/CD 2-30 Patient size

All of the factors we've been talking about are important in producing good radiographs. But don't forget an important variable in the process: the patient. You have to consider the thickness of the part of the body being examined and the composition of that area to get the best possible images. The patient's age and sex are factors, too.

It makes sense that larger patients will need more radiation than smaller ones and thick body parts will absorb more photons than thin ones. Once you measure the thickness of the part of the body you're going to radiograph, you can adjust the mAs or kVp as needed. There are charts to help guide you through this, but the adjustments you make based on your own skilled judgment are what elevate radiography from pure technique to an art.

SLIDE 2-33/CD 2-31 Tissue densities

The type of tissue and thickness of the body part to be radiographed is an important factor as well. Bone absorbs the greatest amount of radiation, followed by muscle, fat, and then air-filled tissues.

The human body is composed of many different tissue types that absorb x-rays at different rates. Some tissues permit x-ray photons to pass through unaffected, some partially absorb them, and others absorb them totally. Attenuation refers to the reduction in number of photons as the x-ray beam passes through matter.

It might be helpful to think of how glass absorbs sunlight. On a bright, sunny day, sunlight streams through the windows in your living room. But you decide the room is too bright and hot, so you draw the blinds tight across the windows so that most of the sun's rays will be deflected and the room stays dark and cool. Later you decide to let some sun in, so you open the blinds a bit. At that point part of the sun's rays are being absorbed. That's attenuation.

An x-ray beam is attenuated when it passes through a patient. Four substances account for different rates of absorption: air, fat, muscle, and bone.

Because the tissue density of air is less than the other substances, tissues that contain air absorb fewer photons as they pass through them. That means more photons reach the film, which makes for greater radiographic density.

Fat and muscle are soft-tissue structures with similar effective atomic numbers. Both are partial attenuators and therefore radiographically exhibit moderate levels of density.

Bone shows clearly on radiographs because it has a high atomic number and tissue density, which means it absorbs more radiation than fat, muscle, or tissues filled with air. Because fewer photons reach the film, there's a lesser degree of density.

SLIDE 2-34/CD 2-32 Effect of pathology

You also need to make adjustments based on the patient's illness or condition. Pathologic conditions such as excess fluid or Paget's disease may require an increase in exposure, although others such as emphysema might necessitate a decrease in exposure. Information in the patient's chart or on the radiographic requisition will help you choose the best technique.

SLIDE 2-35/CD 2-33 Film processing

Once you make a radiographic exposure, the film has to be developed, of course, and that's a process as important in getting a good image as are technique and positioning. Today that's done with automatic processing equipment that greatly cuts down the time it used to take when film was developed manually. The purpose of processing is to convert the latent image to a manifest image by reducing the silver atoms to black metallic silver, which produces the visible density on the film.

Four main steps are involved: developing, fixing, washing, and drying. We'll look at them briefly here and in more depth in a later module.

MORE INFO LEADS TO THIS AUDIO RESPONSE: These days, cost is having an impact on film. Because it is expensive, in some cases it's beginning to be replaced by the digital format used by computers. Radiographic images can be stored on disks and called up on computer screens or printed out on paper. Computer images also allow manipulation and other advantages.

SLIDE 2-36/CD 2-34 Developing

The first step is developing. During developing, exposed silver atoms are reduced to black metallic silver to produce a manifest image in the film emulsion. Density is affected by the developer time and temperature, the concentration of the developer, and the size of the phosphor crystals on the film.

During the exposure of the film, silver atoms migrate to the sensitivity specks in the phosphor crystals. A sensitivity speck is a contaminant, silver sulfide, introduced into the phosphor in the manufacturing process. At least three atoms of silver must have migrated to the sensitivity speck as a result of exposure for the crystals to turn black during developing.

This isn't a perfect process, however. Some crystals that contain a latent image may not be reduced (they stay undeveloped), and some unexposed crystals may be reduced. In both cases, image quality is compromised.

SLIDE 2-37/CD 2-35 Fixing

Next comes fixing, the step when the undeveloped silver halide is removed from the emulsion. In the automatic processor shown here, the film has entered the middle tank for fixing. Once the image is "fixed" on the film, it won't fade and can become a permanent part of the patient's record.

You may hear the term "archival quality." That simply means the film can be stored indefinitely without changing because the fixing step has been properly done.

CD 2-35A Automatic processing

In the days when film was processed by hand, it took about 1 hour to process each film. In 1942, the first automatic processor came along; it then took 40 minutes to process one film.

Eastman Kodak Company introduced the real breakthrough technology in 1956. It was a roller transport system that was used to develop film used with intensifying screens. The machine reduced the amount of time it took to process film to 6 minutes and eliminated all human error.

In 1965, Kodak came out with a new machine that slashed developing time to 90 seconds and could handle 215 films in an hour.

SLIDE 2-38/CD 2-36 Washing

The washing step of the process removes as much of the fixer and developer solutions as possible. The film has entered the third tank from the left. The wash water is usually about 5 degrees cooler than the developer temperature. Washing takes about 20 seconds.

Algae and bacteria can grow when the processor isn't being used, so it may be advisable to drain the tanks if the machine will not be used for an extended period of time.

SLIDE 2-39/CD 2-37 Drying

In drying, hot air is forced over both sides of the film as it comes out of the processor (here, on the right side) and hardens the film so it can be easily handled. The whole development process, from start to finish, takes 90 seconds.

SLIDE 2-40/CD 2-38 Factors in radiographic contrast

You have begun the topic of contrast and the factors that affect it. This subject builds on information covered in the preceding topics of the acceptable range of density and the factors that affect it. If you have not yet worked through those topics, you may want to quit this section now and return later after going through the earlier topics.

Contrast is defined as the density differences on adjacent areas of the radiograph. Contrast is comprised of the blacks, whites, and shades of gray on the image. Proper contrast allows us to see detail of body structures.

Radiographic contrast is a combination of two factors: subject contrast and film contrast. Scatter radiation also directly affects the level of contrast in an image.

SLIDE 2-41/CD 2-39 Subject contrast

Subject contrast refers to the different densities you see on the radiograph as a result of attenuation differences in the body. As you remember from our discussion of density, the density on the film depends on how many x-ray photons, as they pass through the patient, have been absorbed in different body tissues.

Look at this chest radiograph, for example. The ribs and mediastinal area appear white, the heart as a shadow, pulmonary markings as a shade of gray, and the air-filled lungs are darker. The differences occur because the different tissues absorb various amounts of radiation.

The factors that make a difference in the amount of radiation absorbed (and therefore in the subject contrast) are: thickness of the body part, atomic number and density of the tissue, and the energy of the x-ray beam. Thicker body parts, denser tissue, higher atomic number tissues, and low kVp all result in higher absorption.

SLIDE 2-42/CD 2-40 Film contrast

Film contrast is the inherent ability of the film to record a range of densities. It's a quality that's built into the emulsion and therefore is beyond your control.

However, you can choose film that will either enhance or balance the subject contrast. You can get a better idea of film contrast if you think about it in terms of mammography. The differences in breast tissue aren't very great, so it shows up as similar shades of gray on a mammogram and is difficult to read. Using a film with high contrast emulsion produces an image with higher contrast, which makes it easier to see the distinctions. Shown here are radiographs with different contrasts at the same exposure.

SLIDE 2-43/CD 2-41 Scatter radiation and contrast

Scatter radiation negatively affects contrast. Unless it's controlled by some of the techniques you've learned about in this module, it fogs the film (making it gray) and reduces the contrast. The more scatter there is, the lower the contrast.

You can reduce the amount of scatter radiation by lowering the kVp. But even by doing that and using beam-restricting devices, more than half the x-rays that leave the film side of the patient will scatter in all directions.

MORE INFO LEADS TO THIS AUDIO RESPONSE: kVp has to be high enough to penetrate the part of the body under study, but if it's too high, it increases the amount of scatter. To cut down on scatter reaching the film, you can use a grid or try moving the patient farther away from the image receptor.

SLIDE 2-44/CD 2-42 Comparing radiograph contrast

As a radiographer, you should be able to make a distinction between low- and high-contrast radiographs. A radiograph with sharp differences in density is a high-contrast, or short-scale, radiograph. If the density differences aren't very distinct, you have a low-contrast, or long-scale, radiograph.

You can control contrast through kVp, which also controls the penetrating ability of the x-ray beam.

SLIDE 2-45/CD 2-43 Low-contrast radiograph

Low-contrast radiographs are also called long scale because if you piled up the different densities in order of their intensity you'd have a long scale of tones. You want that kind of contrast in some radiographs.

Low-scale contrast may result when high kVp is used.

MORE INFO LEADS TO THIS AUDIO RESPONSE: Imagine taking a radiographic film and cutting it up in lots of different pieces, each one with a different density. Arrange them according to their density, from lightest to darkest. If you end up with lots of pieces with little difference in density, then you have a long scale radiograph.

If you have only a few pieces with large differences in density, you have a short scale radiograph.

SLIDE 2-46/CD 2-44 High-contrast radiograph

On the other hand, high-contrast radiographs are called short scale because if you made the same kind of pile with them you'd see a fairly narrow range of densities. You get high contrast with low kVp because with a lower energy beam, the patient absorbs more x-ray photons. Those that don't run into much tissue density get through to expose the film. The result: a radiograph with very black and very white places and few shades of gray.

You usually see short-scale radiographs when body parts with little subject contrast are examined, such as extremities.

SLIDE 2-47/CD 2-45 Review: density

Several other factors that affect density, as we've seen, also have an impact on contrast.

Grids and close collimation increase contrast by taking away the gray that scatter radiation produces. Contrast increases with small field size collimation and a high grid ratio.

SLIDE 2-48/CD 2-46 Film screen combinations

Generally, an imaging department will use a standard film/screen combination for given examinations. When you use screens with the newer, structured grain x-ray films, you get excellent images with limited patient dose. In fact, using an intensifying screen reduces patient dose by more than 95% compared with examinations not using intensifying screens.

When you use intensifying screens, the images will have higher contrast than when you don't use screens. In theory, you achieve higher contrast with a higher screen speed. In the real world, however, the combination of film and screen is really what determines the contrast.

Shown on the right, for example, is a high-contrast image made using a screen. The film at left was done without a screen and has a lower contrast.

MORE INFO LEADS TO THIS AUDIO RESPONSE: The reason screen-type films are used so much is because they greatly reduce exposure time, and therefore the amount of radiation the patient is exposed to. The thinner emulsions of this type of film are more sensitive to the light of the screens than to x-rays.

SLIDE 2-49/CD 2-47 Foggy radiograph

When unexposed silver halide crystals are developed, you get development fog. It's called that because the image looks dull and washed out and lacks the proper contrast. Development fog is a more common problem in high-speed films.

There are many reasons that fog shows up on a film, but the main ones are development time, temperature, and the concentration of the developer. The level of fog increases as the development time does. In fact, anytime the standard manufacturer recommendations are exceeded on these factors, there will be more fog.

Some other factors can also cause fog. If the developer is chemically contaminated, or if the film is accidentally exposed to radiation or stored under conditions of high temperature and humidity, you're likely to see some fog.

SLIDE 2-50/CD 2-48 SID and contrast

The source-image receptor distance (SID) does not directly impact contrast. That's because the penetrating ability of the x-ray beam, combined with the various rates at which different body parts absorb x-ray photons, are what determine contrast, not the number of x-rays in the primary beam. Distance doesn't change those factors.

Because of the inverse square law, SID affects beam intensity and, ultimately, radiographic density. These changes in density have some effect on contrast.

In actual practice, however, SID is generally standardized at 40 inches for most procedures and 72 inches for chest radiographs. This prevents density and contrast deviations that may result from inconsistent SIDs

SLIDE 2-51/CD 2-49 Use of contrast medium

As we discussed earlier, subject contrast, the difference in density of various parts of the body, is what makes some parts stand out more clearly than others on a radiograph. Bones, for example, absorb more photons and result in higher contrast images.

Other parts of the body, such as kidneys, ureters, the bladder, and the gastrointestinal tract, have very low subject contrast because they absorb fewer photons and do so in a more uniform manner. In order to get diagnostic images of those areas, it's necessary to either have the patient drink a nontoxic substance, called a contrast medium, or have a contrast medium injected intravenously. The common contrast media are air, barium, or iodinated agents. They help to produce radiographs with high subject contrast.

Positive contrast media are those that attenuate the x-rays. By doing so, they decrease density and show light areas on the radiograph. Negative media are the ones that help x-rays pass through the part for a resulting increase in density. In both cases, the images are more diagnostic and easier to read.

MORE INFO LEADS TO THIS AUDIO RESPONSE: Positive contrast agents are liquids that are opaque to x-rays. They make tissues and abnormalities show up on radiographs when they'd otherwise be transparent.

SLIDE 2-52/CD 2-50 Effect of processing factors

Processing has a role to play, too. Processing solutions that are too hot will fog the film. If the film takes too long to develop, the contrast will decrease. The right time and temperature during processing, as well as a solution with the proper concentration, are what help to maintain contrast.

When these factors are off, you get chemical fog. It shows on the radiograph as a constant dull gray.

SLIDE 2-53/CD 2-51 Motion blur

There's another factor that affects image quality. Its effects are not directly related to contrast, but sometimes the effect may resemble or contribute to a contrast problem. This is blur, which results if the patient moves or if the equipment vibrates. Blur, like contrast problems, can greatly diminish the detail of the image. Follow these guidelines to keep motion to a minimum.

1. Use the shortest possible exposure time.

2. Give the patient good instructions or use a restraining device if you have to.

3. Use a large SID.
4. Make sure all locking mechanisms on the equipment are working properly.

SLIDE 2-54/CD 2-52 Positioning patient

To get the best image, remember you have to position the patient so the part of the body to be examined is as close to the image receptor as possible. The center of the x-ray beam should be directed to the center of the part to be studied.

Sometimes, patients need help staying in a difficult position. You may find yourself using immobilization devices like restraining bands, even sandbags, to help them do that.

SLIDE 2-55/CD 2-53 Conclusion

In this module, we've defined radiographic density and contrast and touched on the factors that influence them. Along the way in your studies, you'll learn more about some of these factors, details of how they work, and how they affect the quality of x-ray films.

SLIDE 2-56/CD 2-54 Quiz instructions

THIS AUDIO FOR SLIDE/TAPE ONLY: This concludes the presentation section of this module. If you are not going to work through the self-assessment quiz that follows, you may stop the program at this point and turn off the equipment.

If your instructor has asked you to take this self-assessment quiz on the material you have learned in this module, you should have a piece of paper ready. There will be 10 questions with multiple-choice or short answers. After this self-assessment we will go back through these questions and briefly talk about the reasons for the correct answers. Ready?

THIS AUDIO IN CD ROM LECTURE MODE ONLY: You have reached the self-assessment quiz for this module. Here you will be asked 10 questions to help you assess how well you understand what you have learned in this module. The questions are multiple choice or have short answers. After this self assessment we will go back through these questions and briefly talk about your answers and the reasons for the correct answers. Ready?

THIS AUDIO IN CD ROM STUDENT MODE ONLY: You have reached the self-assessment quiz for this module. Here you will be asked 10 questions to help you assess how well you understand what you have learned in this module. The questions are multiple choice or have short answers. For multiple-choice questions, click on the box next to your answer choice. For those questions that require a short answer, type in your answer at the keyboard and press enter.

After this self-assessment we will go back through these questions and briefly talk about your answers and the reasons for the correct answers.

SLIDE 2-57/CD 2-55 Quiz question 1

1. Radiographic density refers to which of the following?
   a. The amount of white on a radiograph
   b. The amount of overall blackening on a radiograph or a particular part of the radiograph
   c. The amount of radiation that reaches a film
   d. An overexposed radiograph

SLIDE 2-58/CD 2-56 Quiz question 2

2. Radiographic contrast refers to which of the following?
   a. The amount of silver halide deposited on a film during processing
   b. The amount of blackening on a radiograph
   c. The amount of white on a radiograph
   d. The range of the variation in density on a radiograph

SLIDE 2-59/CD 2-57 Quiz question 3

3. What is the primary controlling factor governing exposure and the resulting density of a radiograph?
   a. Milliampere-seconds (mAs)
   b. A combination of time and distance
   c. The thickness of the patient
   d. Kilovoltage (kVp)

SLIDE 2-60/CD 2-58 Quiz question 4

4. Which of the following does mA control?
   a. The penetrating ability of an x-ray beam
   b. The number of x-ray photons produced in the tube, which determines the exposure rate
   c. The quality of the x-ray beam
   d. The length of time of a radiographic examination

SLIDE 2-61/CD 2-58 Quiz question 5

5. The kVp determines which of the following?
   a. The penetrating ability of the x-ray beam and the quality of the beam
   b. The exposure time
   c. Whether a screen should be used or not
   d. The source-image receptor distance

SLIDE 2-62/CD 2-60 Quiz question 6

6. Which of these factors does not affect density?
   a. Intensifying screens
   b. Grids
   c. Restraining devices for patients
   d. Filters

SLIDE 2-63/CD 2-61 Quiz question 7

7. Subject contrast refers to which of the following?
   a. The different densities visible on a radiograph due to patient anatomy
   b. The rate of radiation absorption
   c. An equal proportion of dark and light on a radiograph
   d. The body weight and thickness of the patient

SLIDE 2-64/CD 2-62 Quiz question 8

8. Which of these factors affects contrast?
   a. Grids and collimation
   b. Intensifying screens
   c. Fog
   d. All of the above

SLIDE 2-65/CD 2-63 Quiz question 9

9. Which of the following is true of using a contrast medium?
   a. It helps make the patient more comfortable.
   b. It helps produce a radiograph with a high subject contrast.
   c. It helps produce a radiograph with a high film contrast.
   d. It helps shorten exposure time.

SLIDE 2-66/CD 2-64 Quiz question 10

10. Which of these factors will help reduce blur and improve detail on the radiograph?
    a. Shortest possible exposure time
    b. Clear instructions to the patient
    c. Working lock mechanisms
    d. All of the above

SLIDE 2-67/CD 2-65 Quiz review

That concludes the self-assessment quiz for Module 2: Radiographic Imaging. Let's quickly go back through the questions and see how you did.

SLIDE 2-68/CD 2-66 Review question 1

Question 1 asked you what radiographic density refers to.

The correct answer is b, the amount of overall blackening on a radiograph or a particular part of a radiograph. The other answers involved things that might affect density, but the basic definition of density is the amount of overall blackening.

CD 2-66A Review question 1

Question 1 asked you what radiographic density refers to.

PRESENT THIS AUDIO IF ANSWER WAS b: Yes, you're right. The correct answer is b, the amount of overall blackening on a radiograph or a particular part of a radiograph. The other answers involved things that might affect density, but the basic definition of density is the amount of overall blackening.

PRESENT THIS AUDIO IF ANSWER WAS a, c, or d: No, sorry, your answer is incorrect. The correct answer is b, the amount of overall blackening on a radiograph or a particular part of a radiograph. The other answers involved things that might affect density, but the basic definition of density is the amount of overall blackening.

SLIDE 2-69/CD 2-67 Review question 2

Question 2 asked what radiographic contrast refers to.

The correct answer is d, the range of the variation in density on the radiograph. Other answers, such as the amount of white or the amount of blackening on a radiograph, refer to density, not contrast.

CD 2-67A Review question 2

Question 2 asked you what radiographic contrast refers to.

PRESENT THIS AUDIO IF ANSWER WAS d: Yes, you correctly answered d, the range of the variation in density on the radiograph. Other answers, such as the amount of white or the amount of blackening on a radiograph, refer to density, not contrast.

PRESENT THIS AUDIO IF ANSWER WAS a, b, or c: You answered this one incorrectly. The right answer is d, the range of the variation in density on the radiograph. That is the definition of contrast. Other answers, such as the amount of white or the amount of blackening on a radiograph, refer to density, not contrast.

SLIDE 2-70/CD 2-68 Review question 3
Question 3 asked about the primary controlling factor governing exposure and the resulting density of a radiograph.

The correct answer is a, milliampere-seconds (mAs). You control the exposure through the mAs selection, producing more or fewer x-ray photons. The more photons produced, the more that will reach the film and create more density.

CD 2-68A Review question 3
Question 3 asked about the primary controlling factor governing exposure and the resulting density of a radiograph.

PRESENT THIS AUDIO IF ANSWER WAS a: Yes, you're correct in answering a, milliampere-seconds (mAs). You control the exposure through the mAs selection, producing more or fewer x-ray photons. The more photons produced, the more will reach the film and create more density.

PRESENT THIS AUDIO IF ANSWER WAS b, c, or d: Your answer is incorrect. The right answer is milliampere-seconds (mAs). You control the exposure through the mAs selection, producing more or fewer x-ray photons. The more photons produced, the more will reach the film and create more density.

SLIDE 2-71/CD 2-69 Review question 4
Question 4 asked what mA controls.

The correct answer is b, the number of x-ray photons produced in the tube, which determines the exposure rate. Remember that the mA selection determines how many electrons strike the anode of the x-ray tube, thereby determining how many x-ray photons are produced.

CD 2-69A Review question 4
Question 4 asked what mA controls.

PRESENT THIS AUDIO IF ANSWER WAS b: You're right! mA controls the number of x-ray photons produced in the tube, which determines the exposure rate. Remember that the mA selection determines how many electrons strike the anode of the x-ray tube, thereby determining how many x-ray photons are produced.

PRESENT THIS AUDIO IF ANSWER WAS a, c, or d: Sorry, your answer is wrong. The correct answer is b. mA controls the number x-ray photons produced in the tube, which determines the exposure rate. Remember that the mA selection determines how many electrons strike the anode of the x-ray tube, thereby determining how many x-ray photons are produced.

SLIDE 2-72/CD 2-70 Review question 5
Question 5 asked what kVp determines.

The correct answer is a, the penetrating ability of the x-ray beam and the quality of the beam. Remember that kVp determines the energy levels of the x-ray photons.

CD 2-70A Review question 5
Question 5 asked what kVp determines.

PRESENT THIS AUDIO IF ANSWER WAS a: You're right! The correct answer is a, the penetrating ability of the x-ray beam and the quality of the beam. Remember that the mA selection determines how many electrons strike the anode of the x-ray tube, thereby determining how many x-ray photons are produced.

PRESENT THIS AUDIO IF ANSWER WAS b, c, or d: Sorry, you missed this one. The answer is a, the penetrating ability of the x-ray beam and the quality of the beam. Remember that the mA selection determines how many electrons strike the anode of the x-ray tube, thereby determining how many x-ray photons are produced.

SLIDE 2-73/CD 2-71 Review question 6
Question 6 asked which of the listed factors does not affect density.

The correct answer is c, restraining devices for patients. Such devices may prevent blur caused by patient movement, but this does not affect density. Density is affected, however, by all the other factors: screens, grids, and filters.

CD 2-71A Review question 6
Question 6 asked which of the listed factors does not affect density.

PRESENT THIS AUDIO IF ANSWER WAS c: You chose the correct answer, c, restraining devices for patients. Such devices may prevent blur caused by patient movement, but this does not affect density. Density is affected, however, by all the other factors: screens, grids, and filters.

PRESENT THIS AUDIO IF ANSWER WAS a, b, or d: The right answer is c, restraining devices for patients. Such devices may prevent blur caused by patient movement, but this does not affect density. Density is affected, however, by all the other factors: screens, grids, and filters.

SLIDE 2-74/CD 2-72 Review question 7
Question 7 asked what subject contrast refers to.

The correct answer is a, the different densities visible on a radiograph due to patient anatomy. In essence this is the definition of the term subject contrast.

CD 2-72A Review question 7
Question 7 asked what subject contrast refers to.

PRESENT THIS AUDIO IF ANSWER WAS a: Yes, you were right, the answer is a, the different densities visible on a radiograph, due to patient anatomy. In essence this is the definition of the term subject contrast.

PRESENT THIS AUDIO IF ANSWER WAS b, c, or d: No, you missed it. The correct answer is a, the different densities visible on a radiograph, due to patient anatomy. In essence this is the definition of the term subject contrast.

SLIDE 2-75/CD 2-73 Review question 8
Question 8 asked which of the listed factors affects contrast.

The correct answer is d, all of the factors listed: grids and collimation, intensifying screens, and fog.

CD 2-73A Review question 8
Question 8 asked which of the listed factors affects contrast.

PRESENT THIS AUDIO FOR ANSWER d: Yes, you're correct. The answer is d, all of them: grids and collimation, intensifying screens, and fog.

PRESENT THIS AUDIO IF ANSWER WAS a, b, or c: No, you missed this one. The answer is d, all of them: grids and collimation, intensifying screens, and fog.

SLIDE 2-76/CD 2-74 Review question 9
Question 9 asked which of the listed factors is helped by using a contrast medium.

The correct answer is b. A contrast medium helps to produce radiographic images with high subject contrast. The film contrast and exposure time are unaffected by using a contrast medium.

CD 2-74A Review question 9
Question 9 asked which of the listed factors is helped by using a contrast medium.

PRESENT THIS AUDIO IF ANSWER WAS b: Yes, you're right. The correct answer is b. A contrast medium helps to produce radiographic images with high subject contrast. The film contrast and exposure time are unaffected by using a contrast medium.

PRESENT THIS AUDIO IF ANSWER WAS a, c, or d: Sorry, but you missed it. The correct answer is b. A contrast medium helps to produce radiographic images with high subject contrast. The film contrast and exposure time are unaffected by using a contrast medium.

SLIDE 2-77/CD 2-75 Review question 10
Question 10 asked which of the listed factors will help to reduce blur, thereby producing better detail on a radiograph.

The correct answer is d, all of the factors: shortest possible exposure time, clear instructions to the patient (to help prevent movement), and working lock mechanisms.

CD 2-75A Review question 10
Question 10 asked which of the listed factors will help to reduce blur, thereby producing better detail on the radiograph.

PRESENT THIS AUDIO IF ANSWER WAS d: You're right. All of the factors are important: shortest possible exposure time, clear instructions to the patient (to help prevent movement), and working lock mechanisms.

PRESENT THIS AUDIO IF ANSWER WAS a, b, or c: Sorry, you missed it. The correct answer is that all of the factors are important: shortest possible exposure time, clear instructions to the patient (to help prevent movement), and working lock mechanisms.

SLIDE 2-78/CD 2-76 Quiz conclusion
This concludes the self-assessment quiz. This was not intended as a test, so don't feel bad if you missed some. All that means is that you probably need to review this module or study your textbook more carefully.

CD 2-76A Quiz feedback
FOR SCORE OF 10, THIS AUDIO: You've done an excellent job here with a difficult subject. Clearly you are studying well, and you seem to have worked through the tutorial carefully.

FOR SCORE OF 9, THIS AUDIO: You've done well with a difficult subject. Clearly you are studying and paying attention to the subject. Maybe next time you'll get the perfect score!

FOR SCORE OF 7-8, THIS AUDIO: Your score is about average. I'd suggest you review this material in your textbook. You may also find it helpful, next time, to read the material in your book before coming to the computer to take the tutorial. And don't hesitate to talk to your instructor if you have trouble after both reading the textbook and working through the multimedia tutorial.

FOR SCORE OF 5-6, THIS AUDIO: Your score is below average. You need to review this material in your textbook, and perhaps you should come back and take this tutorial again afterwards. You may have just been unprepared this time, or if you are having trouble after both reading the textbook and working through the multimedia tutorial, be sure to talk to your instructor.

FOR SCORE OF 0-4, THIS AUDIO: Your score is rather low. Don't feel too bad; these are, after all, difficult concepts to grasp. If you tried your best here but are having this much difficulty with the material, you should first go to your textbook and see if you can understand the material there. If it still seems difficult, please ask your instructor for additional study aids.

SLIDE 2-79/CD 2-77 Exam instructions
In the next 7 or 8 minutes you will be presented with 15 multiple-choice questions. Select the one best answer choice. Get ready a blank sheet of paper numbered 1 to 15 down the left side. As you take the examination, write the letter corresponding to your answer choice next to the number for each question. Ready? You will not be asked to perform any complicated calculations.

CD 2-77A More exam instructions
In the next 7 or 8 minutes you will be presented with 15 multiple-choice questions. Select the one best answer choice. This examination covers the material you've been learning about in this tutorial over the last hour or so. It's designed to help you and your instructor determine how well you now grasp this material. You can use scratch paper during the exam if you want, but it shouldn't be necessary for any complicated calculations.

SLIDE 2-80/CD 2-78 Exam question 1

1. The amount of darkening on a radiograph is called the radiographic density. Many factors affect the density of a radiographic image; however, density depends on which of the following?
   a. The size and illness of the patient
   b. The amount of radiation reaching the film and the silver ions deposited at the sensitivity specks
   c. The source-image receptor distance and filtration
   d. Grid ratio

SLIDE 2-81/CD 2-79 Exam question 2

2. What are the two different types of radiographic contrast?
   a. Dark and light areas
   b. Range of density and subject contrast
   c. Subject contrast and film contrast
   d. Film contrast and x-ray penetration

SLIDE 2-82/CD 2-80 Exam question 3

3. What does the prefix milli, as in milliamperes (mA), mean?
   a. 1/100
   b. 1/10
   c. 1
   d. 1/1,000

SLIDE 2-83/CD 2-81 Exam question 4

4. The exposure rate R/sec is directly proportional to mA. For example, when you double the mA, what happens to the x-ray exposure rate?
   a. It doubles.
   b. It is cut in half.
   c. It triples.
   d. It stays the same.

SLIDE 2-84/CD 2-82 Exam question 5

5. You can double the film exposure by increasing the kVp by about how much?
   a. 50%
   b. 10%
   c. 15%
   d. 30%

SLIDE 2-85/CD 2-83 Exam question 6

6. True or false: Development fog comes from unexposed silver halide crystals that develop and make the image look dull and washed out.

SLIDE 2-86/CD 2-84 Exam question 7

7 Which of the following is true when the exposure time is longer?
   a. The mA is higher.
   b. The number of photons emitted by the x-ray tube is larger.
   c. The density is lower.
   d. It is better for the patient.

SLIDE 2-87/CD 2-85 Exam question 8

8. Why are intensifying screens used even though they cause a slight dullness of the image?
   a. They provide less contrast.
   b. They reduce kVp.
   c. They reduce the time a patient is exposed to radiation.
   d. The federal government mandates they be used with new equipment.

SLIDE 2-88/CD 2-86 Exam question 9

9. What are grids used for in radiography?
   a. To shorten exposure time
   b. To reduce scatter radiation reaching the film
   c. To make positioning patients easier
   d. To decrease subject contrast

SLIDE 2-89/CD 2-87 Exam question 10

10. What part of the body absorbs x-rays the best?
   a. Chest
   b. Bone
   c. Kidneys
   d. Gastrointestinal tract

SLIDE 2-90/CD 2-88 Exam question 11

11. Contrast displays a range of densities (white, shades of gray, and dark tones) that make it possible to do which of the following?
   a. Increase recorded detail
   b. Use the lowest kVp possible
   c. Reduce the amount of radiation a patient receives
   d. See the body structures

SLIDE 2-91/CD 2-89 Exam question 12

12. The factors that make a difference in the amount of radiation absorbed, and therefore in the subject contrast, are which of the following?
   a. The thickness of the body part
   b. The tissue's density and atomic number
   c. The energy of the x-ray photons
   d. All of the above

SLIDE 2-92/CD 2-90 Exam question 13

13. A radiograph with sharp differences in density is which of the following?
   a. A low-contrast, or long-scale, radiograph
   b. A high-contrast, or short-scale radiograph
   c. Neutral in terms of contrast
   d. None of the above

SLIDE 2-93/CD 2-91 Exam question 14

14. Why do grids and collimation increase contrast?
    a. Because they help to reduce the amount of scatter produced and that reaching the film
    b. Because they reduce exposure time
    c. Because they increase the energy flow from the x-ray tube
    d. Because they decrease the energy flow from the x-ray tube

SLIDE 2-94/CD 2-92 Exam question 15

15. Which of the following is true of source-image receptor distance?
    a. It has significant impact on contrast.
    b. It affects scatter radiation.
    c. It has no direct impact on contrast.
    d. It cuts down on fog.

SLIDE 2-95/CD 2-93 Conclusion

INSTRUCTOR CD/SLIDE AUDIO: This concludes the examination section of Module 2 of Radiographic Imaging. Please follow your instructor's directions for your answer sheet to the questions.

STUDENT CD AUDIO: This concludes the examination section of Module 2 of Radiographic Imaging. Your score has been saved on the computer. Your instructor will report it to you later.

Answers to the Multimedia Examination

1. b	6. true	11. d
2. c	7. b	12. d
3. d	8. c	13. b
4. a	9. b	14. a
5. c	10. b	15. c

Recorded Detail

3

Overview

Importance of recorded detail
- Measurement of recorded detail

Geometric
- Unsharpness
- Visible Detail
- Magnification
- Effects of SID and OID

Intensifying screens and film speed

Motion unsharpness

This module teaches students about recorded detail and the technical factors related to resolution on radiographs. Because students should, by this time, be familiar with concepts such as SID and OID, film exposure and development, and intensifying screens, the new information in this module builds on the foundation already in place.

After a discussion of why radiographic detail is so important, the concepts of geometric are considered. Focal spot size, SID, and OID are shown as the factors leading to unsharpness caused by blurring. The line focus principle is introduced, and magnification is examined again from the perspective of these geometric variables.

The module then considers intensifying screens and films in relation to recorded detail. The inverse relationship between screen/film speed and recorded detail is explored, along with the effects on patient exposure. The process by which intensifying screens work is explained, and students receive a review of film exposure and development processes.

The final variable discussed in terms of recorded detail is motion unsharpness. Voluntary and involuntary movement is described, along with motion blur caused by vibration or movement of the x-ray equipment. Students learn what they can do to help minimize motion or the blur it causes.

Learning Objectives

Upon completion of this module, the student should be able to do the following:

1. Define all the key terms in the module.
2. Explain the importance of recorded detail for diagnostic radiographs.
3. Explain the concept of geometric unsharpness and why blurring causes unsharpness.
4. List the effects on recorded detail of SID, OID, and focal spot size.
5. Describe how intensifying screens work.
6. List the effects of screen speed and film speed on recorded detail and on patient exposure.
7. List the three causes of motion unsharpness and explain what the radiographer can do to prevent them or minimize their effects.
8. Successfully complete the activities and posttest in the Study Guide.

Key Terms

Blur
Focal spot
Geometric sharpness or unsharpness
Intensifying screen
Involuntary motion
Latent image
Latitude
Line focus principle
Line pair
Magnification
Magnification radiography
Object-to-image receptor distance (OID)
Phosphor
Recorded detail
Sensitivity specks
Source-to-image receptor distance (SID)
Speed
Target
Target angle
Unsharpness
Voluntary motion

Instructional Outline

I. Recorded detail is important for diagnostic quality images.
   A. Recorded detail is the degree of sharpness of structures as recorded in the radiograph.
      1. Recorded detail is also called definition, sharpness, resolution, visible detail, or just detail.
      2. Radiographic quality depends on image sharpness, or recorded detail, along with visibility, resulting from density and contrast.
      3. Unsharpness is lack of recorded detail, or blurring, along the edges of structures; visible detail is the sharp, or unblurred, area within the edges.

B. The amount of recorded detail is determined by the resolution, which is measured in line pairs visible per millimeter.
   1. The human eye can discern up to 5 line pairs per millimeter.
   2. Conventional screen-film combinations can resolve up to about 10 line pairs per millimeter.

II. Geometric unsharpness results from unavoidable geometric factors in how the x-ray beam is produced and interacts with the object being imaged.
   A. Geometric unsharpness occurs because the x-ray beam emerges not from a single spot in the tube but from an area.
      1. Electrons from the cathode strike the target on the anode focal spot where x-rays are produced.
      2. Because of the line focus principle, angling the anode helps decrease the effective focal spot size to improve the recorded detail. The anode is tilted at an average angle of 12 degrees.
   B. Unsharpness occurs because the edge of a structure is imaged by x-rays emerging from all parts of the focal point in the tube, at slightly different angles to the film, producing blur.
   C. Magnification of the image occurs because the x-ray beam continues to disperse and spread out in the distance between the object and the image receptor (the OID).
      1. The magnification factor is calculated by the image size divided by the object's true size, or by dividing the source-to-image receptor distance (SID) by the source-to-object distance (SOD).
      2. Magnification radiography intentionally uses magnification when it is desirable to magnify a structure in a radiograph.
      3. Unsharpness caused by blurring is magnified as well.
   D. Increasing the SID decreases unsharpness because the x-rays from the focal spot do not spread out as far between the object and the film.
      1. Standardized SIDs with acceptable amounts of unsharpness are used for most routine examinations.
      2. Longer SIDs, such as the 72-inch SID used with chest radiographs, decrease unsharpness and the magnification of structures like the heart, providing better recorded detail.
   E. Decreasing the OID to the minimum distance minimizes both the unsharpness and magnification. Except when magnification is intentionally desired, the patient is always positioned as close to the film as possible.

III. Intensifying screens and film also are important for recorded detail.
   A. The speed of film and intensifying screens refers to how much and how quickly they react to the x-ray photons.
   B. Slower film-screen combinations generally produce better recorded detail, but they also involve more patient exposure.
      1. Slower speeds are generally used with extremities, where exposure is not as major a concern.
      2. Faster speeds are used for larger body areas to keep patient dose minimal.
   C. Screens work by converting x-ray photons to light photons to expose the film with less radiation to the patient.
      1. Almost 100% of the exposure of the film results from the light produced in the screen, not the x-ray photons that reach the film, allowing much lower patient doses.
      2. Phosphor crystals inside the screen produce many light photons for each x-ray photon that strikes the crystal.
         a. The screen is composed of a base layer, a reflective layer (to direct all light at the film), the phosphor layer, and a protective coating.
         b. The screen is immediately next to the film, which is exposed by the light photons to create the latent image.

3. Screens are classified by their speed, the rate at which they absorb x-rays. Screen speed is determined by the size of the phosphor crystals and the thickness of the phosphor layer. High-speed screens have larger crystals in thicker layers.
   a. Fast screens reduce motion blur and reduce patient exposure. Because the crystals are larger, recorded detail is less.
   b. Slower screens may be used when very fine detail is needed.

D. The characteristics of the radiographic film also affect recorded detail.
   1. Faster films have thicker emulsion layers and larger silver bromide crystals.
      a. Fast films require less patient exposure but produce less recorded detail.
      b. Slower films require more patient exposure but produce better recorded detail.
   2. Films and screens are used in standardized combinations established for different types of examinations.

IV. Motion unsharpness is blurring in the image produced by movement of the patient during the exposure—just like in photography.
   A. Voluntary motion can be minimized by asking the patient to hold still, to hold his or her breath, using restraints, etc.
   B. Involuntary motion cannot be prevented, such as movement within the gastrointestinal tract or involuntary muscle movement; the radiographer can only try to use short exposures and help the patient remain still with restraints.
   C. Motion of the equipment too must be prevented, so any vibration or damaged equipment should be checked to ensure the unit is working correctly and stays motionless through the examination.

Teaching Tips

Importance of Recorded Detail

It is not difficult to impress upon students the importance of recorded detail in radiographs. This module begins with general explanations of what recorded detail is and why it is so important in the creation of images with diagnostic value. Radiographs are shown that compare good and poor levels of radiographic detail. To help students further realize this importance, you may want to show additional radiographs—either actual films or reproductions in texts—particularly those in which radiographic detail is not good. You may also choose to share with them your own knowledge of problems with recorded detail in practice settings, such as mentioning the number of radiographs that must be repeated because the image did not have enough quality for diagnostic purposes. It is important that students understand that problems can and do occur, and the results may require a second examination or, much worse, a problem in diagnosing the pathology. Most textbooks present such a positive perspective on radiographic technique that students may not realize the consequences of achieving a poor image. If they do understand that problems can occur and that they themselves can do much to prevent such problems, then they will better translate into practice the principles they learn in this and other modules on the imaging process.

At early stages in their education and beginning practice, some students experience confusion about the terminology used. As this module points out, many different terms are used in a manner that is or seems synonymous with "recorded detail," such as resolution, definition, sharpness, visible detail, and so on. In your own teaching you can help students through this difficulty by explaining about these other terms but then being consistent in using only the term "recorded detail" in all the contexts considering the different variables affecting recorded detail.

Finally, to help students truly understand the value of recorded detail, let them experience different degrees of resolution by using samples of line pair measurements. If you have films showing different numbers of line pairs per millimeter, at different levels of recorded detail, let them actually count how many lines they can see with the unaided eye. This helps internalize the reality of what otherwise may seem only a vague concept.

Geometric Sharpness

The underlying concepts of geometric sharpness generally seem very clear to students who have always been "good at math" and difficult for students "bad at math." The actual geometry of focal spot size, SID, OID, and unsharpness on the image is actually fairly simple, except, of course, to those students who are not as successful in visualizing mathematical relationships. In this case a simple classroom demonstration using a flashlight may help. Shine the light at some opaque object so that its shadow appears on a white surface behind it. Manipulate the SID and OID of the flashlight's beam so that students can clearly see the blurring effect around the edges of the shadow. Then refer the students to the diagram showing the cause of this unsharpness. Continue to manipulate the SID and OID to show their effects on the unsharpness.

Magnification is more easily understood by students, but while demonstrating the effects of SID and OID on unsharpness, you can also point out the obvious effects of SID and OID on magnification of the shadow image. Even the formula for calculating the magnification factor can be demonstrated with the flashlight: as the ratio of SID to SOD increases, so will the size of the shadow image. Give students a few examples of numbers for SID, SOD, and either the image size or the object size to give them practice in calculating the unknown object or image size.

Intensifying Screens

The illustrations in this module show how intensifying screens work by converting x-ray photons into light photons, but the limitations of the size of these illustrations may make it difficult for some students to visualize the magnitude of light photons produced in the phosphor crystals. You can demonstrate this in the classroom using a blackboard or other large marker board to sketch out what happens within the layer of phosphor crystals. Use a very large scale sketch to show the size of the crystals, the distance to the film, etc. Trace the path of an x-ray photon into the screen and the multitude of light photons that are produced, emitted in all directions, some reaching the film directly and others in the opposite direction being reflected back to the film. Using a very large sketch like this can help students see not only how the process works but how the light photons emitted in all directions disperse somewhat before they strike the film—thereby reducing recorded detail.

To clarify how technique charts in the radiology department use different film-screen combinations for different types of examinations, you might show the class several examples of technique charts photocopied from the department where your students have their clinical experience.

Voluntary Motion

The concept of blur caused by motion of either the patient or the equipment is easily grasped by students once they realize the situation is analogous to taking photographs of someone who is moving or with the camera jiggling. What students may not realize, however, is that not all patients in all situations can simply "hold still" on command, particularly when the patient is ill or injured, in pain, nervous or apprehensive, or uncomfortably positioned. Explain that radiologic technologists need to be sensitive to these patient variables while still trying to prevent motion blur. To illustrate that it's not always so easy just to "hold still," have several students role play patients in the front of the classroom.

Pose them in positions that are intentionally difficult to maintain (holding one's arm straight out, standing on one foot, etc.), explaining that these positions may not be realistic because you're exaggerating to make the point. Pose the students and ask them to "hold still" as long as they can. If you do this in a light, almost joking manner, others in the class may be commenting on these "patients" or trying to make them move by laughing—and invariably the students will not be able to hold the poses long without moving. Let the students enjoy this little game, and then bring them back to the serious message behind it: lots of things can make it difficult for a patient to hold perfectly still, and you always need to be sensitive to the patient's feelings and do whatever you can to ensure they are comfortable and have all body parts supported adequately.

If time permits, you may also discuss the "problem patients" encountered in emergency rooms: those who are semiconscious or severely disoriented, in great pain or hysterics, or intoxicated. Pose the question for students: what can you do to prevent these patients from moving? Let them talk about it and soon they will realize how complex this issue can become. Share any of your own experiences with such patients along with any tips for helping overcome these problems of motion.

Workbook Posttest Answers and Rationales

1. The average human eye can discern up to how many line pairs per millimeter?
   a. 1
   b. 2
   c. 5—This is simply a matter of how much detail the eye can see in a small space without magnification; the eye can see up to 5 line pairs per millimeter in sharp resolution, and a radiograph can resolve up to 10 line pairs per mm.
   d. 10

2. What can be done to prevent geometric unsharpness?
   a. Increase the kVp
   b. Increase the mAs
   c. Use a higher-ratio grid
   d. None of the above—Geometric unsharpness results from the fact that the focal spot is an area rather than a single point, and this fact cannot be avoided, regardless of the kVp, mAs, or grid use; the area of unsharpness can be reduced by increasing the SID, reducing the focal spot size, and reducing the OID.

3. Why does unsharpness occur?
   a. With high kVp the central beam is too powerful and "spills over" at the edges.
   b. The edges of a structure are imaged by x-rays from both sides of the focal spot. This is a geometric reality caused by x-ray photons emerging from different areas, thereby imaging the same body structure at different angles to the film.
   c. Poor collimation does not restrict the edges of the beam.
   d. All of the above are true.

4. Why does magnification occur in all radiographs?
   a. **The x-ray beam continues to spread out after passing through the patient.** This is an unavoidable geometric factor, since the object being imaged is always at some small distance from the film; thus the beam continues to spread out between the structure and the film.
   b. The focal spot is an area rather than a point.
   c. This is an unavoidable aspect of film emulsions.
   d. Light photons from the intensifying screen spread out before they reach the film.

5. The magnification factor is calculated as which of the following?
   a. The image size divided by the object's true size
   b. The SID divided by the SOD
   c. **Both of the above**—Because of the geometric variables involved, these two calculations result in the same answer; the magnification factor is how much bigger the image size is than the object's actual size.
   d. Neither of the above

6. Why is a 72-inch SID for chest radiographs standard?
   a. A longer SID decreases unsharpness.
   b. A longer SID decreases magnification of structures such as the heart.
   c. This longer SID provides better recorded detail.
   d. **All of the above**—Unsharpness always decreases with longer SID because of geometric relationships; assuming the OID stays the same, increasing the SID always decreases magnification; with decreased unsharpness, recorded detail is better.
   e. None of the above is true.

7. If magnification was desired in a radiograph, what change would likely be made?
   a. Increase the SID
   b. **Increase the OID**—This increases the magnification, because the x-ray beam will continue to spread out in the increased distance between the patient and the image receptor.
   c. Increase the SOD
   d. Any of the above
   e. None of the above

8. Which of the following is true of slower speed intensifying screens?
   a. **They generally produce more recorded detail than faster speed screens.** The phosphor crystals in slow speed screens are smaller and in thinner layers in the screen, thus providing higher resolution; the patient dose is higher, however, and therefore slow screens are used with extremities, not larger body areas, because of the concern for patient exposure.
   b. They generally produce less recorded detail than faster speed screens.
   c. They involve lower patient exposures.
   d. They are generally used for large body areas.

9. What percentage of the film exposure results from light photons from the intensifying screen, rather than from x-ray photons from the beam?
   a. About 1%
   b. 10%
   c. 50%
   d. Almost 100%—This demonstrates the powerful effect of the screen in producing many light photons for each x-ray photon, so that the exposure to the patient can be minimized.

10. What are the advantages of high-speed screens?
   a. Lower patient exposure and reduced motion blur—High-speed screens need less radiation to make the exposure, thus decreasing the total exposure to the patient and the length of the exposure (reducing motion blur); recorded detail is less, however; contrast and density are determined more by other factors.
   b. Lower patient exposure and more recorded detail
   c. More recorded detail and better contrast
   d. Better contrast and density

11. Which of these best describes the composition of slow-speed intensifying screens?
   a. Larger phosphor crystals, thicker layer of crystals
   b. Larger phosphor crystals, thinner layer of crystals
   c. Smaller phosphor crystals, thinner layer of crystals—This is why the exposure is somewhat slower, because there are fewer, smaller crystals to interact with the x-ray photons; this results, however, in finer resolution in the image.
   d. Smaller phosphor crystals, thicker layer of crystals

12. Which of these best describes the composition of slow-speed films?
   a. Larger silver halide crystals, thicker layer of crystals
   b. Larger silver halide crystals, thinner layer of crystals
   c. Smaller silver halide crystals, thinner layer of crystals—This is why the exposure is somewhat slower, because there are fewer, smaller crystals to interact with the light and x-ray photons; this results, however, in finer resolution in the image; this situation is analogous to intensifying screen speed.
   d. Smaller silver halide crystals, thicker layer of crystals

13. What could help minimize blur caused by involuntary patient movement?
   a. Ask the patient to hold still
   b. Ask the patient to hold his or her breath
   c. Use short exposure times—Short exposure times can help minimize the blur caused by involuntary motion such as movement of gastrointestinal fluids; asking for patient cooperation has no effect because the motion is beyond the patient's control.
   d. All of the above
   e. None of the above

14. Motion blur can be caused by which of the following?
   a. The patient breathing
   b. The patient's heart beating
   c. Vibration of the x-ray tube
   d. **All of the above**—These are all types of motion blur, which occurs whenever there is movement in either the tube or the patient relative to the film.
   e. None of the above

15. Which of the following is true of film-screen combinations?
   a. **They are standardized for standard examinations.** Film-screen combinations are standardized for different exams, allowing the radiographer to set exposure factors following technique charts for different patient sizes and other variables.
   b. They are established individually for each examination.
   c. They depend on the size of the patient.
   d. They are used only with very high kVp selections.

Testbank Questions

1. The degree of sharpness in a radiograph is which of the following?
   a. Contrast
   b. Density
   c. Recorded detail
   d. Speed

2. The blurring caused by geometric factors at edges of structures on a radiograph is which of the following?
   a. Unsharpness
   b. Visible detail
   c. Focal point blur
   d. Fog

3. Where is the most visible detail on a radiograph found?
   a. The recorded detail area
   b. The unsharpness area
   c. Both the recorded detail and unsharpness areas
   d. Neither the recorded detail nor unsharpness areas

4. How is resolution on a radiograph measured?
   a. Line pairs per millimeter
   b. Exposed film crystals per millimeter
   c. The percentage of phosphor crystals that fluoresce
   d. None of the above

5. The average human eye on the average can discern which of the following?
   a. More line pairs per millimeter than can be resolved in most radiographs
   b. Fewer line pairs per millimeter than can be resolved in most radiographs
   c. The answer depends on the kVp selection
   d. The answer depends on the mAs selection

6. The three factors that affect geometric sharpness are the SID, the OID, and which of the following?
   a. Size of the silver halide crystals in the film
   b. Size of the phosphor crystals in the screen
   c. Size of the strips of lead in the grid
   d. Size of the focal spot

7. The term "target" refers to which of the following?
   a. The area of the patient being radiographed
   b. The cross hairs in the light image projected by the collimator light
   c. The area of the anode struck by electrons from the cathode
   d. The film or other image receptor struck by x-ray photons that penetrate the patient

8. What is the disadvantage of angling the anode?
   a. The film size that can be used is limited.
   b. The exposure to the patient increases.
   c. The contrast is lower.
   d. The recorded detail is diminished.

9. Generally, what is the range of target angles in x-ray tubes?
   a. 2 to 5 degrees
   b. 7 to 17 degrees
   c. 17 to 27 degrees
   d. 30 to 45 degrees

10. The magnification factor is calculated by dividing what by the SOD?
    a. SID
    b. OID
    c. Object size
    d. Image size

11. Compared with a 72-inch SID used in a chest radiograph, the standard 40-inch SID for other examinations results in which of the following?
    a. More recorded detail
    b. Less recorded detail
    c. The same recorded detail
    d. Cannot determine from information provided

12. Why is it always important to position the patient as close as possible to the image receptor?
    a. Less unsharpness
    b. More recorded detail
    c. Less magnification
    d. All of the above
    e. None of the above

13. Slow film/screen combinations provide excellent recorded detail and are used more commonly with examinations of which of the following?
    a. Chest
    b. Pelvis
    c. Abdomen
    d. Extremities

14. When an intensifying screens is used, which of the following is true?
    a. Fewer x-ray photons are needed to create the image.
    b. More x-ray photons are needed to create the image.
    c. The same number of x-ray photons are needed to create the image.

15. X-ray photons cause phosphor crystals to do which of the following?
    a. Change into metallic silver
    b. Explode
    c. Fluoresce
    d. Absorb scatter radiation

16. How are light photons emitted from phosphor crystals?
    a. In all directions
    b. In the direction of the film only
    c. Against the reflective layer only
    d. None of the above

17. High-speed screens may be used for which of the following?
    a. Mammographic screening
    b. Scoliosis screening
    c. Radiographs of extremities
    d. All of the above

18. Which image is formed first on radiographic film?
    a. The latent image
    b. The diagnostic image
    c. The manifest image
    d. The developed image

19. Restraining devices are used to prevent which of the following?
    a. Unnecessary patient exposure
    b. Motion blur
    c. Patient nausea
    d. Poor positioning of the part being examined

20. Poor recorded detail can be caused by which of the following?
    a. A damaged Bucky lock assembly
    b. Rotating anodes with damaged bear assemblies
    c. An unbalanced tube suspension system
    d. All of the above
    e. None of the above

Answers to Testbank Questions

1. c	6. d	11. b	16. a
2. a	7. c	12. d	17. b
3. a	8. a	13. d	18. a
4. a	9. b	14. a	19. b
5. b	10. a	15. c	20. d

Audiovisual Script

SLIDE 3-1/CD 3-i Welcome
Welcome to Mosby's Radiographic Instructional Series.

SLIDE 3-2/CD 3-ii Recorded detail
The module you are about to experience is the third of eight in the Radiographic Imaging program: Recorded Detail.

This module will help you understand recorded detail and the several factors that affect recorded detail.

SLIDE 3-3/CD 3-1 Introduction
Knowing what recorded detail is and understanding the factors that affect it will give you a broader knowledge of the radiographic imaging process. The more you know about ways to achieve high-quality images, the better prepared you will be to perform radiographic examinations that are of significant diagnostic value to a radiologist.

We'll begin this module by defining recorded detail.

SLIDE 3-4/CD 3-2 Patient diagnosis
Radiography has important consequences for the health and well-being of patients. As a radiographer, you're one of the crucial links in the chain of information that will determine the treatment a particular patient receives. Although the time you spend with a patient is short and you don't participate in analyzing the results of the radiographs you produce, doctors would be incapable of practicing modern medicine without the information you provide.

When you thoroughly understand the radiographic process and equipment, you'll be better prepared to take top-quality images. Radiography is an art as well as a science, and the decisions you make as you work affect the quality of the images you get. High-quality images help a physician diagnose disease and prescribe treatment. Poor-quality images don't provide much diagnostic help and can even lead physicians to make incorrect treatment decisions.

MORE INFO LEADS TO THIS ADDITIONAL AUDIO RESPONSE: There's another danger of taking poor-quality images: if they can't be read accurately, they may need to be retaken, and that exposes the patient to unnecessary additional radiation.

SLIDE 3-5/CD 3-3 Good recorded detail

Achieving good radiographic quality means there must be a balance between how well you can see structural details on a radiograph (body parts such as bone structure and small pulmonary vessels) and how sharp those details appear.

In this module, we'll study recorded detail, which means the degree of sharpness of structures actually recorded on the radiograph. We'll also take a look at the factors that influence it. The many terms that are interchangeable with recorded detail, such as definition, sharpness, resolution, visible detail, or just plain detail, can be very confusing. To avoid that, we'll call it recorded detail.

SLIDE 3-6/CD 3-4 Detail and unsharpness

In radiography recorded detail is evaluated by how sharp the anatomic structures are recorded on the radiograph. The structures of interest must be well defined without any blur or unsharpness to them. You can see the difference in sharpness between these two radiographs, for example. One demonstrates the anatomic structures sharply, the other has quite a bit of blur.

Generally, when you think about the meaning of recorded detail, think about how sharply recorded the structures of interest are. Many factors influence this.

MORE INFO LEADS TO THIS ADDITIONAL AUDIO RESPONSE: Good detail can exist although you might not be able to see it very well because the contrast and/or the density are poor. However, it's one of the easiest technical factors to adjust.

SLIDE 3-7/CD 3-5 Radiographic quality

Radiographic quality results from two different sets of factors: sharpness and visibility.

Image sharpness depends on several geometric factors, which you'll learn about in the next section. Image visibility depends on the photographic properties of the image: on contrast and density.

SLIDE 3-8/CD 3-6 Unsharpness

The opposite of sharp recorded detail is poor recorded detail, and it's very common at the edges of radiographic images. This kind of blur is called unsharpness. And, in fact, you can't take a radiograph without recording some degree of unsharpness around the edges.

The amount of recorded detail that does (or does not) show up on a radiograph depends on focal spot size, object-to-image receptor distance, and source-to-image receptor distance. All of those factors can be manipulated to decrease the amount of unsharpness.

MORE INFO LEADS TO THIS ADDITIONAL AUDIO RESPONSE: Scientists borrowed the terms penumbra and geometric unsharpness from the scientific disciplines of astronomy and mathematics. Some contemporary scientists believe those terms are becoming outdated and choose not to use them.

SLIDE 3-9/CD 3-7 Detail

The opposite of unsharpness, or blur, is recorded detail. Recorded detail refers to the area of structures that shows up as sharp on radiographs. There are ways to produce a higher level of recorded detail, or less unsharpness. We'll get into that in the next section of this module.

SLIDE 3-10/CD 3-8 Resolution grid

As you get more involved in radiography, you'll also hear the term resolution, which describes the amount of recorded detail, or information, on a radiograph. It's expressed in line pairs per millimeter, or lp/mm.

A line pair is an easy concept to remember. It's just a line and a space. The more line pairs per millimeter that can clearly be visualized, the greater the recorded detail.

SLIDE 3-11/CD 3-9 Resolution: line pairs

A resolution tool is a device used to measure the detail on a radiograph. The human eye can discern up to 5 lp/mm. Conventional screen film systems can resolve up to about 10 lp/mm, which is beyond the range of human visualization. That's good detail.

With that basic understanding of recorded detail in mind, let's move on to the factors that affect it. But before we do, let's review for a moment.

Recorded detail is one of the factors that determines radiographic quality. Recorded detail can be called a number of things, including definition and resolution. Fill in the blank in the following sentence. These terms refer to how ________ body structures are shown on the radiograph.

Type in your answer now.

With so many terms being thrown around to describe recorded detail, it's easy to get confused. But recorded detail and the other synonyms all refer to the degree of sharpness with which body parts are shown on the radiograph.

PRESENT THIS AUDIO IF ANSWER WAS sharp or sharply: Yes, you're correct. With so many terms being thrown around to describe recorded detail, it's easy to get confused. But they all refer to the degree of sharpness with which body parts are shown on the radiograph.

PRESENT THIS AUDIO IS ANSWER WAS anything else: No, you didn't get this one. With so many terms being thrown around to describe recorded detail, it's easy to get confused. But recorded detail and the other synonyms all refer to the degree of sharpness with which body parts are shown on the radiograph.

SLIDE 3-12/CD 3-10 Factors affecting detail

Blurring is a natural part of radiography. Because radiographs are images of the interior anatomy of the body, the x-ray beam has to pass through an outer level of tissue to reach them. That alone causes some blurring on the film. As a result, all radiographs record somewhat less detail than the object being examined actually possesses. That means you can never see every single segment of the body part being examined with absolute clarity.

We say radiography is an art as well as a science because even though unsharpness will occur, you can control the degree of it so that it doesn't unnecessarily obscure the image and make diagnosis difficult.

SLIDE 3-13/CD 3-11 Unsharpness

You have begun the topic of geometric unsharpness, which is one of the factors that affects recorded detail. This subject builds on information covered in the preceding section, including the definition of recorded detail. If you have not yet worked through the earlier topic, you may want to quit this section now and return later after going through the earlier topic.

Now let's take a closer look at blur, or unsharpness, and the factors that contribute to it. The three factors are geometry, motion, and materials (such as intensifying screens). In this section, we'll discuss geometric unsharpness.

CD 3-11A Geometric principles

You remember geometry from high school, don't you? If you recall, it's the mathematics of the properties, measurement, and relationships of points, lines, angles, and surfaces. Well, try not to let that formal definition shake your confidence, because now we'll be talking about the way geometry influences unsharpness on radiographs.

SLIDE 3-14/CD 3-12 Focal spot geometry

The amount of unsharpness related to geometric relationships depends on three factors: the focal spot of the x-ray beam, the location of the x-ray tube, and the distance of the body part being examined in relation to the placement of the image receptor.

SLIDE 3-15/CD 3-13 OID and SID

More specifically, the factors that affect geometric sharpness are: the size of the focal spot, the distance between the x-ray source and the image receptor (SID), and the distance between the part of the body to be examined and the image receptor (OID).

SLIDE 3-16/CD 3-14 Sharpness and unsharpness

The focal spot is the portion of the anode in the x-ray tube where x-ray photons are produced by bombardment of electrons from the cathode. Actually, it's not just one tiny spot, but an area that usually measures from a small focal spot of less than 1 mm to a large focal spot of 2 mm.

It would be ideal if it were possible to produce x-rays from just one specific point rather than from a larger area. If they came from a single point source you could produce sharply-defined images. But in reality, x-ray photons come from the entire surface of the focal spot and pass over the borders of the body structures, and that creates a degree of unsharpness.

SLIDE 3-17/CD 3-15 Focal spot size

The electrons that flow from the cathode in the x-ray tube are focused on a small portion of the anode, called the target or focal spot. A smaller focal spot will produce a sharper image. There will be less blurring of the image, resulting in better recorded detail.

SLIDE 3-18/CD 3-16 Line focus principle

Modern x-ray tube anodes use something called the line-focus principle to achieve the best recorded detail. The actual focal spot size is the area of the anode bombarded by electrons, and the effective focal spot size is the area projected onto the patient or image receptor. By angling the anode, the effective focal spot size is reduced. This is the line focus principle, which helps improve recorded detail.

The average angle of the anode on a diagnostic tube is 12 degrees, although they are available with angles ranging from 7 to 17 degrees.

By using a steeper target angle, resolution capabilities are increased. One big disadvantage, however, is that using a steeper angle limits the film size you can use.

MORE INFO LEADS TO THIS ADDITIONAL AUDIO RESPONSE: In order to get an idea of this principle, imagine lying on a table and looking up at the target. The focus would look to you like a square rather than a rectangle. In other words, it's foreshortened, or smaller.

CD 3-16A Focal spot and angulation
Try this to get a better idea of the line-focus principle. Hold a pencil straight up and then angle it toward and away from yourself. See how your perceived dimensions of the pencil change as the angle changes?

A similar thing happens when the angle changes in the x-ray tube. Doing that changes the effective focal spot.

SLIDE 3-19/CD 3-17 Standard target angles
In many radiography procedures, the standard target angle is 12 degrees. A 12 degree target angle will cover a 14" X 17" field size. But there are also tubes that range from angles of 7 to 17 degrees.

The disadvantage of a steeper angle is that it limits your choices in film size because it covers a smaller area.

Usually, you'll use a steeper angle only in special procedures. As you can see, although such an angle will get much better recorded detail, the size of the target area is quite limited.

SLIDE 3-20/CD 3-18 Magnification
If it seems that your eyes can play tricks on you in radiography, you aren't just imagining things. X-ray equipment can alter more than your perceptions. Just as there is always a degree of unsharpness, it's also true that all images recorded on a radiograph are larger than the actual object they represent. This phenomenon is called magnification. Like a magnifying glass, the radiographic process makes things just a little bit bigger.

Most of the time you want as little magnification as possible. Sometimes, however, you might want objects to be even larger than they appear with natural magnification, and you can plan for this. This kind of exam is called magnification radiography.

MORE INFO LEADS TO THIS ADDITIONAL AUDIO RESPONSE: When the x-ray beam comes out from the tube's focal spot, it naturally fans out. One of the tube's characteristics is that it allows only the useful x-ray beam to emanate through the window in the tube housing, producing a shaped beam. As that beam moves out, it becomes broader. And just as would happen if you shone a flashlight in a dark woods, objects close by within the path of the beam appear to be larger than those farther away.

SLIDE 3-21/CD 3-19 Magnification formula
You can learn to measure magnification to get the true size of a body part. Use this formula: MF = Image size divided by object size.

Most radiographs taken at an SID of 100 cm (40 inches) will result in a magnification factor of 1.1. Those taken at an SID of 180 cm (72 inches) would be about 1.05.

SLIDE 3-22/CD 3-20 Calculating magnification

You can't measure the precise size of a body part in a regular examination, but there are times you will need to do this from the radiograph that results. You can figure out the magnification factor by using this formula: MF = SID divided by SOD.

SLIDE 3-23/CD 3-21 SID and OID and magnification

Two geometric factors, source-to-image receptor distance (SID) and object-to-image receptor distance (OID), control the amount that an image is magnified. They magnify the unsharpness as well. Let's take a look at the degree of blurring, which depends to a certain extent on the distance between the focal spot and the image receptor.

SLIDE 3-24/CD 3-22 Changing SID and sharpness

A change in SID (the distance between the x-ray tube and the film cassette) changes the intensity of the beam that reaches the image receptor. If you increase the distance between the x-ray source and the object to be examined (and keep the object-to-image distance the same) the x-rays from the focal spot spread less after they pass the object on their way to the film. Increasing the SID, then, cuts down on blurring and improves the recorded detail.

SLIDE 3-25/CD 3-23 Standard 40-inch SID

A 40-inch SID is standard for most routine radiographic procedures. At this distance, it's possible to get good detail and a magnification level that is acceptable for diagnosis. As previously illustrated, a longer SID results in less magnification and less unsharpness, and therefore better detail. Some radiology departments are now adopting a 48-inch SID standard to take advantage of this.

SLIDE 3-26/CD 3-24 Unsharpness and sharpness

Some routine exams, such as a chest radiograph, maintain an SID of 72 inches. That allows for a good look at the chest and decreases the magnification of the heart. Once again, this results in less unsharpness around the image, and therefore sharper images result.

SLIDE 3-27/CD 3-25 SID for chest radiograph

Although it's important to understand the effects of SID on magnification and detail, it isn't a factor in most radiographic exams. That's because in most radiography departments, examinations use the same SID; it isn't changed routinely. It is more practical to create and use a technique chart when SID remains constant.

SLIDE 3-28/CD 3-26 OID and unsharpness

Magnification can also be decreased by decreasing the OID while keeping the SID and the focal spot size constant. Unsharpness is decreased when the object to be examined is positioned close to the film, which improves the recorded detail.

That's why it's important to always position the patient as close to the film as possible. However, because you'll never be able to put the body part directly on the film inside the cassette, there will always be some unsharpness.

SLIDE 3-29/CD 3-27 Review: geometric factors

Okay, let's sum up these three influencing geometric factors. Two of them are here; can you remember the third? Try filling in the blank. You get better recorded detail with: (1) a long source-to-image receptor distance; (2) a short object-to-image receptor distance; and (3) ________.

Type in your answer now.

The correct answer is a small focal spot. That's one of the influencing geometric factors. The smaller the focal spot, the sharper the image. For the best results, also use the longest SID and try for the shortest OID by placing the part to be radiographed as close to the film as you can.

PRESENT THIS AUDIO IF ANSWER INCLUDES a small focal spot: You're right that a small focal spot is one of the influencing geometric factors. The smaller the focal spot, the sharper the image. For the best results, also use the longest SID and try for the shortest OID by placing the part to be radiographed as close to the film as you can.

PRESENT THIS AUDIO IF ANSWER WAS anything else: All of these terms can be a bit confusing, but you're wrong. The correct answer is a small focal spot. That's one of the influencing geometric factors. The smaller the focal spot, the sharper the image. For the best results, also use the longest SID and try for the shortest OID by placing the part to be radiographed as close to the film as you can.

SLIDE 3-30/CD 3-28 Conclusion: geometric factors

This concludes the discussion of one of the factors that affects recorded detail: geometric unsharpness. You may find yourself a bit confused by all the "initial" terms like SID and OID, but as you study more and get used to using radiographic equipment, they'll become easy to remember.

SLIDE 3-31/CD 3-29 Screens and film

You have begun the topic of two other factors that affect recorded detail: screens and film, and motion unsharpness. This subject builds on information covered in the preceding sections: recorded detail and geometric unsharpness. If you have not yet worked through those topics, you may want to quit this section now and return later after going through the earlier ones.

We'll begin this section by discussing the equipment that affects unsharpness. The two major ones are intensifying screens and the film you choose to use with them.

SLIDE 3-32/CD 3-30 Variations in screens

Once you've optimized all the factors to reduce geometric unsharpness, the next consideration for recorded detail is the film/screen combination. Such combinations are generally classified by speed. A slow film/screen system will give you better detail than a fast one.

Most radiography departments maintain at least two standardized film/screen combinations. Slow film/screen combinations are used to radiograph extremities and provide excellent detail. Faster film/screen combinations are used for larger body parts to reduce patient exposure. Radiation exposure to the extremities is less of a concern than to the rest of the body.

SLIDE 3-33/CD 3-31 Cassette and screens

Although they're used in combination, it's worth discussing screens and film separately. Let's begin with intensifying screens. Shown here is a cross-section of a film cassette showing the screens in place.

There is one major reason for using intensifying screens. They decrease the patient radiation dose. With the use of screens, fewer x-ray photons are needed to create the image. This lowers the patient's exposure.

CD 3-31A Screen use vs no screen

Thomas Edison came up with the idea of intensifying screens in 1896, although they weren't used very much until World War I. He discovered that when x-rays strike screens, they produce a great deal of light photons. Although less than one third of the x-ray photons that hit the cassette interact with the screen, they still intensify the beam's latent imaging power.

Nearly 100% of the latent image is formed by light from the intensifying screens; less than 1% is contributed by direct x-ray photon interaction. That means that by using a screen, patient exposure can be drastically decreased while still obtaining a high-quality image. There's a small decrease in detail with the use of screens, but new technology is making this less and less of a problem.

MORE INFO LEADS TO THIS ADDITIONAL AUDIO RESPONSE: If radiographic equipment depended solely on film to get images, that would be an extremely inefficient process. Less than 1% of x-rays produced react with the film to produce a latent image. Screens are called "intensifying" screens because the x-ray beam causes the screens to fluoresce, producing visible light that enhances or "intensifies" the action of the x-ray beam on the film. The light interacts with the film to create the image.

SLIDE 3-34/CD 3-32 Screen cross section

Intensifying screens have bases composed of polyester plastic or cardboard. They're coated with phosphors that emit light when struck by x-ray photons. Most systems use two screens with the film placed between them, in a lightproof cassette. The radiographic film has emulsion on both sides to absorb the light emitted by the two screens.

SLIDE 3-35/CD 3-33 Phosphors

Phosphors are materials that can absorb the energy of an x-ray photon and then emit light photons. They have one purpose in radiography: to harness the energy of the beam to produce visible light. You may remember from an earlier module that the German physicist, Wilhelm Roentgen, the "father" of x-rays, made his great discovery accidentally in the late nineteenth century when he saw barium platinocyanide, a phosphor, glow on a piece of cardboard in his lab.

CD 3-33A Function of phosphors

When an intensifying screen is exposed to x-ray photons, it glows. The material that makes it react this way (the phosphor) must have these characteristics:

1. It must have a high atomic number so it will interact well with the x-ray photon.
2. It should emit a lot of light when it interacts with the x-ray photon.
3. The wavelength of the light should match the sensitivity of the film.
4. It should not continue to emit light after the exposure has stopped.

SLIDE 3-36/CD 3-34 Composition of screens

Screens are made of a base, a reflective layer, a phosphor layer, and a protective coat.

The base, usually made of plastic, supports the other layers. It's permanently mounted on the front and back of the film holder.

The reflective layer guides the light rays that are striking it back toward the film. It increases the screen's speed by allowing more light to reach the film. That creates more density with less radiation exposure than would otherwise be needed.

The phosphor layer, coated onto the base, emits light energy in all directions when x-rays activate it.

And the protective layer guards the phosphor layer from moisture, stains, and abrasions that can damage the screen when it is being used and cleaned.

SLIDE 3-37/CD 3-35 High speed screens
Screens are classified by their speed (the rate at which they absorb x-rays) and by how efficient they are in converting x-ray energy into light energy. As shown here high-speed screens have certain advantages.

For many years calcium tungstate was the phosphor of choice for intensifying screens. Since the early 1970s, rare earth elements have been used, and the majority of screens manufactured now use these elements.

Rare earth elements are those that are not found in abundance in nature. They are incorporated into phosphors such as gadolinium oxysulfide and lanthanum oxybromide.

MORE INFO LEADS TO THIS ADDITIONAL AUDIO RESPONSE: At about the time of World War I, when film screen combinations started to be used fairly often, calcium tungstate was the phosphor of choice. Barium lead sulfate and zinc sulfate were popular for a while, but calcium tungstate proved to be the long distance winner until the 1970s. Rare earth screens have been more popular since then because they're faster.

SLIDE 3-38/CD 3-36 Ultra high-speed screens
You may also hear screen/film combinations referred to by their speed in many radiography departments. What speed you decide to use will depend on what kind of exam is needed for a particular patient, how much resolution, or degree of recorded detail, is necessary, and the equipment you have to work with. Ultra high-speed screens, for example, have a number of advantages.

MORE INFO LEADS TO THIS ADDITIONAL AUDIO RESPONSE: Many companies manufacture intensifying screens and they all use their own terms to describe them. Screen speed is a relative number that indicates how efficiently x-rays are converted into light.

Par screens are the standard by which other screens are rated; they have a value of 100.
High-speed screens range in speed from 200 to 1200.
Fine-detail screens have a speed of about 50.

SLIDE 3-39/CD 3-37 Screens: mobile radiography
For example, high-speed screens are used when you want to limit dose and when fine detail is not a consideration. Exams using high-speed screens may include scoliosis screening, many pediatric exams, and portable imaging.

Special screens have been developed to use in cases where it's important to have as much sharpness as possible, such as in mammography.

SLIDE 3-40/CD 3-38 Review: screens in cassettes
Let's stop for a moment and review. Here is a view of the intensifying screens in a cassette positioned on both sides of the film. You've learned about the purpose of screens and how they're made. You've also learned that screens are rated by two things. One is speed. Now, fill in the blank in the following sentence. The other is how efficiently screens convert x-ray energy into ________.

Type in your answer now.

The answer is light energy. The speed of screens is the rate at which they absorb x-rays. And the other way screens are rated is how efficiently they convert x-ray energy into light energy.

PRESENT THIS AUDIO IF ANSWER WAS light energy: You got this one right. The speed of screens is the rate at which they absorb x-rays. And the other way screens are rated is how efficiently they convert x-ray energy into light energy.

PRESENT THIS AUDIO IF ANSWER WAS anything else: Better think this one over. The speed of screens is the rate at which they absorb x-rays. And the other way screens are rated is how efficiently they convert x-ray energy into light energy.

SLIDE 3-41/CD 3-39 Screens and resolution
Overall, screens decrease resolution, when compared with using direct exposure film. However, several factors affect the resolution of a particular screen. These include the size of the phosphor crystals, the thickness of the phosphor layer, and conversion efficiency. High-speed screens typically have larger phosphors in a thicker layer, resulting in lower patient dose but reduced resolution.

SLIDE 3-42/CD 3-40 Exposure adjustments
To get better resolution, you need to use slow speed screens, which increases the patient radiation dose, and that, of course, is a classic dilemma in radiography. Opting for better detail or more exposure is a decision that often comes down to you, the radiographer, so you have to be familiar with the pros and cons every time you make a decision.

SLIDE 3-43/CD 3-41 Radiographic film
Now let's take a look at radiographic film. There are many medical uses for it, from dentistry to mammography. Most of it has this common structure: a transparent base coated with a radiation-sensitive emulsion, an adhesive subcoating, and a protective coating. The emulsion, the most important part of the film, is that part that's sensitive to light and x-rays. It contains the latent image before processing and the image that's visible once the film is processed.

The image that is formed on the film after exposure to radiation but before processing is referred to as the latent image. The latent image becomes the manifest image (the one we can view) after processing.

MORE INFO LEADS TO THIS ADDITIONAL AUDIO RESPONSE: Film emulsions are made with varying sensitivity and speed in responding to light or x-ray photons. The film speed depends on the concentration of the halide crystals and the imperfections in the crystal structure, the "sensitivity specks."

SLIDE 3-44/CD 3-42 Film changes

As shown in this illustration, it takes several steps to produce the latent image. When an x-ray photon strikes a crystal in the film, electrons are released and move to the sensitivity speck. Positive silver ions are attracted to this negative charge. When several silver ions have moved to the speck, that crystal is said to have a latent image. Processing converts the silver ions to black metallic silver, thereby converting the latent image to a manifest image.

Films can be stored indefinitely with little degradation of the image. The drawback to film storage is the amount of space needed. New technologies, such as computed radiography, have greatly reduced storage problems. Computed tomography (CT) and magnetic resonance imaging (MRI) also use images stored on computer disks.

CD 3-42A CT unit

A CT scanner doesn't contain film and doesn't take conventional images. Instead, a detector measures radiation and transmits that information to a computer. The computer analyzes the data and transforms it into an image you can see on a monitor screen. Printed copies can also be made.

SLIDE 3-45/CD 3-43 Film speed

How film is evaluated depends on two things: its ability to respond to radiation and its latitude (how well it can show different shades of gray, from light to black). In the long run, of course, what really counts is the film's capacity to form visible images that are useful to radiologists.

Faster films generally have a thicker emulsion layer and larger silver bromide crystals.

SLIDE 3-46/CD 3-44 Film/screen combinations

As discussed earlier, film and intensifying screens are usually considered in combination. Because screens are so commonly used, the film's response is mainly from light rays the screens emit.

SLIDE 3-47/CD 3-45 Motion unsharpness

The last factor that affects recorded detail is motion. This is the biggest problem in producing radiographs with sharply recorded detail. No matter how careful you are in positioning the patient and no matter how good the equipment is, if the patient moves, or if some parts of the patient's body move involuntarily, the image can be blurred and the detail compromised. This forces you to repeat the examination, which exposes the patient to more radiation.

But there are steps you can take to cut down on patient motion.

SLIDE 3-48/CD 3-46 Controlling motion

When radiographers talk about patient motion, they categorize it as voluntary or involuntary. When patients move their bodies, arms or legs, or breathe during the exam, that's considered voluntary movement.

Voluntary movement is the easiest for you to control. A few well placed words to the patient, like the familiar "Take a big breath, hold it, and stay still," can do the job. But patients are usually anxious during an exam and they can end up moving even though they don't mean to. You can decrease the possibility of motion by using restraining devices such as sandbags and angle sponges.

MORE INFO LEADS TO THIS ADDITIONAL AUDIO RESPONSE: When you're radiographing some parts of the body, such as the head, go ahead and use some kind of restraint to minimize the possibility of having to repeat exposures. Some radiographers put a strip of tape across the patient's forehead for this reason.

SLIDE 3-49/CD 3-47 Decreasing blur

When motion is involuntary, it's more difficult for you to control because it's not something the patient can control either. It can happen in the gastrointestinal tract or the cardiovascular system. Or you might have an unconscious patient who can't hold his breath for the length of the exposure.

In these cases, use the shortest possible exposure times. Try helping the patient to stay still by using items such as compression bands, foam pads, and sand-bags. Most radiography departments will have special restraints to use with children.

SLIDE 3-50/CD 3-48 Movement: suspension system

Patient motion is usually, but not always, the cause of blur. The equipment can sometimes be the problem. The x-ray tube can vibrate and cause blur. If a Bucky lock assembly is damaged, it can create motion in the Bucky tray and cassette. Rotating anodes with damaged bearing assemblies can vibrate. An unbalanced tube suspension system can drift. Check your equipment before you perform an exam to make sure it's in good working order.

This concludes this section on materials and motion unsharpness.

SLIDE 3-51/CD 3-49 Quiz instructions

THIS AUDIO FOR SLIDE/TAPE ONLY, NOT IN CD ROM VERSION: This concludes the presentation section of this module. If you are not going to work through the self-assessment quiz that follows, you may stop the program at this point and turn off the equipment.

If your instructor has asked you to take this self-assessment quiz on the material you have learned in this module, you should have a piece of paper ready. There will be 10 questions with multiple-choice or short answers. After this self-assessment we will go back through these questions and briefly talk about the reasons for the correct answers. Ready?

THIS AUDIO IN CD ROM LECTURE MODE ONLY: You have reached the self-assessment quiz for this module. Here you will be asked 10 questions to help you assess how well you understand what you have learned in this module. The questions are multiple choice or have short answers. After this self assessment we will go back through these questions and briefly talk about your answers and the reasons for the correct answers.

Ready?

THIS AUDIO IN CD ROM STUDENT MODE ONLY: You have reached the self-assessment quiz for this module. Here you will be asked 10 questions to help you assess how well you understand what you have learned in this module. The questions are multiple choice or have short answers. For multiple-choice questions, click on the box next to your answer choice. For those questions that require a short answer, type in your answer at the keyboard and press enter.

After this self-assessment we will go back through these questions and briefly talk about your answers and the reasons for the correct answers.

SLIDE 3-52/CD 3-50 Quiz question 1

1. What does the term "recorded detail" mean?
   a. The amount of blur on a radiograph
   b. The degree of sharpness on the edges of structures recorded on a radiograph
   c. Penumbra
   d. The amount of density in a radiograph

SLIDE 3-53/CD 3-51 Quiz question 2

2. To what does the term "unsharpness" refer?
   a. The amount of poor recorded detail at the edges of structures that shows up on a radiograph
   b. The amount of sharpness at the edges of structures that shows up on a radiograph
   c. The way detail is produced on a radiograph
   d. The amount of recorded detail on a radiograph

SLIDE 3-54/CD 3-52 Quiz question 3

3. Which of the following is true of the focal spot (which is where x-rays originate)?
   a. The smaller the focal spot, the more unsharpness on the radiograph.
   b. The smaller the focal spot, the greater the penumbra.
   c. The smaller the focal spot, the less unsharpness on the radiograph.
   d. The smaller the focal spot, the less recorded detail.

SLIDE 3-55/CD 3-53 Quiz question 4

4. Which three geometric factors affect recorded detail?
   a. The size of the focal spot, magnification, and source-to-image receptor distance (SID)
   b. The size of the focal spot, resolution, and object-to-image receptor distance (OID)
   c. The size of the focal spot, SID, and penumbra
   d. The size of the focal spot, SID, and OID

SLIDE 3-56/CD 3-54 Quiz question 5

5. Which of the following is a reason to use intensifying screens?
   a. To screen out blur
   b. To reduce patient exposure to radiation
   c. To be able to use a lower film speed
   d. To make images sharper

SLIDE 3-57/CD 3-55 Quiz question 6

6. Besides being classified by how efficient they are in converting x-ray energy into light energy, how else are screens classified?
   a. By the type of plastic they use
   b. By the amount of contrast resulting on the radiograph
   c. By their speed
   d. By the film they are combined with

SLIDE 3-58/CD 3-56 Quiz question 7

7. Besides how well it responds to radiation, how else is film evaluated?
   a. By how long it can be stored
   b. By its color
   c. By its response to gamma radiation
   d. By its contrast capabilities

SLIDE 3-59/CD 3-57 Quiz question 8

8. When film is discussed, it is invariably paired with which of the following?
   a. Intensifying screens
   b. The degree of recorded detail it produces
   c. Its geometric properties
   d. Its photographic properties

SLIDE 3-60/CD 3-58 Quiz question 9

9. What is the biggest obstacle to producing radiographs with sharp recorded details?
   a. Figuring out the proper film speed
   b. Matching the proper SID and OID
   c. Motion
   d. Determining the proper focal spot size

SLIDE 3-61/CD 3-59 Quiz question 10

10. Which of the following will provide the best results in a radiographic examination?
   a. The smallest focal spot possible
   b. The longest SID
   c. The shortest OID
   d. All of the above

SLIDE 3-62/CD 3-60 Quiz review

That concludes the self-assessment quiz for Module 3: Recorded Detail. Let's quickly go back through the questions and see how you did.

SLIDE 3-63/CD 3-61 Review question 1

Question 1 asked you the definition of recorded detail.

The correct answer is b, the degree of sharpness on the edges of structures recorded on a radiograph. Congratulate yourself if you got it right! The other answers, such as blur, density, and penumbra, all relate to detail in different ways, but recorded detail is defined in terms of the sharpness at the edges of structures recorded in the image.

CD 3-61A Review question 1

Question 1 asked you the definition of recorded detail.

PRESENT THIS AUDIO IF ANSWER WAS b: Congratulations on getting it right! The correct answer is the degree of sharpness on the edges of structures recorded on a radiograph.

PRESENT THIS AUDIO IF ANSWER WAS a, c, or d: No, your answer is incorrect. The correct answer is b, the degree of sharpness on the edges of structures recorded on a radiograph. The other answers, such as blur, density, and penumbra all relate to detail in different ways, but recorded detail is defined in terms of the sharpness at the edges of structures recorded in the image.

SLIDE 3-64/CD 3-62 Review question 2
Question 2 asked what the term "unsharpness" refers to.

The correct answer is a, the amount of poor recorded detail at the edges of structures that shows up on a radiograph. The other answer choices all relate to sharpness and detail, true, but not specifically to the unsharpness at the edges of structures.

CD 3-62A Review question 2
Question 2 asked you what the term "unsharpness" refers to.

PRESENT THIS AUDIO IF ANSWER WAS a: Yes, you correctly answered that unsharpness is the amount of poor recorded detail at the edges of structures that shows up on a radiograph. The other answer choices all relate to sharpness and detail, true, but not specifically to the unsharpness at the edges of structures.

PRESENT THIS AUDIO IF ANSWER WAS b, c, or d: You incorrectly answered this one. The correct answer is a. Unsharpness is the amount of poor recorded detail at the edges of structures that shows up on a radiograph. The other answer choices all relate to sharpness and detail, true, but not specifically to the unsharpness at the edges of structures.

SLIDE 3-65/CD 3-63 Review question 3
Question 3 stated that the focal spot is where x-rays originate and asked you what the result of a smaller focal spot was.

The correct answer is c, less unsharpness on the radiograph. The other answer choices were all wrong because the opposite of each is true: there is less unsharpness, not more; the penumbra is smaller, not larger; and there is more recorded detail, not less.

CD 3-63A Review question 3
Question 3 stated that the focal spot is where x-rays originate and asked what the result of a smaller focal spot was.

PRESENT THIS AUDIO IF ANSWER WAS c: Yes, you're correct in answering less unsharpness on the radiograph.

PRESENT THIS AUDIO IF ANSWER WAS a, b, or d: Your answer was incorrect. The correct answer is c, less unsharpness on the radiograph. The other answer choices were all wrong because the opposite of each is true: there is less unsharpness, not more; the penumbra is smaller, not larger; and there is more recorded detail, not less.

SLIDE 3-66/CD 3-64 Review question 4
Question 4 asked what three geometric factors affect recorded detail.

The correct answer is d, the size of the focal spot, SID, and OID.

CD 3-64A Review question 4
Question 4 asked what three geometric factors affect recorded detail.

PRESENT THIS AUDIO IF ANSWER WAS d: Your answer is right! The size of the focal spot, SID, and OID.

PRESENT THIS AUDIO IF ANSWER WAS a, b, or c: Sorry, your answer is wrong. The best answer is d, the size of the focal spot, SID, and OID.

SLIDE 3-67/CD 3-65 Review question 5
Question 5 asked the reason for using intensifying screens.

The correct answer is b, to reduce patient exposure to radiation. This is the main purpose for which screens were developed. Screens do not decrease blur or make images sharper.

CD 3-65A Review question 5
Question 5 asked the reason for using intensifying screens.

PRESENT THIS AUDIO IF ANSWER WAS b: Yes, the correct answer is b, to reduce patient exposure to radiation. This is the main purpose for which screens were developed. Screens do not decrease blur or make images sharper.

PRESENT THIS AUDIO IF ANSWER WAS a, c, or d: No, the correct answer is b, to reduce patient exposure to radiation. This is the main purpose for which screens were developed. Screens do not decrease blur or make images sharper.

SLIDE 3-68/CD 3-66 Review question 6
Question 6 asked how else screens are classified, besides being classified by how efficient they are in converting x-ray energy into light energy.

The correct answer is c, their speed (the rate at which they absorb x-rays).

CD 3-66A Review question 6
Question 6 asked how screens are classified, besides being classified by how efficient they are in converting x-ray energy into light energy.

PRESENT THIS AUDIO IF ANSWER WAS c: That's right, the correct answer is c, their speed (the rate at which they absorb x-rays).

PRESENT THIS AUDIO IF ANSWER WAS a, b, or d: You missed this one. The correct answer is c, their speed (the rate at which they absorb x-rays).

SLIDE 3-69/CD 3-67 Review question 7
Question 7 asked how film is evaluated (besides how well it responds to radiation).

The correct answer is d, the film's contrast capabilities. Other answer choices should have seemed obviously wrong: film does have a storage life, but this is not relevant to its rating or uses; film has no actual color; and how it responds to gamma radiation is irrelevant in radiography.

CD 3-67A Review question 7
Question 7 asked how film is evaluated (besides how well it responds to radiation).

PRESENT THIS AUDIO IF ANSWER WAS d: Yes, the correct answer is d, the film's contrast capabilities.

PRESENT THIS AUDIO IF ANSWER WAS a, b, or c: No, you missed this one. The correct answer is d, the film's contrast capabilities. Other answer choices should have seemed obviously wrong: film does have a storage life, but this is not relevant to its rating or uses; film has no actual color; and how it responds to gamma radiation is irrelevant in radiography.

SLIDE 3-70/CD 3-68 Review question 8
Question 8 stated that when discussing film, it is almost always paired with what.

The correct answer is a, intensifying screens. This is because the type and speed of the film must be matched with the type and speed of the screen for different types of examinations.

CD 3-68A Review question 8
Question 8 stated that when discussing film, it is almost always paired with what.

PRESENT THIS AUDIO FOR ANSWER a: Yes, your answer was correct: intensifying screens. This is because the type and speed of the film must be matched with the type and speed of the screen for different types of examinations.

PRESENT THIS AUDIO IF ANSWER WAS b, c, or d: Sorry, you missed it. The correct answer is a, intensifying screens. This is because the type and speed of the film must be matched with the type and speed of the screen for different types of examinations.

SLIDE 3-71/CD 3-69 Review question 9
Question 9 asked about the biggest obstacle to producing radiographs with sharp recorded details.

The correct answer is c, motion. Other factors can be controlled more easily by the radiologic technologist, but you cannot always prevent patient motion.

CD 3-69A Review question 9
Question 9 asked about the biggest obstacle to producing radiographs with sharp recorded details.

PRESENT THIS AUDIO IF ANSWER WAS c: Yes, you're right. The correct answer is c, motion. Other factors can be controlled more easily by the radiologic technologist; but you cannot always prevent patient motion.

PRESENT THIS AUDIO IF ANSWER WAS a, b, or d: Sorry, but you missed it. The correct answer is c, motion. Other factors can be controlled more easily by the radiologic technologist; but you cannot always prevent patient motion.

SLIDE 3-72/CD 3-70 Review question 10
Question 10 asked which factors provide the best results in a radiographic examination.

The correct answer is d, all of the elements listed: the smallest focal spot possible, the longest SID, and the shortest OID. All of these contribute to producing the best image.

CD 3-70A Review question 10

Question 10 asked which factors provide the best results in a radiographic examination.

PRESENT THIS AUDIO IF ANSWER WAS d: You're right, it's all of the things listed. They are the smallest focal spot possible, the longest SID, and the shortest OID.

PRESENT THIS AUDIO IF ANSWER WAS a, b, or c: Sorry, you missed it. The correct answer is d, all of the things listed. They are the smallest focal spot possible, the longest SID, and the shortest OID. Your choice was correct, but so were the other factors. All of these contribute to producing the best image.

SLIDE 3-73/CD 3-71 Quiz conclusion

This concludes the self-assessment quiz. This was not intended as a test, so don't feel bad if you missed some. All that means is that you probably need to review this module or study your textbook more carefully.

CD 3-71A Quiz feedback

FOR SCORE OF 10, THIS AUDIO: You've done an excellent job here with a difficult subject. Clearly you are studying well, and you seem to have worked through the tutorial carefully.

FOR SCORE OF 9, THIS AUDIO: You've done well with a difficult subject. Clearly you are studying and paying attention to the subject. Maybe next time you'll get the perfect score!

FOR SCORE OF 7-8, THIS AUDIO: Your score is about average. I'd suggest you review this material in your textbook. You may also find it helpful, next time, to read the material in your book before coming to the computer to take the tutorial. And don't hesitate to talk to your instructor if you have trouble after both reading the textbook and working through the multimedia tutorial.

FOR SCORE OF 5-6, THIS AUDIO: Your score is below average. You need to review this material in your textbook, and perhaps you should come back and take this tutorial again afterwards. You may have just been unprepared this time, or if you are having trouble after both reading the textbook and working through the multimedia tutorial, be sure to talk to your instructor.

FOR SCORE OF 0-4, THIS AUDIO: Your score is rather low. Don't feel too bad; these are, after all, difficult concepts to grasp. If you tried your best here but are having this much difficulty with the material, you should first go to your textbook and see if you can understand the material there. If it still seems difficult, please ask your instructor for additional study aids.

SLIDE 3-74/CD 3-72 Exam instructions

In the next 7 or 8 minutes you will be presented with 15 multiple-choice questions. Select the one best answer choice. Get ready a blank sheet of paper, numbered 1 to 15 down the left side. As you take the examination, write the letter corresponding to your answer choice next to the number for each question.

Ready? You will not be asked to perform any complicated calculations.

CD 3-72A More exam instructions

In the next 7 or 8 minutes you will be presented with 15 multiple-choice questions. Select the one best answer choice. This examination covers the material you've been learning about in this tutorial over the last hour or so. It is designed to help you and your instructor determine how well you now grasp this material. You can use scratch paper during the exam if you want, but it shouldn't be necessary for any complicated calculations.

SLIDE 3-75/CD 3-73 Exam question 1

1. High quality in radiography means there must be a balance between how well you see structural details on a radiograph and which of the following?
   a. The degrees of gray on the radiograph
   b. The degree of penumbra
   c. How sharp the details appear on the radiograph
   d. The geometric factors that affect recorded detail

SLIDE 3-76/CD 3-74 Exam question 2

2. What should you be most concerned about when evaluating radiographs for recorded detail?
   a. How sharply the anatomic structures are recorded
   b. The degree of penumbra
   c. The size of the focal spot that was used in the exam
   d. The SID and OID used in taking the image

SLIDE 3-77/CD 3-75 Exam question 3

3. Standardized radiographic examinations are designed to produce the best image by arranging for which of the following?
   a. Long SID and long OID
   b. Short SID and short OID
   c. Short SID and long OID
   d. Long SID and short OID

SLIDE 3-78/CD 3-76 Exam question 4

4. Unsharpness is common at the edges of structures on radiographs. Which of the following factors does not affect unsharpness?
   a. Focal spot size
   b. The source-to-image receptor distance (SID)
   c. Film speed
   d. The object-to-image receptor distance (OID)

SLIDE 3-79/CD 3-77 Exam question 5

5. Resolution, the amount of recorded detail on a radiograph, is measured in line pairs per millimeter, or lp/mm. Generally, which of the following occurs with a higher number of lp/mm?
   a. More blur
   b. Poor resolution
   c. Lower contrast
   d. More diagnostic information

SLIDE 3-80/CD 3-78 Exam question 6

6. Which of the following items does not affect the degree of unsharpness on radiographs?
   a. Geometry
   b. The type of radiographic equipment being used
   c. Motion
   d. Materials

SLIDE 3-81/CD 3-79 Exam question 7

7. Which of these factors affects the amount of unsharpness in an image?
   a. The focal spot
   b. The part of the body being examined
   c. The film being used
   d. All of the above

SLIDE 3-82/CD 3-80 Exam question 8

8. A smaller focal spot will produce which of the following?
   a. A larger extent of unsharpness
   b. Less unsharpness
   c. Increased radiation to the patient
   d. Images that are difficult for the human eye to see

SLIDE 3-83/CD 3-81 Exam question 9

9. What happens when you use an anode with a steeper target angle than the standard 12 degrees generally used in radiography departments?
   a. It limits the size of film you can use.
   b. It decreases resolution.
   c. It endangers the patient.
   d. It limits the kinds of equipment you can use.

SLIDE 3-84/CD 3-82 Exam question 10

10. To what does SID refer?
    a. The distance between the x-ray tube and the object
    b. The distance between the x-ray tube and the film cassette
    c. The distance between the equipment and the patient
    d. The distance between the x-ray tube and the examining table

SLIDE 3-85/CD 3-83 Exam question 11

11. What are the two major materials that affect the unsharpness on a radiograph?
    a. Intensifying screens and the film cassette
    b. Film and the film cassette
    c. Intensifying screens and film
    d. Film and grids

SLIDE 3-86/CD 3-84 Exam question 12

12. In many radiography departments, you'll hear screen/film combinations categorized by which of the following?
    a. Screen speed
    b. Film speed
    c. Resolution speed
    d. Standard combinations

SLIDE 3-87/CD 3-85 Exam question 13

13. Screens affect resolution, the amount of recorded detail on a radiograph. The extent of the affect depends on which of the following?
    a. Phosphor crystal size
    b. Phosphor layer thickness
    c. Phosphor conversion efficiency
    d. All of the above

SLIDE 3-88/CD 3-86 Exam question 14

14. New advances in digital electronics, television systems, and computers have captured radiographic images on materials other than film. Which of these statements is true of computerized images and film images?
    a. Computer images are permanent, whereas film fades.
    b. Less storage space is needed for computer images.
    c. Film has better contrast than computer images.
    d. All of the above are true.

SLIDE 3-89/CD 3-87 Exam question 15

15. Patient motion is the biggest challenge facing the radiographer trying to produce radiographs with sharp recorded detail because motion causes blur. What is the most serious consequence of a blurry film?
    a. The need to redo the exam and expose the patient to more radiation
    b. Too much of the radiographer's time being wasted
    c. A waste of film
    d. Patient anxiety

SLIDE 3-90/CD 3-88 Conclusion

INSTRUCTOR CD/SLIDE AUDIO: This concludes the examination section of Module 3 of Radiographic Imaging. Please follow your instructor's directions for your answer sheet to the questions.

STUDENT CD AUDIO: This concludes the examination section of Module 3 of Radiographic Imaging. Your score has been saved on the computer. Your instructor will report it to you later.

Answers to the Multimedia Examination

1. c	6. b	11. c
2. a	7. d	12. a
3. d	8. b	13. d
4. c	9. a	14. b
5. d	10. b	15. a

Distortion

4

Overview

Distortion inevitable
Magnification
- Effect of SID
- Effect of OID
- Calculating magnification factor
- Magnification technique

Shape distortion
- Foreshortening and elongation
- Evaluating shape distortion

Minimizing distortion by positioning of patient and equipment
Obtaining accurate size measurements

Understanding the factors that cause size and shape distortion will help students obtain more diagnostic images, particularly as they gain appreciation for factors under their control. In this module they will learn why the patient and equipment must be positioned carefully and accurately to minimize size distortion and control for shape distortion as much as possible.

Students learn first that size distortion is inevitable because of the geometric properties involved. The effects of SID and OID on magnification are described and explored, and students learn how to calculate magnification factor and use it to determine the actual size of a body structure when the image size, SID, and SOD are known. Students also see how magnification can intentionally be used when imaging very small structures.

Shape distortion results from a number of factors involved in the position of the central ray, image receptor, and patient structure. Some factors can be controlled by the radiologic technologist, whereas others are geometric realities that cannot. Students learn the importance of positioning the patient with the central ray centered on the anatomy being examined, the anatomy being parallel to the image receptor, and the x-ray beam being perpendicular to the image receptor.

Learning Objectives

Upon completion of this module, the student should be able to do the following:

1. Define all the key terms in the module.
2. Explain distortion as a geometric characteristic.
3. Describe the factors responsible for size distortion (magnification) and explain why this is inevitable on all images.
4. State the effects of changes in SID and OID on the amount of magnification that occurs.
5. Explain when and why magnification technique might be used purposefully.
6. Describe how each of the following situations can result in increased shape distortion:
   - Thicker structures
   - Central ray not perpendicular to image receptor
   - Body part being imaged not parallel to image receptor
   - Central ray not centered on body part being imaged
   - X-ray beam angled
7. List two things a radiologic technologist can do, in addition to correct positioning, to minimize shape distortion or to obtain an accurate measurement on an image.
8. Successfully complete the activities and posttest in the Study Guide.

Key Terms

Angulation
Central ray
Distortion
Elongation
Focal spot
Foreshortening
Inverse square law
Magnification
Magnification factor
Magnification radiography
Object-to-image receptor distance (OID)
Recorded detail
Shape distortion
Size distortion
Source-to-image receptor distance (SID)
Unsharpness

Instructional Outline

I. Distortion is a misrepresentation of the size or shape of a part of the body in a radiographic image.
   A. Like recorded detail, distortion is a geometric property of the image affecting image detail.
   B. Size distortion occurs to some extent in all images because of the unavoidable magnification caused by the diverging x-ray beam.

C. Shape distortion causes the image of the body part to be shaped differently from the object. Some degree of shape distortion is also inevitable.

II. Size distortion is magnification.
  A. Magnification occurs because the x-ray beam spreads out as it travels farther out from the focal point. The image becomes larger, just as shadows are always larger than the objects making them.
  B. The x-ray beam spreads out following the inverse square law.
  C. The degree of magnification depends on the source-to-image receptor distance (SID) and the object-to-image receptor distance (OID).
    1. The greater the SID, the less the magnification.
      a. Because the SID is usually fixed (e.g., at 40 inches), increasing it can be impractical.
    2. The smaller the OID, the less the magnification.
      a. The patient is almost always positioned as close to the image receptor as possible to reduce magnification.
      b. With mammography, breast tissue compression will help reduce magnification of calcifications and vessels located farther from the film.
      c. When grids are used for thick body parts to reduce scatter, the grid increases the OID and thus increases magnification.
      d. Body structures farther from the image receptor are magnified more than other structures closer to the image receptor in the same radiographic image.
    3. The magnification factor is a measurement of how much bigger the image size is than the object's size.
      a. Magnification factor is the ratio of the image size to the object's size.
      b. Because of the geometric principle of similar triangles, the magnification factor can be calculated as the source-to-image receptor distance (SID) divided by the source-to-object distance (SOD).
    4. Magnification radiography is the intentional use of magnification to enlarge smaller structures in an image.
      a. A small focal spot is used to reduce the amount of unsharpness that could affect the magnified structure.
      b. Grids are not used with magnification radiography because the air gap diverts much of the scatter radiation before it reaches the image receptor.

III. Shape distortion arises from several factors and takes different forms.
  A. Shape distortion occurs as either elongation or foreshortening of a structure.
    1. Elongation is shape distortion in which the object appears longer than it really is.
    2. Foreshortening is shape distortion in which the object appears shorter than it really is.
  B. Evaluating shape distortion is more subjective and depends on understanding human anatomy and the normal appearances of body parts.
  C. Because of geometric factors, shape distortion results from a number of factors.
    1. Thicker objects or structures cause more distortion because the greater distance from the top to the bottom in relation to the distance to the image receptor results in the diverging x-ray beam striking these aspects of the structure at different angles.
    2. Distortion results if the central ray is not perpendicular to the image receptor.
    3. Distortion results if the body part is not positioned parallel to the image receptor.
    4. Distortion results if the central ray is not centered on the anatomy being imaged, because off centering causes uneven divergence of the x-ray beam through the different parts of the structure; the farther a part is from the central ray, the greater the distortion.
      a. The divergence of the x-ray beam can be used to advantage in some exams such as lumbar spine exams visualizing intervertebral disk spaces.
    5. Distortion results if the image receptor is not perpendicular to the central ray and parallel to the part being examined, or is off-center.

6. Angling the x-ray beam causes distortion but may be done intentionally for better imaging of a certain structure.

D. Special techniques can minimize shape distortion or its effects.
   1. Radiopaque rulers positioned alongside a structure can provide a true measurement even when shape (and size) distortion occur.
   2. Using several spot exposures along an extremity, each with the central ray perpendicular to the structure, can involve less distortion than one larger image with more distortion.

Teaching Tips

Introduction to Distortion

Because many students today are visual learners, this unit on distortion can be enjoyable to teach. Most of the concepts here can be visually illustrated in classroom demonstrations, as described below, and even those students who usually have difficulty with geometrical relationships can come to grasp the principles involved because they can see them in action.

Before going too far into the details of what distortion is and how it results from various factors, you would do well to establish the importance of this topic in the practice of radiography and radiology. If you have some radiographs with greatly distorted images you can show to the class, discuss how such distortion can make diagnostic interpretation difficult or impossible, or potentially contribute to misdiagnosis. Explain to students that incorrect positioning can cause so much distortion that the image may not be usable, and remind them that repeat radiographs cause unnecessary patient exposure. Positioning the patient and equipment are just as important as other skills of the radiologic technologist, such as mAs and kVp selection, because they contribute to obtaining the best possible diagnostic images.

Once students grasp the fundamental goal of preventing or minimizing distortion, they are then ready to understand the individual factors that affect size and shape distortion and factors the technologist can control.

Size Distortion

Size distortion, or magnification, is a simple concept for students to grasp once they can visualize what is happening with the geometric factors involved. The best way to illustrate magnification is by making shadows on the wall from a point light source such as a single bulb. Students will immediately see how OID affects magnification. Demonstrating the effect of SID is not as dramatically obvious but is still possible with a light source casting a shadow from a fixed object onto the wall as the source moves closer and farther from the object.

It is even possible to demonstrate the formula for calculating the magnification factor. Give one student a 12-inch ruler to measure the shadow cast on the wall, and another student a yardstick or tape measure to measure the SID and SOD. At first, use simple ratios quickly understood without having to use a calculator. For example, use an SID of 20 inches and an SOD of virtually 20 inches (a flat object touching the wall), and measure the shadow (which will show almost no magnification); then move the object back halfway to the light to produce an SOD of 10 inches for the same SID of 20 inches. With a magnification factor of 2, the shadow's measurement should be twice what it was at first.

Students will quickly visualize the geometry involved and then can be presented with a number of problems for using the formula. Because SID and SOD can usually be easily measured, as can the image size on the resulting radiograph, explain that this formula is most useful for calculating the object's size, the one unknown because a structure inside the body cannot be directly measured from the outside. Let them have some practice doing the math.

Here is a question that might provoke some interesting class discussion. Why would it generally be better to use magnification radiography with a larger OID to enlarge the size of a small structure on a radiographic image, than to use the usual smallest possible OID and then look at the resulting image with a magnifying glass? Students who can think this through either on their own or in a class discussion will have a better grasp not only of the geometry of magnification but of the principles involved in recorded detail.

Shape Distortion

Shape distortion is not as intuitive to most students, but the concept can be introduced best by again using shadowgraphs on the wall. Preparing a progressive series of demonstrations can be very effective for helping students grasp the factors involved in shape distortion as well as an enjoyable classroom activity. If possible, have some actual bones or models in the room to use for casting the shadows. First, clarify the basics of elongation and foreshortening. This can be done simply with a uniformly shaped object such as a 12-inch ruler. Manipulate its position in between a light source and the wall so that its image size is drastically foreshortened. Then show how off-centering the ruler (parallel to wall) affects shape, making the end farther from the light wider, along with elongation. Then show the effects of not having the ruler parallel to the wall (image receptor)—how the distortion varies this way. Using a ruler is a good way to start because students know it "should" have an even width in the shadow image, and it is easy to demonstrate how the width and length can vary.

Once students become familiar with the various types of distortion you are producing with the ruler and shadow images, encourage them to imagine what kind of distortion will occur in various situations. Have a student turn the light source on and off at your request. Position the ruler in a particular way relative to the light and wall, with the light source off, and ask students to describe what image will appear when the light (the "x-ray beam") is turned on. After this is done a number of times with different configurations of positioning, students should become adept at understanding and predicting the distortion that will occur in different positions.

At this point you can help students further apply this understanding of distortion to human anatomy. Use bones or models, or other models of organs, to demonstrate distortion that can occur in these shadow images. By experimenting with different models and different ways to position them for great distortion, the results can be dramatic: if you can position yourself and the light in a way that students cannot see the actual bone or model you are imaging, it should be possible to create shadows that students will not be able to recognize at all—this effectively makes the point about the problems of distortion.

Depending on the point in the curriculum your students have reached, you can expand this exercise even further. For example, students may have their anatomy text open and be looking at the skeletal system while you present distorted images of various bones or other organs. Have students identify what they are seeing. You may even have students describe or demonstrate in the room the appropriate patient positions to be used to image certain body areas to avoid distortion.

Workbook Posttest Answers and Rationales

1. Which statement is true about distortion?
   a. Distortion can be eliminated by careful positioning.
   b. Distortion can be reduced by careful positioning. Because of necessary geometrical factors, distortion such as magnification can never be completely eliminated, but careful positioning of the tube, patient, and image receptor can minimize it.
   c. Distortion can be eliminated by controlling exposure factors.
   d. Distortion can be reduced by controlling exposure factors.

2. What is the effect of scatter radiation on distortion?
   a. Scatter increases distortion.
   b. Scatter decreases distortion.
   c. Scatter and distortion are unrelated. Scatter causes fog and a generalized darkening of an image, but this is unrelated to distortion caused by geometric factors.
   d. The effect of scatter on distortion depends on other factors.

3. Which statement is true?
   a. Magnification always occurs. This is true because the OID can never be reduced to zero, meaning that the x-ray beam always continues to spread out between the object and the image receptor.
   b. Magnification occurs only with elongation.
   c. Magnification occurs only when you increase the OID to image small structures
   d. Magnification occurs only with an SID shorter than standard SIDs used.

4. The SID divided by the SOD equals which of the following?
   a. The SOD plus the OID
   b. The OID divided by the SOD
   c. The image size divided by the object size—This is the magnification factor; the ratio of the SID to SOD is the same as the ratio of the image to the object size.
   d. The object size divided by the image size

5. How can the formula for calculating the magnification factor be used?
   a. To calculate object size when image size, SID, and SOD are known.
   b. To calculate image size when object size, SID, and OID are known.
   c. To calculate SOD when image size, object size, and SID are known.
   d. All of the above are true. Knowing any three of these variables allows you to calculate the fourth; note that although the formula uses SID along with SOD rather than OID, if you know SID and OID you can subtract OID from SID to find the value of SOD to use in the formula.
   e. None of the above is true.

6. Which statement is true about using a grid?
   a. **Size distortion increases.** This occurs because the grid increases the distance between the patient and the image receptor, thereby increasing the OID and the magnification.
   b. Size distortion decreases.
   c. Shape distortion increases.
   d. Shape distortion decreases.

7. Positioning an extremity parallel to the image receptor and perpendicular to the x-ray beam helps minimize what?
   a. Elongation
   b. Foreshortening
   c. Angulation
   d. **All of the above**—All of these are forms of shape distortion that may result when there is not good alignment of the tube, body part, and image receptor; correct positioning helps minimize all of them.
   e. None of the above

8. In an exam of the arm from elbow to fingertips, where does the greatest image distortion occur when positioning the central ray over the wrist?
   a. The fingertips
   b. The wrist
   c. **The elbow**—The elbow will be distorted the most because it is farthest from the central ray, and the x-rays reaching it are more angled than those reaching the other areas, resulting in more distortion.
   d. The distortion is the same for all.

9. With all other factors being equal, which structure will be most distorted on an image?
   a. Dense bone
   b. Less dense muscle tissue
   c. Air-filled lungs
   d. **All distorted equally**—Distortion is a geometric property, unaffected by tissue density.
   e. None distorted

10. A radiopaque ruler can be used to do which of the following?
   a. Measure the amount of recorded detail
   b. Measure density of adjacent image areas
   c. Measure OID when positioning the patient
   d. **Determine the true size of a structure in an image**—Because there is always some magnification in an image, the most accurate measurement of a structure can be made with a radiopaque ruler.

11. Which statement is true?
    a. **Avoid angulation of the x-ray tube except for a special purpose.** Any angulation could increase distortion; the tube needs to be perpendicular to both the body part and the image receptor.
    b. Angulation of the x-ray tube has no effect as long as the body part and image receptor are parallel.
    c. Angulation of the x-ray tube has no effect as long as the central ray is perpendicular to the body part.
    d. All of the above are true.
    e. None of the above is true.

12. When imaging some internal structures (for example, the intestines) that cannot be positioned in a parallel plane perpendicular to the central ray, how can distortion best be evaluated?
    a. **An understanding of anatomy**—With such irregular shapes and distances from the image receptor and tube, the distortion can be better evaluated by comparing the image with normal anatomy.
    b. Using similar triangles to calculate distances and thus distortion
    c. The formulas for calculating the magnification factor
    d. None of the above

13. Why might off-centering the central ray from the anatomy being examined be done intentionally?
    a. To magnify small vessels
    b. To increase contrast when a grid is being used
    c. To compensate for tissue density differences
    d. All of the above
    e. **None of the above**—Off-centering the central ray will increase distortion and may cause the image not to show all the anatomy required; it does not have any of the effects listed here and would not be done intentionally for these reasons.

14. A radiograph taken with a child lying on his back shows the images of two pennies the child has swallowed. What can be known about the penny that looks smaller?
    a. It has been in the stomach longer.
    b. **It is closer to the image receptor.** The smaller the OID, the less the magnification.
    c. It is farther from the image receptor.
    d. None of the above is true.

15. Assuming the central ray is perpendicular to the image receptor and passes through the center of a long bone, in which of these situations will the long bone's image be the longest?
    a. **With the long bone parallel to the image receptor**—In either of the other two situations, foreshortening will occur.
    b. With the long bone perpendicular to the image receptor
    c. With the long bone angled midway between the image receptor and the central beam
    d. All are the same.

Testbank Questions

1. Increasing exposure factors (mAs and kVp) has what effect on distortion?
   a. Increases both size and shape distortion
   b. Increases size distortion only
   c. Increases shape distortion only
   d. Increases neither size nor shape distortion

2. Why is there some magnification in all radiographs?
   a. OID cannot be reduced to zero.
   b. SID cannot exceed 72 inches.
   c. Screens must always be used to minimize patient exposure.
   d. All of the above are true.

3. The inverse square law applies to the x-ray beam with which of the following conditions?
   a. Only with large focal spots
   b. Only with small focal spots
   c. With both small and large focal spots
   d. With neither small nor large focal spots

4. A radiologic technologist can take steps to eliminate or minimize which of the following?
   a. Elongation distortion only
   b. Foreshortening distortion only
   c. All shape distortion
   d. No shape distortion

5. You can use a formula to calculate the amount of which of the following?
   a. Elongation
   b. Foreshortening
   c. Magnification
   d. All of the above

6. What is the problem with magnification?
   a. Inaccurate size of the image
   b. More unsharpness
   c. Both of the above
   d. Neither of the above

7. Magnification is minimal with which of the following?
   a. Large OID and small SID
   b. Small OID and large SID
   c. Large OID and large SID
   d. Small OID and small SID

8. At the standard 40-inch SID used for many examinations, which of the following is true?
   a. Detail is good, patient exposure is relatively low, but there is too much magnification.
   b. Detail is good, patient exposure is relatively low, and magnification is minimal.
   c. Detail is good, magnification is minimal, but patient exposure is high.
   d. Magnification is minimal, patient exposure is relatively low, but detail is compromised.

9. For imaging a patient's anatomic structure 1 inch from the image receptor, what is the effect of increasing the SID from 40 inches to 72 inches?
   a. At 72 inches the magnification factor is roughly half of what it was at 40 inches.
   b. At 72 inches the magnification factor is roughly double what it was at 40 inches.
   c. The magnification factor does not change at all as long as the OID remains the same.
   d. The magnification factor decreases by only a small fraction.

10. Compression of breast tissue in mammography will do which of the following?
    a. Minimize magnification of structures farther from the image receptor
    b. Increase magnification of small vessels in the breast
    c. Decrease the patient exposure
    d. Prevent shape distortion

11. In a lateral (side view) radiograph of the skull and jaw, which statement is true about the size of the teeth in the image?
    a. The teeth on the side closer to the image receptor will look bigger than the equivalent teeth on the other side.
    b. The teeth on the side closer to the image receptor will look smaller than the equivalent teeth on the other side.
    c. The teeth on the side closer to the image receptor will look the same size as the equivalent teeth on the other side.
    d. Answer depends on which tooth the central ray is centered.

12. Use a calculator or scrap paper to calculate the correct answer. The SID is 40 inches. The OID is 2 inches. The width of a bone on the image is 1.7 inches. What is the true width of that bone?
    a. 1.48 inches
    b. 1.54 inches
    c. 1.62 inches
    d. 1.68 inches

13. When is distortion kept to a minimum?
    a. When the anatomy and image receptor are parallel
    b. When the anatomy and the x-ray beam are perpendicular
    c. When the image receptor and the x-ray beam are perpendicular
    d. All of the above
    e. None of the above

14. When is the central ray intentionally off-centered?
   a. When using magnification technique
   b. When it is crucial to prevent foreshortening
   c. When tissue densities vary significantly
   d. All of the above
   e. None of the above

15. Which of the following is true when distortion increases?
   a. Distortion increases in the exact center of the central ray.
   b. Distortion increases a close distance from the central ray.
   c. Distortion increases a farther distance from the central ray.
   d. Distortion is not related to position of central ray.

16. To obtain radiographic images that would accurately show any difference in the length of the right and left legs, which choice would make the most sense?
   a. Take two images, one of each leg, and measure each to compare.
   b. Take a series of spot films along each leg, and add up the measurements on all the images to compare.
   c. Take one image with the central ray centered halfway between the legs and measure each on this image.
   d. All of the above will produce equivalent results.

17. Magnification technique is sometimes used for imaging which of the following?
   a. Soft tissues
   b. Blood vessels
   c. The gastrointestinal system
   d. Finger bones

18. Magnification technique typically uses which of the following?
   a. A smaller focal spot
   b. A larger focal spot
   c. A larger focal spot for bones, otherwise smaller
   d. Any size focal sport

19. The air gap technique used with magnification radiography eliminates the need for which of the following?
   a. A grid
   b. An intensifying screen
   c. Controlling for shape distortion
   d. All of the above
   e. None of the above

20. The x-ray tube might intentionally be angled for what purpose?
   a. To correct for off-centering a body structure
   b. To avoid superimposing one body structure over another in an image
   c. To improve density and contrast in certain body areas
   d. All of the above
   e. None of the above

Answers to Testbank Questions

1. d	6. c	11. b	16. c
2. a	7. b	12. c	17. b
3. c	8. b	13. d	18. a
4. c	9. d	14. e	19. a
5. c	10. a	15. c	20. b

Audiovisual Script

SLIDE 4-1/CD 4-i Welcome
Welcome to Mosby's Radiographic Instructional Series.

SLIDE 4-2/CD 4-ii Distortion
The module you are about to experience is the fourth of eight in the Radiographic Imaging program: Distortion. This module will help you understand distortion and the difference between size and shape distortion. It will also analyze the relationships of factors that affect distortion.

SLIDE 4-3/CD 4-1 Introduction
In Module 3 you learned about some of the photographic and geometric factors that affect the quality of radiographs. That knowledge will help you understand how images are created. It will also allow you to manipulate the variables involved in performing exams so you can get the best quality results while limiting the radiation exposure to the patient as much as possible.

We'll begin this module by briefly reviewing recorded detail, one of the two geometric factors that affect the quality of radiographic images. You'll also learn about the second geometric factor, distortion, and more about magnification, which we touched on briefly in Module 3.

SLIDE 4-4/CD 4-2 Radiographic recorded detail
To begin, let's take a second look at the one geometric factor you studied in Module 3: recorded detail. Recorded detail, you remember, means the degree of sharpness of structures actually recorded on the radiographic film. Contrast and density, the photographic properties that also affect the radiographic image quality, affect how visible the overall image is.

Achieving good radiographic quality means there must be a balance between these two factors: how well you can see structural details on a radiograph (such as bone structure and small pulmonary vessels) and how sharp those details appear to the naked eye.

Recorded detail is one of the two geometric factors that affect image quality. The other is distortion, the misrepresentation of the size or shape of the part of the body under examination. There's an inverse relationship between detail and distortion: less distortion produces better detail.

SLIDE 4-5/CD 4-3 Photographic detail
Let's go over that distinction again. The photographic properties of contrast and density control how visible the detail is. The geometric properties (recorded detail and distortion) control the actual detail.

Maybe thinking of it this way will help to make the difference clearer. After a snowstorm, you can look out the window of your kitchen and see the white stuff covering your yard like a blanket. But if you go outside and put a little bit of snow in your palm, you can see that the blanket you observed is really composed of individual flakes (millions and millions of them). They're the beautiful details that make up the pile you're going to have to shovel, and you can see them clearly when you look at them one by one.

In the world of radiography, photographic properties control the blanket, while geometric properties control those tiny flakes.

SLIDE 4-6/CD 4-4 Distortion
Now let's consider that second geometric property. When you distort something, you change its form or character. In radiography, when a body part appears on a radiograph shaped differently from what it really is, or when it appears bigger than it really is, you have distortion. There are two kinds: size distortion (also called magnification), and shape distortion.

Distortion occurs to some degree on every radiograph. As you learned in Module 3, images will always be magnified a little and will never be recorded as their actual size. As x-ray photons exit the body they spread out en route to the film, causing each body part to be somewhat increased in size.

CD 4-4A Cause of magnification
Size distortion happens this way. As x-rays leave the tube, they naturally spread out in all directions. As they encounter a body part, they cause the resultant image to be spread out on the film. This causes both magnification and a resultant loss of detail.

SLIDE 4-7/CD 4-5 Magnification
If it seems like your eyes can play tricks on you in radiography, you aren't just imagining things. The manner in which the patient and equipment are positioned can alter the resulting image. There will always be some degree of unsharpness on the image and all images will in fact be larger than the actual objects they represent. This phenomenon is called magnification (or size distortion). Like a magnifying glass, radiography makes things appear just a little bit bigger.

Most of the time you want as little magnification as possible, and you can control this. Sometimes, though, you might want objects to be even larger than they appear with natural magnification, and you can plan for this, as well. We'll talk more about magnification, and about magnification radiography (aimed at achieving a higher degree of magnification) a little later.

MORE INFO LEADS TO THIS AUDIO RESPONSE: Some distortion is a fact of life, and while it can take away from the quality of the radiograph, there's no point in fighting it. Getting rid of it entirely is as impossible as trying to capture the splendor of the Grand Canyon in a snapshot: a radiographic image is a two-dimensional look at a three-dimensional object. And unlike the way you usually see things, in radiography, objects farther away from the film appear larger than those that are closest to it.

SLIDE 4-8/CD 4-6 Foreshortening and elongation

The second kind of distortion, shape distortion, results in the image of the body part being shaped differently than it really is. If the x-ray tube, patient, and image receptor are not aligned properly, the shape of the structure can be distorted.

Shape distortion is manifested as elongation, the object appearing longer than it really is, or foreshortening, appearing to be shorter than the actual size.

MORE INFO LEADS TO THIS AUDIO RESPONSE: It can be difficult to avoid shape distortion when you're examining some areas of the body. Body parts frequently do not lie parallel to the film or image receptor. This causes shape distortion.

SLIDE 4-9/CD 4-7 Elongation in radiograph

Shape distortion, as you can see, is pretty much what it sounds like. Because it is magnified unevenly, the body part shows up on the radiograph shaped somewhat differently than it is in real life. That happens when x-rays pass through the body at the wrong angle, when the plane of the film is tilted, or when the body part is tilted.

Shape distortion is common because parts of the body frequently do not lie parallel to the film or image receptor. It also happens when the x-ray beam is not centered over the anatomy or when the x-ray beam is improperly angled.

Evaluating shape distortion is more subjective than evaluating size distortion. There's no formula you can use to check shape distortion, as there is with the magnification factor when you're assessing size distortion. In the end, it comes down to how well you understand human anatomy and how body parts should look.

SLIDE 4-10/CD 4-8 Recorded detail

Let's stop for a minute to review before we move on to the next section. You learned at the beginning of this section that there are two geometric properties that affect image quality: recorded detail and distortion.

Those two factors are related. As the level of magnification (or size distortion) decreases, what happens to recorded detail?

Type in a one-word answer.

SLIDE 4-11/CD 4-9 Less distortion, better detail

It improves, of course! If a radiograph shows structures that have been magnified only a little bit, that means the variables that control size distortion have been controlled properly. If they have not, there will be more magnification and a resulting loss of detail.

PRESENT THIS AUDIO IF ANSWER WAS increases, increase, increased, sharpens: you're absolutely right. It increases. You understand the principles at work here. The less magnification, the better the level of detail.

PRESENT THIS AUDIO IF ANSWER WAS anything else: No, think through this again. Remember that the less magnification, the better the level of recorded detail. If a radiograph shows structures that have been magnified only a little bit, that means the variables that control size distortion have been controlled properly. If they have not, there will be more magnification and a resulting loss of detail.

SLIDE 4-12/CD 4-10 Distortion: conclusion

This concludes the section that defines distortion, the second geometric factor that affects the quality of radiographs. There are many variables that can produce distortion that we'll study as you move along in this module.

SLIDE 4-13/CD 4-11 Distortion radiographs:

You have begun the topic of size distortion. This section builds on information covered in the preceding section. If you have not yet worked through the earlier topic, you may want to quit this section now and return later after going through it.

We'll begin this section by taking another look at magnification.

SLIDE 4-14/CD 4-12 Shadowgraph

To understand how magnification works, think back to slide shows your family staged at home, or back to junior high when your social studies teacher showed lots of film strips and movies in class. Between slides, or when the reel was being changed, there was always someone who stuck his fingers up to the source of light and made shadowy hand puppets, turning plain old fingers and thumbs into exotic rabbits and cats.

Do you remember how those shadows changed depending on where the fingers were in relation to the light? They were biggest and fuzziest when the fingers were close to the light; the shadows became smaller and more sharply defined the farther away the fingers moved from the light toward the white screen.

SLIDE 4-15/CD 4-13 Distance

What is happening is that the image-forming light rays in the beam diverge as they move away from their source. When the distance between the source of light and the object is small, you'll see magnification and blur. On the other hand, when the distance between the object and the image receptor is small (in the case of shadow puppets, the screen is the image receptor), the amount of magnification is relatively small.

Let's put this in radiographic terms. Source-to-image receptor distance (SID) and object-to-image receptor distance (OID) affect the degree of magnification. As a general rule, a long SID and a short OID will keep magnification to a minimum.

MORE INFO LEADS TO THIS AUDIO RESPONSE: Keep in mind the inverse square law. It states that the intensity of radiation is inversely proportional to the square of the distance from the source of radiation. At a longer SID, the intensity of radiation lessens.

SLIDE 4-16/CD 4-14 SID and OID

It's possible, then, to cut down on size distortion by doing one of two things. You can increase the SID or reduce the OID.

Changing the SID has an impact on magnification. Increasing the distance between the source of radiation and the patient will minimize magnification, but doing that also decreases the intensity of radiation reaching the patient and the image receptor.

Over the years, a distance of 100 cm (40 inches) has emerged as the standard for many radiographic procedures. At this distance, there is a good balance of relatively low radiation exposure with good detail and minimal magnification.

The standard is 180 cm (72 inches) in chest imaging, where a horizontal beam and a longer SID keep magnification of the heart shadow to a minimum. There's rarely a situation where a SID of more than 180 cm (72 inches) would be in order.

CD 4-14A Different SIDs

There are a couple of other standards for special procedures. Many dentists now use 40 cm (16 inches) for tooth examinations rather than the old standard of 20 cm (8 inches). Radiography units designed solely for mammography use 50 to 80 cm (20 to 32 inches), which is rather short, but the intensity of the radiation is relatively low. These machines compress the breast, which minimizes magnification.

SLIDE 4-17/CD 4-15 SID and magnification

The closer the patient is to the source of radiation, the more radiation he or she receives. That's because the x-ray beam is most intense as it leaves the tube and becomes less intense the farther away it moves. With a short SID, there is more magnification as well as more intense radiation.

Increasing the SID will decrease magnification, but it will lower the amount of radiation being transmitted to the patient as well, so exposure factors have to be increased.

SLIDE 4-18/CD 4-16 Variable OID

The OID is the other important distance to keep in mind. The shorter the distance between the object and the image receptor, the less magnification you'll get. That's why it's important to position the patient as close to the x-ray film as possible. That's relatively easy to do with a table top exam when you can put the part to be examined right on the film cassette.

It becomes more difficult to maintain that short distance when you're dealing with thick body parts or a part that can't be placed directly on the cassette. Thick body parts require a Bucky grid, and using that will cause some magnification because the grid increases the OID.

SLIDE 4-19/CD 4-17 OID and magnification

When body parts are at different levels, their images will be magnified at different rates. This phenomenon is like depth perception, or the way your eyes perceive objects at different distances. With depth perception, smaller objects seem farther away than closer ones.

One way to visualize this is to go back to our discussion of shadowy finger puppets at a slide show. Shadows of fingers held up to the light change size depending on where they are in relation to the light and the screen. Close to the light and farther from the screen, fingers become large shadows. When those fingers move away from the light and closer to the screen, they become smaller shadows.

It's just the same with radiographic images. Body parts that are closer to the x-ray tube and farther from the image receptor will appear to be larger than those farther from the tube and closer to the receptor. On a PA (postero-anterior) chest radiograph, for example, the posterior ribs will appear wider than the anterior ones. As a radiographer, you'll have to get used to a new way of seeing things.

SLIDE 4-20/CD 4-18 Review: distance

Okay, it's time to stop for a second and review what you've just learned. All this talk of seeing things in a different way can be pretty confusing. But once you understand the basic concept and make it a part of your knowledge, you won't have any problem in your work as a radiographer.

Think back to our discussion of shadowgraphs. To understand how shadows look larger when they're close to the source of light and smaller when they're farther away from it, try this little experiment. Take a pencil and a piece of white paper. Line them up to a light, positioning the pencil between the light and the paper. Hold the light source and the paper in steady positions while you move the pencil around and see how its shadow on the paper changes size.

At what point does the pencil's shadow appear to be largest?

Yes, that's right. The pencil's shadow appears to be largest when it's closer to the light source.

SLIDE 4-21/CD 4-19 Review question: SID

Now apply this concept to radiography. You can change the SID and the OID to alter the degree of magnification that appears on a radiograph. When you increase the SID, what happens to the degree of magnification?

Type in a one-word answer.

SLIDE 4-22/CD 4-20 Answer: SID

You're right on target if you said that making the SID longer decreases the degree of magnification. Of course if you do lengthen the SID, you need to adjust the exposure factors.

PRESENT THIS AUDIO IF THE ANSWER WAS decrease, decreases, or decreased: Yes, you're right. Making the SID longer decreases the degree of magnification. Of course if you do lengthen the SID, you need to adjust the exposure factors.

PRESENT THIS AUDIO IF THE ANSWER WAS anything else: Go back and do that pencil experiment again. You'll see that increasing the distance from the light source to the paper makes the pencil shadow look smaller. Making the SID longer decreases the degree of magnification. In radiography, if you do lengthen the SID, you need to adjust the exposure factors.

SLIDE 4-23/CD 4-21 Magnification defined

You've seen that you can manipulate SID and OID to alter the degree of magnification. It's often important for diagnosis to know how much magnification is occurring.

First, let's consider how magnification is defined. The amount of magnification, sometimes called the magnification factor, is a measurement of how much bigger the image size is than the true object size.

For example, if a heart measurement that is actually 11 cm at its widest point measures 12.5 cm on the radiograph, then the magnification is 1.136, or 12.5 divided by 11.

SLIDE 4-24/CD 4-22 Measuring magnification

But you can't actually measure a heart, or any other part of the body that's hidden from view. So to find the amount of magnification, the magnification factor, you use measurements that geometrically determine the magnification. The source-to-image receptor distance (SID) divided by the source-to-object distance (SOD) gives you the magnification factor, as shown in this illustration.

You can measure the SID, and you can estimate the SOD if you have a good grasp of anatomy. Then you have to fall back to geometry and the relationship between similar triangles to figure out the ratio between those distances. When two right triangles share a hypotenuse, they will have the same ratio of height to base.

SLIDE 4-25/CD 4-23 Similar triangles

These similar triangles are shaped exactly the same but they are of different sizes. The corresponding sides are proportional and the corresponding angles are equal. This can help you figure out some important information about the size of objects and their images.

Take a triangle and draw a line within that triangle, parallel to its base. You'll see two similar triangles, one superimposed on the other. It's even easier to see these similar triangles when you separate them, as you can see in this illustration.

SLIDE 4-26/CD 4-24 Image size and object size

Now you can use that concept to calculate the size of objects and their images in radiography. Think of placing an object in the path of light. The shadow it casts (or its image, in radiographic terms), is larger than the object itself. When you know how far the object and the image are from the source of light, and you know the size of the image, you can calculate the size of the object.

That's where the similar triangles come in. You take this proportion:

$$\frac{\text{Image size}}{\text{Object size}} = \frac{\text{source-to-image receptor distance}}{\text{source-to-object distance}}$$

If you know any three values, you can easily calculate the fourth.

SLIDE 4-27/CD 4-25 Formula: magnification

Let's figure this out with real numbers. Say an object is 15 inches in diameter and lies 10 inches above the film. The SID is 40 inches. How do you determine the magnification (the image size)?

Using the formula:

$$\frac{\text{image size}}{\text{object size}} = \frac{\text{SID}}{\text{SOD}}$$

You calculate it this way:

$$\frac{\text{image size}}{15} = \frac{40}{30}$$

Therefore the size of the image is 20 inches.

MORE INFO LEADS TO THIS AUDIO RESPONSE: As you can see, there's a lot to visualize and figure when you're trying to determine the extent of magnification. Always draw a sketch for yourself so you can see the calculations you're making.

SLIDE 4-28/CD 4-26 Magnification calculation
Using the numbers from the previous example, you can figure out the magnification factor in this way:

$$MF = \frac{20 \text{ (image width)}}{15 \text{ (object width)}}$$

$$= 1.33$$

In this example, then, the object is magnified $1\frac{1}{3}$ times.

SLIDE 4-29/CD 4-27 Geometry
Let's pause for a moment to digest this information about magnification factors. You can show the rate of magnification either in a ratio or a percentage by using the calculations you've just learned. Just keep a few things in mind.

You've seen that the concept of similar triangles is important in radiography. Because their corresponding sides are proportional and their corresponding angles are equal, you can find information that's important in diagnosis. If you don't know the object size but you do know the size of the image, the SID, and the SOD, what is the formula for finding the object size?

SLIDE 4-30/CD 4-28 Magnification formula
Did you say image size divided by object size equals SID divided by SOD?

That's the right formula, just as you see in this illustration. You can easily measure the SID and the SOD, and once you find the size of the image it's a quick jump to calculating the size of the object.

You see that a firm grasp of the concept of similar triangles helps to better understand this.

SLIDE 4-31/CD 4-29 Distortion radiographs
This concludes the section on size distortion and how it can appear on radiographs. With a firm understanding of size distortion, you'll be in good shape to go on to study other factors that can affect radiographic quality.

SLIDE 4-32/CD 4-30 Distortion variables
You have begun the topic of the factors that affect shape distortion. This subject builds on information covered in the preceding topics on distortion. If you have not yet worked through those topics, you may want to quit this section now and return later after going through the earlier topics.

Now let's talk about the factors that affect shape distortion and the ways those factors relate to one another. Take a close look at this illustration. Do you see that the bone at the fracture site appears a little bit different in each radiograph? Depending on the alignment of the tube, bone, and film, the fracture site seems to be somewhat larger and slightly more distorted than its true size and shape.

SLIDE 4-33/CD 4-31 Shape distortion
You learned in the previous section that distance plays a large part in determining how much an object is magnified. How far the object is from the source of radiation and how close it is to the film cassette are variables that you can control.

There are several factors that affect shape distortion (also referred to as true distortion) as well. They include the thickness of the object being examined, its position on the examining table, the angle of the x-ray tube, and the position of the film. Because there is more uneven magnification with thick objects, there is more shape distortion, too.

SLIDE 4-34/CD 4-32 Thickness of part
If the object you were examining were as thin as a dime, you wouldn't see much shape distortion. But the human body is made up of irregularly shaped parts that range from thin to thick. When you try to examine the thick ones, the distance from their tops to bottoms in relation to the film cassette will vary. The x-ray beam will diverge and hit the part at different angles, causing distortion.

MORE INFO LEADS TO THIS AUDIO RESPONSE: As you determine the rate of magnification, you'll be relying on geometry again to adjust things in order to cut down on shape distortion. The relationship of the positioning of the x-ray beam, the part, and the film are crucial. So is your knowledge of how different parts of the body usually look.

SLIDE 4-35/CD 4-33 Misalignment of central ray
Look closely at this illustration to see what happens when the central ray, the body part, and the film are not properly aligned. Do you see how the images will be distorted?

The correct way to perform an x-ray examination is to first line up the central ray, the part of the body under examination, and the film cassette. The central ray should be at right angles to the part and the film. The part and the film should be parallel. When these elements are in alignment, distortion is kept to a minimum.

Of course, that's not always easy to achieve. You may need to utilize creative patient positioning in order to get the part as parallel to the film as possible.

CD 4-33A Distortion and off-centering
If you have even one of these three factors out of kilter, that's enough to cause some distortion. Always check to make sure the central ray is perpendicular and that the film is parallel to the part. If the film is off center you'll get some distortion.

It's also likely that off-centering will result in some of the essential anatomy not being included on the image. This will require you to perform another exposure.

SLIDE 4-36/CD 4-34 More distortion

The central ray is the exact center of the x-ray beam as it exits the tube from the focal spot. As you know, the focal spot is more of a square than a single spot, and the x-ray beam begins to diverge as it exits from it. In the best of all worlds, that beam is projected perpendicular to the part and the film. When it isn't, you get some degree of distortion.

But not all body parts can be placed parallel to the film or directly centered in the central ray. When they aren't, or when only a portion is, the beam divergence causes some distortion. As you might suspect, there's more distortion the farther away the part is from the central ray. This is true whether the distance is longitudinal (in the direction of the long axis of the object), or transverse (at right angles to the long axis).

CD 4-34A Beam divergence

If the central ray is off (not directed to the desired anatomical landmark), it will create the same effect as angling the tube. The resulting image may be distorted.

The divergence of the x-ray beam can be used to advantage for certain radiographic examinations. For example, the lumbar spine is naturally curved. The divergent x-ray beam naturally follows the path of the curved lumbar spine and allows for better visualization of the intervertebral disk spaces.

SLIDE 4-37/CD 4-35 Counteracting distortion

Other parts of the body present particular radiography problems. Because of their size, getting accurate measurements of long bones in one x-ray exam is difficult. The farther away from the central ray the end of the bone lies, the greater the degree of distortion.

So different procedures have been developed to counter the natural tendency towards distortion. For example, it's common to place a radiopaque ruler along the extremity from hip to ankle to get accurate measurements. Rather than take one image of the total length of the extremity, you take spot exposures at the hip, knee, and ankle joints, positioning the central ray perpendicular to the joint space. That way you get an accurate measurement of leg length with minimal distortion.

SLIDE 4-38/CD 4-36 Alignment

Okay, time for a quick review. Putting the body part, tube, and film in the right position is everything when you're trying to keep distortion to a minimum. That means the central ray must be perpendicular to the part being examined.

How do you position the part in relation to the film?

Type in your answer.

SLIDE 4-39/CD 4-37 Misalignment

You place it parallel to the film cassette, or as close to parallel as you can get. Sometimes, that calls for some creativity in the way you position the patient. In radiography, proper positioning is crucial. If any of the variables are out of alignment, you will get imperfect images and increase the likelihood of having to do the exam over again, exposing the patient to more radiation. That's something you must always try to avoid.

ADD THIS AUDIO IF THE ANSWER WAS parallel or parallel to the film cassette: Great, you've been paying attention. You place it parallel to the film cassette, or as close to parallel as you can get. Sometimes, that calls for some creativity in they way you position the patient. In radiography, proper positioning is crucial. If any of the variables are out of alignment, you will get imperfect images and increase the likelihood of having to do the exam over again, exposing the patient to more radiation. That's something you must always try to avoid.

ADD THIS AUDIO IF THE ANSWER WAS anything else: No, think again. The part and the film cassette must be parallel, or as close to parallel as you can make them. Sometimes, that calls for some creativity in they way you position the patient. In radiography, proper positioning is crucial. If any of the variables are out of alignment, you will get imperfect images and increase the likelihood of having to do the exam over again, exposing the patient to more radiation. That's something you must always try to avoid.

SLIDE 4-40/CD 4-38 Distortion: part

You've seen that the part of the body to be examined must be placed perpendicular to the central ray and parallel to the film.

But there is another consideration in placement you need to think about. The body part should be placed along its long axis. If it isn't, there will be foreshortening (and magnification too).

SLIDE 4-41/CD 4-39 Distortion: film

The last element in the lineup is the image receptor, the film cassette. As you know, it should be parallel to the part being examined. Even when it is, you can still have a problem if the part is parallel but off center. You may not get an image of the entire part and will have to repeat the exposure.

The bigger problem comes in the form of serious shape distortion if the film cassette isn't parallel to the part. A similar result will show up if the central ray isn't centered to the part.

SLIDE 4-42/CD 4-40 Radiograph: distortion

You've seen how important it is for the tube to be perpendicular to the part being examined. When it's not, when it's at something other than 90 degrees and directed somewhere other than at the center of the part, that's called angulation. The result, as you might be able to predict, is distortion.

There are times when you will want to place the tube at a different angle because you want a certain result. That's usually when you want to avoid body parts being superimposed on one another and appearing distorted on the film. (Through angulation distortion can be controlled to help in making a better diagnostic image. Keep in mind that when you angle the tube, you need to make sure the SID remains constant.

SLIDE 4-43/CD 4-41 Magnification radiography

You may recall that we mentioned magnification radiography at the beginning of this module. This is a special application in radiography that you might also hear referred to as macroradiography or the magnification technique. It's a technique usually used to diagnose vascular or neurological conditions by making fine vessels and bony structures appear larger on the radiograph than they are in reality.

In magnification radiography, the object is not placed as close to the film as you can position it, but rather at a distance from it so that it will be purposefully magnified.

SLIDE 4-44/CD 4-42 Intentional magnification

Think back to what you've already learned about calculating the magnification factor. Do you remember the formula?

$$MF = \frac{SID}{SOD}$$

SID, you recall, is the source-to-image receptor distance, and SOD is the source-to-object distance.

MORE INFO LEADS TO THIS AUDIO RESPONSE: Let's try an example to illustrate this formula. Assume you take a magnified radiograph of an object situated 30 mm from the film. The magnified image is 10 mm in diameter. The SID is 80 mm. Subtract the object distance from the SID to get the SOD, which is 50 mm. MF = 80 divided by 50, or 1.6

Then, to get the actual size of the object, you calculate this way:

$$\frac{\text{image size}}{\text{object size}} = MF$$

$$\text{Object size} = \frac{\text{image size}}{MF}$$

$$= \frac{10}{1.6}$$

$$= 6.25 \text{ mm}$$

SLIDE 4-45/CD 4-43 Unsharpness

The key to taking a magnified radiograph is using a small focal spot. A large focal spot will produce so much blur that the radiograph won't be of much diagnostic use. As a matter of fact, if you were to use a focal spot that's bigger than what you're imaging, tiny blood vessels for example, the amount of blur produced could actually wipe out the object's image.

SLIDE 4-46/CD 4-44 Air gap

Grids usually aren't used with magnification radiography because the larger OID creates an air gap that diverts scatter radiation and prevents it from reaching the film. There's a relationship here: the larger the OID, the smaller the amount of scatter radiation that reaches the film.

SLIDE 4-47/CD 4-45 Using magnification

Magnification radiography can produce clearer images of small body parts. In this illustration, for example, the hand is being magnified to show small vessels. But there's a downside to that, higher levels of radiation reach the patient, always something you try to avoid.

To double the magnification factor, you must position the patient midway between the radiation source and the film. Since the intensity of radiation is related to the square of the distance, the radiation dose to the patient is actually four times the amount of a normal exam. That's why such exams are performed only when necessary.

SLIDE 4-48/CD 4-46 Quiz instructions

THIS AUDIO FOR SLIDE ONLY: This concludes the presentation section of this module. If you are not going to work through the self-assessment quiz that follows, you may stop the program at this point and turn off the equipment.

If your instructor has asked you to take this self-assessment quiz on the material you have learned in this module, you should have a piece of paper ready. There will be 10 questions with multiple-choice or short answers. After this self-assessment we will go back through these questions and briefly talk about the reasons for the correct answers. Ready?

THIS AUDIO IN CD ROM LECTURE MODE ONLY: You have reached the self-assessment quiz for this module. Here you will be asked 10 questions to help you assess how well you understand what you have learned in this module. The questions are multiple choice or have short answers. After this self assessment we will go back through these questions and briefly talk about your answers and the reasons for the correct answers. Ready?

THIS AUDIO IN CD ROM STUDENT MODE ONLY: You have reached the self-assessment quiz for this module. Here you will be asked 10 questions to help you assess how well you understand what you have learned in this module. The questions are multiple choice or have short answers. For multiple-choice questions, click on the box next to your answer choice. For those questions that require a short answer, type in your answer at the keyboard and press enter.

After this self-assessment we will go back through these questions and briefly talk about your answers and the reasons for the correct answers.

SLIDE 4-49/CD 4-47 Quiz question 1

1. What is it called when the image of a radiographed object or a part of the body is misrepresented either in size or shape?

SLIDE 4-50/CD 4-48 Quiz question 2

2. What kind of distortion is caused when parts of the body do not lie parallel to the film or are of different thicknesses?

SLIDE 4-51/CD 4-49 Quiz question 3

3. Generally, which of the following is true of a long SID (source-to-image receptor distance) and a short OID (object-to-image receptor distance)?
   a. They will maximize shape distortion.
   b. They will minimize magnification.
   c. They will not affect distortion.
   d. They will cause only elongation.

SLIDE 4-52/CD 4-50 Quiz question 4

4. What is the standard SID for most radiographic procedures?
   a. 180 cm (72 inches)
   b. 72 cm (29 inches)
   c. 100 cm (40 inches)
   d. 40 cm (16 inches)

SLIDE 4-53/CD 4-51 Quiz question 5

5. You need to know the magnification factor to make the best diagnostic use of a radiograph. To find it, divide the size of the image by which of the following?
   a. The size of the object
   b. The size of the SID
   c. The size of the SOD
   d. The size of the OID

SLIDE 4-54/CD 4-52 Quiz question 6

6. If the size of an object's radiographic image is 20 inches in diameter, and it lies 10 inches above the film with the SID at 40 inches, what is the actual size of the object?
   a. 12 inches
   b. 15 inches
   c. 18 inches
   d. 16 inches

SLIDE 4-55/CD 4-53 Quiz question 7

7. What is affected by the thickness of the object, its position, the angle of the x-ray tube, and the position of the film?

SLIDE 4-56/CD 4-54 Quiz question 8

8. In taking radiographs, it's important to position the body part parallel to the film cassette and as close to it as possible. True or false?

SLIDE 4-57/CD 4-55 Quiz question 9

9. In magnification radiography, the object is to magnify blood vessels or bone structures. To do that, the body part must be placed as close to the film as possible. True or false?

SLIDE 4-58/CD 4-56 Quiz question 10

10. To get radiographs with as little distortion as possible, what three elements must be aligned?

SLIDE 4-59/CD 4-57 Quiz review

That concludes the self-assessment quiz for Module 4: Distortion. Let's quickly go back through the questions and see how you did.

SLIDE 4-60/CD 4-58 Review question 1

Question 1 asked what is the term for a radiographed image of an object or body part misrepresented either in size or shape.

The correct answer is distortion. Congratulate yourself if you got it right!

Size distortion means that the image of an object is magnified and appears larger than its actual size. Shape distortion means an object appears longer or shorter than it really is.

CD 4-58A Review question 1
Question 1 asked what is the term for a radiographed image of an object or body part misrepresented either in size or shape.

PRESENT THIS AUDIO IF ANSWER WAS distortion OR size and shape distortion:

Yes, you're right. Actually there are two kinds of distortion, but we refer to both simply as distortion. Size distortion means that the image of an object is magnified and appears larger than its actual size. Shape distortion means an object appears longer or shorter than it really is.

PRESENT THIS AUDIO IF ANSWER WAS magnification: No, the correct answer is distortion. Actually there are two kinds of distortion, but we refer to both simply as distortion. Size distortion means that the image of an object is magnified and appears larger than its actual size. Shape distortion means an object appears longer or shorter than it really is.

Magnification refers to an image that appears larger than the object or body part, but not larger and in a different shape.

PRESENT THIS AUDIO IF ANSWER WAS anything else: No, you didn't get this one. The correct answer is distortion. Actually there are two kinds of distortion, but we refer to both as simply distortion. Size distortion means that the image of an object is magnified and appears larger than its actual size. Shape distortion means an object appears longer or shorter than it really is.

SLIDE 4-61/CD 4-59 Review question 2
Question 2 asked what kind of distortion is created when body parts do not lie parallel to the film or are of different thicknesses.

The correct answer is shape distortion. Body parts or objects that differ in thicknesses or that do not lie parallel to the film are magnified at varying rates, which is called shape distortion.

CD 4-59A Review question 2
Question 2 asked you what kind of distortion is created when body parts do not lie parallel to the film or are of different thicknesses.

PRESENT THIS AUDIO IF ANSWER WAS shape or shape distortion: Yes, you correctly answered this one as shape distortion. Body parts or objects that differ in thicknesses or that do not lie parallel to the film are magnified at varying rates, which is called shape distortion.

PRESENT THIS AUDIO IF ANSWER WAS size distortion: No, the correct answer is shape distortion. Body parts or objects that differ in thicknesses or that do not lie parallel to the film are magnified at varying rates, which is called shape distortion. Those conditions cause the part to appear shaped differently than they are in real life.

PRESENT THIS AUDIO IF ANSWER WAS magnification: Well, you're partly right, but the correct answer is shape distortion. Body parts or objects that differ in thicknesses or that do not lie parallel to the film are magnified at varying rates, which is called shape distortion. Those conditions cause the part to appear shaped differently than they are in real life as well as magnified.

PRESENT THIS AUDIO IF ANSWER WAS anything else: No, the correct answer is shape distortion. Body parts or objects that differ in thicknesses or that do not lie parallel to the film are magnified at varying rates, which is called shape distortion. Those conditions cause the part to appear shaped differently than they are in real life.

SLIDE 4-62/CD 4-60 Review question 3
Question 3 asked what happens with distortion when you use a long SID and a short OID.

The correct answer is b, minimizes magnification. Think back to the shadowgraphs. The image-forming light rays in the beam diverge as they move away from their source. A small distance between the source and the object causes magnification. A short distance between the object and the image receptor creates relatively little magnification. A long distance from the source to the object minimizes magnification.

CD 4-60A Review question 3
Question 3 asked what happens with distortion when you use a long SID and a short OID.

PRESENT THIS AUDIO IF ANSWER WAS b: Yes, you're correct in answering b, that it minimizes magnification. Think back to the shadowgraphs. Image-forming light rays in the x-ray beam diverge as they move away from their source. When there is a short distance between the light source and the object, there is magnification and blur. When the distance between the object and the image receptor is small and the distance between the source and the object is large, there is relatively little magnification.

PRESENT THIS AUDIO IF ANSWER WAS a, c, or d: The correct answer is b, minimizes magnification. Think back to the shadowgraphs. The image-forming light rays in the beam diverge as they move away from their source. A small distance between the source and the object causes magnification. A short distance between the object and the image receptor creates relatively little magnification. A long distance from the source to the object minimizes magnification.

SLIDE 4-63/CD 4-61 Review question 4
Question 4 asked what is the standard SID for most radiographic procedures.

The correct answer is c, 100 cm or 40 inches, that standard has developed over time as knowledge and technology has changed.

CD 4-61A Review question 4
Question 4 asked what is the standard SID for most radiographic procedures

PRESENT THIS AUDIO IF ANSWER WAS c: You're right! The correct answer is c, 100 cm or 40 inches, that standard has developed over time as knowledge and technology has changed.

PRESENT THIS AUDIO IF ANSWER WAS a, b, or d: Sorry, you're answer is wrong. The correct answer is c, 100 cm or 40 inches, that standard has developed over time as knowledge and technology has changed.

SLIDE 4-64/CD 4-62 Review question 5
Question 5 asked what do you divide the image size by in determining the magnification factor.

The correct answer is that you divide the image size by the size of the object to find the magnification factor.

CD 4-62A Review question 5
Question 5 asked what do you divide the image size by in determining the magnification factor.

PRESENT THIS AUDIO IF ANSWER WAS a: You're right! The correct answer is a, you divide the image size by the object size to find the magnification factor.

PRESENT THIS AUDIO IF ANSWER WAS b, c, or d: Sorry, you missed this one. The correct answer is a, you divide the image size by the object size to find the magnification factor.

SLIDE 4-65/CD 4-63 Review question 6
Question 6 asked you to find the actual size of an object when its radiographic image, its position, and the SID are known.

The correct answer is 15. You arrive at that number by using this formula:

$$\frac{\text{image size}}{\text{object size}} = \frac{\text{source-to-image receptor distance (SID)}}{\text{source-to-object distance (SOD)}}$$

CD 4-63A Review question 6
Question 6 asked you to find the actual size of an object when its radiographic image, its position, and the SID are known.

PRESENT THIS AUDIO IF ANSWER WAS b: Good, you got the correct answer b, 15. You arrive at that number by using this formula:

$$\frac{\text{image size}}{\text{object size}} = \frac{\text{source-to-image receptor distance (SID)}}{\text{source-to-object distance (SOD)}}$$

PRESENT THIS AUDIO IF ANSWER WAS a, c, or d: Oops, you missed it. The correct answer is b, 15. You arrive at that number by using this formula:

$$\frac{\text{image size}}{\text{object size}} = \frac{\text{source-to-image receptor distance (SID)}}{\text{source-to-object distance (SOD)}}$$

SLIDE 4-66/CD 4-64 Review question 7
Question 7 asked what is affected by the thickness of the object, its position, the angle of the x-ray tube, and the position of the film.

The correct answer is shape distortion. Unless each of these factors are correctly anticipated and planned for, you will have some distortion.

CD 4-64A Review question 7
Question 7 asked what is affected by the thickness of the object, its position, the angle of the x-ray tube, and the position of the film.

PRESENT THIS AUDIO IF ANSWER WAS shape distortion: Yes, you were right, the answer is shape distortion. Unless each of these factors is correctly anticipated and planned for, you will have some distortion.

PRESENT THIS AUDIO IF ANSWER WAS magnification: No, you missed it. Magnification can also be present. But the correct answer is shape distortion. Even having one of these factors not anticipated or planned for will cause shape distortion.

PRESENT THIS AUDIO IF ANSWER WAS anything else: No, you missed it. The correct answer is shape distortion. Even having one of these factors not anticipated or planned for will cause shape distortion.

SLIDE 4-67/CD 4-65 Review question 8
Question 8 asked if it is true or false that in taking radiographs, it's important to position the body part parallel to the film cassette and as close to it as possible.

The correct answer is true. In order for the x-ray beams to penetrate the part at the proper angle and to minimize magnification, positioning the part correctly is crucial.

CD 4-65A Review question 8
Question 8 asked if it is true or false that in taking radiographs, it's important to position the body part parallel to the film cassette and as close to it as possible.

PRESENT THIS AUDIO IF ANSWER WAS true: Yes, of course you're correct. The answer is true. In order for the x-ray beams to penetrate the part at the proper angle and to minimize magnification, positioning the part correctly is crucial.

PRESENT THIS AUDIO IF ANSWER WAS false: No, you missed this one. The answer is true. In order for the x-ray beams to penetrate the part at the proper angle and to minimize magnification, positioning the part correctly is crucial.

SLIDE 4-68/CD 4-66 Review question 9
Question 9 asked whether it is true or false that in magnification radiography, the body part must be placed as close to the film as possible.

The correct answer is false. In this specialty, the object is to see tiny blood vessels or bone structures as clearly as possible, and that is done when they are purposefully magnified. To do that, they are placed closer to the source of radiation. In regular procedures, you do want the part close to the film.

CD 4-66A Review question 9
Question 9 asked whether it is true or false that in magnification radiography, the body part must be placed as close to the film as possible.

PRESENT THIS AUDIO IF ANSWER WAS false: Great, you've been paying attention. The correct answer is that in this specialty, the object is to see tiny blood vessels or bone structures as clearly as possible, and that is done when they are purposefully magnified. To do that, they are placed closer to the source of radiation. In regular procedures, you do want the part close to the film.

PRESENT THIS AUDIO IF ANSWER WAS true: Sorry, but you missed it. You answered true. The correct answer is that in this specialty, the object is to see tiny blood vessels or bone structures as clearly as possible, and that is done when they are purposefully magnified. To do that, they are placed closer to the source of radiation. In regular procedures, you do want the part close to the film.

SLIDE 4-69/CD 4-67 Review question 10
Question 10 asked what three things had to be properly aligned in order to get as little distortion as possible.

The correct answer is the central ray, the body part, and the film. The central ray must be perpendicular to the part and the film, which are parallel to each other.

CD 4-67A Review question 10
Question 10 asked what three things had to be properly aligned in order to get as little distortion as possible.

PRESENT THIS AUDIO IF ANSWER WAS the central (OR primary) ray (OR x-ray), the part (OR body part OR object), and the film (OR film cassette OR cassette) with or without the articles "the" & "and": Well, you're right. The central ray must be perpendicular to the part and the film, which are parallel to each other.

PRESENT THIS AUDIO IF ANSWER WAS anything else: Sorry, you missed it. The correct answer is that the central ray must be perpendicular to the part and the film, which are parallel to each other. It's very important that these elements are aligned properly.

SLIDE 4-70/CD 4-68 Quiz conclusion
This concludes the self-assessment quiz. This was not intended as a test, so don't feel bad if you missed some. All that means is that you probably need to review this module or study your textbook more carefully.

CD 4-68A Quiz feedback
FOR SCORE OF 10, THIS AUDIO: You've done an excellent job here with a difficult subject. Clearly you are studying well, and you seem to have worked through the tutorial carefully.

FOR SCORE OF 9, THIS AUDIO: You've done well with a difficult subject. Clearly you are studying and paying attention to the subject. Maybe next time you'll get the perfect score!

FOR SCORE OF 7-8, THIS AUDIO: Your score is about average. I'd suggest you review this material in your textbook. You may also find it helpful, next time, to read the material in your book before coming to the computer to take the tutorial. And don't hesitate to talk to your instructor if you have trouble after both reading the textbook and working through the multimedia tutorial.

FOR SCORE OF 5-6, THIS AUDIO: Your score is below average. You need to review this material in your textbook, and perhaps you should come back and take this tutorial again afterwards. You may have just been unprepared this time, or if you are having trouble after both reading the textbook and working through the multimedia tutorial, be sure to talk to your instructor.

FOR SCORE OF 0-4, THIS AUDIO: Your score is rather low. Don't feel too bad; these are, after all, difficult concepts to grasp. If you tried your best here but are having this much difficulty with the material, you should first go to your textbook and see if you can understand the material there. If it still seems difficult, please ask your instructor for additional study aids.

SLIDE 4-71/CD 4-69 Exam instructions

In the next 7 or 8 minutes you will be presented with 15 multiple-choice questions. Select the one best answer choice. Get ready a blank sheet of paper numbered 1 to 15 down the left side. As you take the examination, write the letter corresponding to your answer choice next to the number for each question. Ready? You will not be asked to perform any complicated calculations.

CD 4-69A More exam instructions

In the next 7 or 8 minutes you will be presented with 15 multiple-choice questions. Select the one best answer choice. This examination covers the material you've been learning about in this tutorial over the last hour or so. It is designed to help you and your instructor determine how well you now grasp this material. You can use scratch paper during the exam if you want, but it shouldn't be necessary for any complicated calculations.

SLIDE 4-72/CD 4-70 Exam question 1

1. In this module you learned about distortion, one of the two geometric factors that affect the quality of radiographic images. What is the second?
   a. Magnification
   b. Recorded detail
   c. Contrast
   d. Resolution

SLIDE 4-73/CD 4-71 Exam question 2

2. What do the two geometric factors that affect radiographic quality control?
   a. Contrast
   b. Density
   c. The visibility of detail
   d. The actual detail

SLIDE 4-74/CD 4-72 Exam question 3

3. Magnification is also referred to as which of the following?
   a. Size distortion
   b. Elongation
   c. Shape distortion
   d. Foreshortening

SLIDE 4-75/CD 4-73 Exam question 4

4. When is an object magnified more?
   a. When it is closest to the image receptor
   b. When it is closest to the central ray
   c. When it is perpendicular to the image receptor
   d. When it is closest to the source

SLIDE 4-76/CD 4-74 Exam question 5

5. As the level of detail on a radiograph improves, what happens to the magnification?
   a. It increases.
   b. It decreases.
   c. It stays the same.
   d. It doubles.

SLIDE 4-77/CD 4-75 Exam question 6

6. In radiography, how will body parts that are positioned farther away from the image receptor appear, as compared with those closer to it?
   a. Smaller
   b. The same
   c. Larger
   d. Elongated

SLIDE 4-78/CD 4-76 Exam question 7

7. How can the magnification factor be expressed?
   a. In whole numbers only
   b. In a percentage only
   c. In whole numbers or a percentage

SLIDE 4-79/CD 4-77 Exam question 8

8. When referring to shape distortion, what does elongation mean?
   a. An image is lengthened or extended.
   b. An image is shorter than it is in reality.
   c. An image is at least twice its normal size.
   d. An image can take any kind of new shape.

SLIDE 4-80/CD 4-78 Exam question 9

9. To get a good quality radiograph, how must the central ray be positioned in relation to the object and film?
   a. At less than 90 degrees
   b. Parallel
   c. Perpendicular

SLIDE 4-81/CD 4-79 Exam question 10

10. If the body part being radiographed is not placed along its long axis, in addition to magnification, there will be which of the following?
    a. Elongation
    b. Foreshortening
    c. No distortion

SLIDE 4-82/CD 4-80 Exam question 11

11. If the film cassette is placed parallel to the object but is off center, what might be the result?
    a. Partial imaging
    b. Foreshortening
    c. Elongation
    d. Magnification

SLIDE 4-83/CD 4-81 Exam question 12

12. What is the term for an x-ray tube that is placed other than perpendicular to the object and is directed somewhere other than at the center of the part?
    a. Macroradiography
    b. Angulation
    c. Magnification technique

SLIDE 4-84/CD 4-82 Exam question 13

13. What is the key to purposefully taking a magnified radiograph?
    a. A large focal spot
    b. An angulated x-ray beam
    c. A short OID
    d. A small focal spot

SLIDE 4-85/CD 4-83 Exam question 14

14. In magnification radiography, to double the magnification factor, where must the patient be positioned in relation to the radiation source and the film?
    a. One-third of the way between the film and the source
    b. Closer to the film
    c. Midway between the film and the source
    d. Closer to the radiation source

SLIDE 4-86/CD 4-84 Exam question 15

15. When the part hasn't been aligned properly, the result is uneven magnification. What is a second result?
    a. Foreshortening
    b. Elongation
    c. Poor recorded detail

SLIDE 4-87/CD 4-85 Exam conclusion

This concludes the examination section of Module 4 of Radiographic Imaging. Please follow your instructor's directions for your answer sheet to the questions.

SLIDE 4-85A Exam conclusion

This concludes the examination section of Module 4 of Radiographic Imaging. Your score has been saved on the computer. Your instructor will report it to you later.

Answers to the Multimedia Examination

1. b	5. b	9. c	13. d
2. d	6. c	10. b	14. c
3. a	7. c	11. a	15. a
4. d	8. a	12. b	

Beam Limitation and Filtration

5

Overview

- Scatter radiation
  - Reducing field size to reduce scatter
- Early beam-restricting devices
  - Aperture diaphragms
  - Cones and cylinders
- Collimators
  - Shutters
  - Light localizing system
  - Advantages of collimators
- Filtration
  - Inherent filtration
  - Added filtration
  - Compensating filters

This module introduces students to the key concepts of beam-restricting devices and filtration—two of the ways the radiologic technologist controls the x-ray beam.

The module begins with a discussion of scatter radiation, which leads into an important rationale for limiting the field size: to minimize scatter and its effects on the image.

After it is explained why field size should be controlled, early beam-restricting devices are illustrated and described. Students learn how aperture diaphragms, cones, and cylinders work, as well as their inherent limitations.

Collimators are then discussed in greater detail, from the inner workings of the pairs of shutters to the function of the light localizing system. The advantages of collimators over the earlier beam-restricting devices are described.

The final section of the module examines filtration and the benefits of hardening the beam and using compensating filters appropriately to compensate for density differences.

Learning Objectives

Upon completion of this module, the student should be able to do the following:

1. Define all the key terms in the module.
2. Explain why beam-restricting devices are used.
3. Describe how aperture diaphragms, cones, and cylinders work.
4. Describe how collimators work, and list three benefits of using collimators rather than aperture diaphragms.
5. Explain why the x-ray beam is filtered and the standards of aluminum equivalence for measuring filtration.
6. Describe how compensating filters function and give two examples of when they are used.
7. Successfully complete the activities and posttest in the Study Guide.

Key Terms

Added filtration
Aluminum equivalency
Aperture diaphragm
Beam limitation technique
Central ray
Collimator
Compensating filter
Compton scatter, Compton effect
Cone
Cone cutting
Contrast
Cross hairs
Cylinder
Density
Field size
Filtration
Focal spot
Fog
Half-value layer
Hardening
Inherent filtration
Lead blocker
Light localizer
Off-focus radiation
Positive beam limitation device (PBL)
Scatter radiation
Shutters
Stem radiation
Total filtration
Trough filter
Unsharpness
Wedge filter

Instructional Outline

I. The x-ray beam is limited and filtered to get the best possible images.
  A. Scatter radiation produced in the body adds fog to the image.
    1. Scatter radiation occurs as a result of Compton interactions of x-ray photons and atoms in the body.
    2. Scatter radiation that reaches the image receptor causes a generalized increase in density, which also diminishes contrast in the image.

B. Scatter can be reduced by various techniques.
   1. Because thinner body areas produce less scatter, compressing tissue when practical causes less scatter to be produced.
   2. Decreasing kVp tends to reduce scatter, but if kVp is too low, the low-energy photons will be absorbed in the body, increasing patient dose, without contributing to the image.
   3. The smaller the field size, the less scatter radiation is produced inside the patient, and consequently the less fog there is in the image. Therefore beam-restricting devices are used to control the field size.

II. Early beam-restricting devices included aperture diaphragms, cones, and cylinders.
   A. A fixed aperture diaphragm is a flat lead plate with a hole in it through which the x-ray beam passes; the aperture diaphragm is attached to the x-ray tube housing.
      1. Aperture diaphragms can be of any size or shape.
      2. Aperture diaphragms are easy to use but have several disadvantages.
         a. Because they are mounted close to the tube, they produce more unsharpness in the image.
         b. They allow some off-focus radiation to reach the film, producing image shadows.
         c. Unlike collimators, aperture diaphragms do not have a light guide to aid in positioning the patient.
   B. Cones and cylinders are types of aperture diaphragms shaped for specific applications.
      1. Cones and cylinders are used in dental radiography and for certain types of examinations.
      2. A problem called cone cutting can occur if the equipment is not properly aligned and the cylinder or cone blocks a part of the x-ray beam needed for the image.

III. Collimators are the most commonly used beam-limiting devices today.
   A. Also called variable-aperture collimators, these devices have advantages over aperture diaphragms.
      1. Collimators do a better job of controlling field size to protect the patient from unnecessary radiation and to control scatter radiation.
      2. They include a light system to aid in patient positioning.
      3. They are quick and easy to use.
   B. Two pairs of shutters control the field size.
      1. The entrance shutters closest to the tube control for off-focus radiation that can cause image shadows.
      2. The second-stage shutters are farther from the tube and therefore reduce the unsharpness and restrict the field size.
      3. The shutters are easily controlled to a precise field size.
      4. Collimator settings are typically predetermined for standard examinations.
   C. The light localizer system within a collimator aids in patient positioning.
      1. A light within the collimator reflects from a mirror to project a light beam in the same area as the x-ray beam.
      2. Cross hairs show the exact position of the central ray.
   D. A positive beam limitation device (PBL) has been required in all fixed radiographic equipment since 1974.
      1. The PBL automatically adjusts the collimator shutters to ensure that the field size is appropriate for the size of the film cassette.
      2. Even with the PBL, the radiologic technologist must ensure the appropriate field size is chosen for the particular examination.

IV. Filtration removes some of the x-ray photons from the beam.
   A. Filtration is desirable to eliminate some of the low-energy x-ray photons that do not contribute to the image but are most likely absorbed by the body, increasing the patient dose. This is called hardening the beam.

B. Inherent filtration is that inherent in the radiographic equipment: the filtration provided by the glass tube and the insulating oil.

C. Added filtration, usually in the form of aluminum sheets, can be added to further filter the beam.

  1. Filtering capacity is typically measured in aluminum equivalency or half-value layer—the thickness of the aluminum to reduce the intensity of the beam by half.
  2. The National Council on Radiation Protection (NCRP) sets standards for minimum levels of total filtration.

D. Compensating filters are used in some situations to produce better diagnostic images by evening out the density when there are great variations in tissue densities.

  1. Wedge filters filter more at one end than the other, as might be used with a foot exam.
  2. Trough filters filter more at the edges and less down the middle, as might be used in a spine exam.
  3. Other specialized filters include bowtie and conic filters, and lead-impregnated Plexiglas filters.

Teaching Tips

Scatter

Before beginning this module students should already know what scatter radiation is and its possible detrimental effects on images. If it has been a while since your students studied the Compton effect, you might wish to review the basic concepts with students before moving on to the topic of beam limitation, as reducing scatter is one of the primary reasons to be concerned with field size. A simple blackboard sketch showing how a high-energy x-ray photon is scattered in an atom and then strikes the film from an oblique angle should be enough to remind students how fog results from scatter. The same diagram can be used to illustrate how reducing the field size reduces scatter, thus helping students through the transition from familiar concepts to the first major subject of the module: beam-restricting devices. (At the same time, be sure to explain also how beam limitation reduces patient dose by not exposing tissues outside the area of examination.)

Beam-restricting devices

The concept of controlling the x-ray beam by restricting it to the size of a "window" through which it passes is quite simple, although some students may lose sight of this basic concept when immersed in new vocabulary and learning types of equipment. A classroom demonstration of how the beam can be controlled in different ways is well worth the time needed to set it up. (If you performed demonstrations earlier to show the geometric principles involved in SID, OID, magnification, and size distortion [Module 4], the same materials can be used now to demonstrate beam limitation principles).

Use a light source positioned a suitable distance from the "image" receptor—usually a blank section of wall. If convenient, bring actual aperture diaphragms, cones, and cylinders into the classroom and demonstrate how they restrict the field size of the "x-ray beam" from the light; if unavailable, make several sizes from cardboard. If the room can be darkened sufficiently, you should be able to demonstrate how the unsharpness is greater when the aperture is moved closer to the light: the edges of the field will become blurrier.

You need not construct actual shutters to demonstrate how a collimator offers better control than aperture diaphragms. Use two aperture diaphragms made of cardboard, with openings of appropriate size for the demonstration, to illustrate how unsharpness is reduced (compared with a single aperture diaphragm positioned closer to the light bulb).

You can also show how off-focus radiation is better controlled with a collimator: position a second light bulb of a different color immediately next to the original bulb to represent radiation produced in the tube elsewhere than at the focal point. With an appropriately sized aperture diaphragm positioned the right distance from both bulbs, colored light from the off-focus bulb should be visible in the image, adding a kind of shadowy confusion to the image. Then use two aperture diaphragm cardboard positioned such that the off-focus radiation (the colored light) cannot pass through both pairs of "shutters" to reach the image receptor.

Once students grasp the mechanics and geometry of beam restriction devices, they may gain from examining images that show the effects of scatter and the benefits of decreasing field size. Using actual radiographs or book reproductions, have students form small groups to analyze a range of images for fog resulting from scatter radiation. Show other images where scatter has been reduced by tight collimation and have students compare them.

Filters

Demonstrating the effects of filtration on the x-ray beam can be done in the classroom but is more complicated and may require special materials. A translucent material such as waxed paper or very thin white cloth can be held before the light bulb to show how some but not all light gets through this "filter" to reach the wall. Making graduated "filters" to illustrate different filtering capacities or compensating filters can be rather complex, however. It may be more useful to bring actual radiographic filters into the classroom and discuss their use while students see and handle them. The use of compensating filters, such as a wedge filter positioned over the foot, can be demonstrated easily while you talk about how the beam is being filtered as it passes through the filter.

As suggested above for collimation, have students form small groups and analyze radiographs made using filters.

Workbook Posttest Answers and Rationales

1. What is the main problem with scatter radiation?
   a. The required long exposures
   b. Increased patient radiation dose
   c. Fog on the image—Scatter radiation that strikes the film does not contribute to the image but increases the overall density.
   d. All of the above
   e. None of the above

2. What affects how much scatter is produced?
   a. The size and thickness of the body area examined
   b. The tissue density of the body area examined
   c. The kVp selection
   d. All of the above
   e. None of the above

3. kVp can be lowered to reduce scatter, but this also causes which of the following?
   a. Reduced density—With lower kVp, fewer x-ray photons penetrate the body to reach the film.
   b. More penumbra
   c. Smaller field size
   d. All of the above
   e. None of the above

4. Aperture diaphragms have what shape?
   a. Round
   b. Square
   c. Rectangular
   d. All of the above—They may be in any shape.
   e. None of the above

5. Limitations of aperture diaphragms include which of the following?
   a. They cause unsharpness.
   b. They allow off-focus radiation to reach the film.
   c. They do not provide light to guide positioning.
   d. All of the above—These result from using aperture diaphragms but not from collimators.
   e. None of the above

6. What are the basic parts of a collimator?
   a. Light source, mirror, and shutters
   b. Light source, shutters, and lead blockers
   c. Light source, aperture diaphragm, and lead blockers
   d. Light source, mirror, and aperture diaphragm

7. The second stage shutters (farther from the tube) reduce which of the following?
   a. Off-focus radiation
   b. Unsharpness—Because of the geometrical factors involved with the second stage shutters being farther from the tube, the unsharpness is reduced.
   c. Low-energy x-rays
   d. All of the above
   e. None of the above

8. The mirror inside the collimator does which of the following?
   a. Focuses the x-ray beam
   b. Redirects the x-ray beam to the proper field
   c. Reflects the light beam to the same area as the radiation beam—The mirror thus redirects the light beam in exactly the same path as the x-ray beam.
   d. Redirects the light beam so the tube can be better seen

9. The position of the central ray is determined by which of the following?
   a. **The collimator's cross hairs**—The cross hairs indicate the exact center of the beam.
   b. Measuring downward from the x-ray tube
   c. The red dot projected from the collimator
   d. None of the above

10. Which of the following is true of a positive beam limitation (PBL) device?
    a. It is required on all new fixed radiographic equipment.
    b. It ensures the field size is never larger than the image receptor.
    c. It works automatically to determine film size being used.
    d. **All of the above**—A PBL works automatically to match the field size to the image receptor and has been required on all new fixed equipment since 1974.
    e. None of the above is true.

11. Which statement is true about how a radiologic technologist can control a collimator?
    a. One set of shutters can be moved to control the width of the field.
    b. One set of shutters can be moved to control the length of the field.
    c. **Both sets of shutters can be moved to control both width and length.** All collimators adjust both width and length of the field.
    d. Some equipment allows controlling both sets of shutters, while others allow control of only one.

12. Compensating filters compensate for which of the following?
    a. **Uneven rates at which body parts absorb x-rays**—These filters are used to even out density on the image when needed because of greatly differing areas of body tissue density.
    b. The broad spectrum of x-ray photon energy levels in the beam
    c. Using different field sizes
    d. The anode heel effect

13. "Inherent filtration" refers to which of the following?
    a. Compensating filters
    b. Aluminum filters added in the beam
    c. Wedge filters
    d. All of the above
    e. **None of the above**—Inherent filtration refers to unavoidable filtration caused by the equipment, such as the filtration by the glass portal of the x-ray tube; the types of filters listed here are all added filtration, not inherent filtration.

14. "Aluminum equivalency" refers to which of the following?
    a. **The amount of filtering**—The amount of filtering provided by other filter materials is measured against the standard provided by aluminum.
    b. The density of a body structure
    c. Materials used in collimator shutters
    d. The x-ray tube housing

15. Which of the following are compensating filters?
    a. Wedge filters
    b. Trough filters
    c. Step-wedge filters
    d. All of the above—These are all compensating filters with shapes developed for specific body areas in particular types of exams.
    e. None of the above

Testbank Questions

1. Which of the following is the phenomenon named for the American physicist Compton?
    a. Scatter radiation
    b. The photoelectric effect
    c. The inverse square law
    d. Attenuation

2. Compressing breast tissue for a mammographic exam reduces magnification and also does which of the following?
    a. Increases the contrast on the image
    b. Decreases the contrast on the image
    c. Increases the density on the image
    d. Reduces the amount of scatter

3. What do aperture diaphragms control?
    a. Beam intensity
    b. Field size
    c. Leakage radiation
    d. All of the above
    e. None of the above

4. The field size created by an aperture diaphragm should be which of the following?
    a. A little smaller than the film size
    b. A little larger than the film size
    c. The same size as the film
    d. Any of the above

5. What is a common use for cones and cylinders?
    a. Dental exams
    b. Extremity exams
    c. Chest exams
    d. All of the above
    e. None of the above

6. To what does "cone cutting" refer?
   a. Making a cone from a sheet of lead
   b. The technique for attaching the cone to the tube housing
   c. The edge of a cone obstructing part of the x-ray beam
   d. None of the above

7. What is a lead blocker?
   a. A lead sheet positioned on the patient to help control scatter
   b. Part of the shutters in a collimator
   c. Part of the x-ray tube housing
   d. None of the above

8. In most radiographic examinations the use of aperture diaphragms has been replaced by which of the following?
   a. Cones
   b. Cylinders
   c. Collimators
   d. Lead blockers

9. Collimators do a better job than aperture diaphragms of limiting which of the following?
   a. Leakage radiation
   b. Off-focus radiation
   c. High-energy photons
   d. All of the above
   e. None of the above

10. Which beam-limiting devices use cross hairs to show the position of the central ray?
    a. Collimators
    b. Aperture diaphragms
    c. Cones and cylinders
    d. Both collimators and aperture diaphragms

11. Even when using a positive beam limitation device, what must the radiologic technologist determine?
    a. The field size and film are limited to the area being examined.
    b. The collimator is set correctly.
    c. A cone is being used.
    d. All of the above are true.
    e. None of the above is true.

12. "Hardening" refers to which of the following?
    a. Limiting the field size with a collimator
    b. Using an intensifying screen to increase the film exposure
    c. Raising the average energy level of the x-ray beam with a filter
    d. None of the above

13. The half-value layer refers to the thickness of which of the following?
    a. Anodes
    b. Aperture diaphragms
    c. Filters
    d. Collimator shutters

14. The National Council on Radiation Protection (NCRP) recommends which of the following?
    a. Maximum levels of total filtration
    b. Minimum levels of total filtration
    c. Average levels of total filtration
    d. All of the above

15. Filtration results from which of the following?
    a. The silver on a collimator mirror
    b. A cone
    c. An aperture diaphragm
    d. All of the above
    e. None of the above

Answers to Testbank Questions

1. a	5. a	9. b	13. c
2. d	6. c	10. a	14. b
3. b	7. a	11. a	15. a
4. a	8. c	12. c	

Audiovisual Script

SLIDE 5-1/CD 5-i Welcome
Welcome to Mosby's Radiographic Instructional Series.

SLIDE 5-2/CD 5-ii Beam limitation and filtration
The module you are about to experience is the fifth of eight in the Radiographic Imaging program: Beam Limitation and Filtration.

This module will help you understand why beam-limiting devices are used in radiography, the different kinds of devices, and how and when they're used. You'll also learn about filtration and its many applications. You'll learn the rationale for limiting and filtering x-ray beams, as well as the devices that have been invented to accomplish those purposes. The modules you've already completed in this series will give you a good background for understanding this material.

SLIDE 5-3/CD 5-1 Introduction

Think back to what you've already learned about the path x-ray photons take when they leave the focal spot and travel towards the patient. Several things can happen.

Some photons pass directly through the patient and don't interact with the body at all. Others are absorbed by the body. And still others reach the patient and then scatter in many directions, some away from the film, some toward the film, and others within the body itself.

SLIDE 5-4/CD 5-2 Scatter radiation

Of those possibilities, two are important in determining contrast, density, and the overall image on a radiograph. They involve the photons that pass through the patient and those that interact with some portion of the body, scatter within it, and then exit the patient. Both, called remnant x-rays, make contact with the film and produce the radiograph.

X-ray photons that have scattered are usually more oblique, or angled, than those that have not interacted with parts of the body. They may also travel through longer paths in the body than primary radiation. Scatter radiation contributes to the fog that appears on radiographs, although it is not the only cause. The same thing can happen when the film has been handled or stored improperly or when there are problems in processing the film.

CD 5-2A Radiograph fogged by scatter

The American physicist Arthur H. Compton discovered, in the first part of the twentieth century, how x-rays produce scatter radiation. The term "Compton effect" or "Compton scatter" is used to describe that phenomenon.

Compton saw that when a high-energy photon strikes an electron in an outer shell, the high-energy photon can be deflected from its path and lose energy. The term "Compton effect" is used to describe that scattered, lower-energy photon.

SLIDE 5-5/CD 5-3 Radiographs comparing fog

Three things affect the amount of scatter radiation that will be produced in a radiographic exam. They are the thickness of the patient and the density of the patient's tissue, the size of the area under examination, and the kilovoltage level.

Let's take each of these one at a time, beginning with the thickness and density of the patient. More scatter radiation is produced in examinations of "thicker" patients, or body parts, than thinner ones because there is more area for the photons to interact with. A 250-pound man, for example, will generate more scatter than a 115-pound woman just because there's more of him to expose.

It's also true that x-rays penetrating fluid-filled tissues or denser parts of the body, such as the abdomen or chest, will produce more scatter than those penetrating a bony part of the body such as fingers or toes. You can see the fog produced by this scatter in the radiograph at the left.

CD 5-3A Compression reduces scatter

There are ways to position a patient so you can decrease the amount of scatter. For example, a person's abdomen is compressed when he or she is lying down rather than standing, making that part of the body seem less "thick." So you radiograph the patient in a recumbent position and reduce scatter and chance of fog.

You can also use compression devices to do the same thing. As you see in this image, such a device is incorporated into a mammography machine. A woman's breast is compressed until it is nearly flat so that it becomes more uniform in thickness and can be placed closer to the film cassette. This has to be done because the breast is thicker at the chest wall than it is at the nipple; taking a radiograph without compression would increase the amount of scatter produced in the thicker part of the breast tissue.

SLIDE 5-6/CD 5-4 Effect of field size

Another factor that makes a difference in how much scatter is produced is the size of the area being examined. That's called the field size. The bigger the field, the more scatter radiation that's likely to be produced. And more scatter, as you recall, means a radiograph with more fog and lower contrast.

In the images here, the intent was to get a clear look at the vertebral column. As you can see, the radiograph on the left shows the vertebral column and the abdominal tissue around it. The radiograph on the right focuses in on the vertebral column only. Because this is a smaller field size, less scatter radiation is produced and the contrast is greater, providing a better diagnostic image.

SLIDE 5-7/CD 5-5 kVp and scatter

The third factor that affects the amount of scatter radiation created is the kVp. When the kVp is increased, more photons are transmitted through the body without interaction and a greater percentage of scatter radiation will reach the film or image receptor. The amount of radiation absorbed photoelectrically is decreased.

You might assume that using a low kVp all the time makes sense because it reduces the amount of scatter contributing to the image. However, doing so will not only increase the patient dose but will also affect contrast on the film.

Fewer x-rays reach the film at a low kVp, so to compensate, you may choose to increase the mAs (the total number of photons produced by the x-ray tube during an exposure). But that's not a good idea either, because that will expose the patient to an even higher dose of radiation.

MORE INFO LEADS TO THIS AUDIO RESPONSE: As we move on, you'll learn how to modify kVp and mAs to get the right balance of radiation exposure and high-quality radiographs. But keep this in mind as a general rule: on balance, it's better to keep the kVp high because that means a lower radiation dose to the patient.

SLIDE 5-8/CD 5-6 Minimizing scatter

You've seen the factors that make a difference in the amount of scatter radiation produced during a radiographic exposure. You can understand now why you would want to know how to keep scatter to a minimum while you keep exposure to the patient as low as you can.

The best way is to produce as little radiation as possible and still get a good diagnostic radiograph. The second practical step is to try to limit the amount of radiation that reaches the patient. You do that through what's called "beam limitation" techniques, which we'll look at next.

Before we do, let's review for a moment. Think back to what you've just learned. What are the factors that affect the amount of scatter radiation produced during an x-ray exposure?

a. Patient thickness and density of tissue
b. Field size
c. kVp
d. All of the above

Click on the box next to your answer choice.

SLIDE 5-9/CD 5-7 Factors affecting scatter

The correct answer is the thickness of the patient and density of the tissue, the field size, and the kVp.

PRESENT THIS AUDIO IF ANSWER WAS d: Yes, you're right. All of these things play a part in determining the amount of scatter produced.

PRESENT THIS AUDIO IF ANSWER WAS a, b, or c: No, take another look back at what's involved. The thickness of the patient and density of the tissue, the field size (or size of the area to be examined), and the kVp all determine the amount of scatter produced.

SLIDE 5-10/CD 5-8 Aperture diaphragm

There are several ways to control x-rays as they emerge from the x-ray tube in order to limit the number that reach the patient. One of the earliest and simplest beam restriction devices invented was the fixed aperture diaphragm.

The aperture diaphragm controls the size of the x-ray beam that is emitted from the x-ray tube. The diaphragm is a flat plate made of lead, or lined with it, that attaches to the port of the x-ray tube. An opening, or aperture, in the diaphragm allows the primary beam to pass through to the patient. Aperture diaphragms can be of any shape: rectangular, square, or circular, for example. Someone in the radiology department can make these kinds of diaphragms, or they can be bought commercially.

MORE INFO LEADS TO THIS AUDIO RESPONSE: You've probably heard the term aperture used in photography. It's a hole that controls the amount of light that gets to the film. In radiography, the aperture diaphragm is the opening that controls the size of the x-ray beam that is emitted.

SLIDE 5-11/CD 5-9 Aperture diaphragm 2

The opening in the aperture diaphragm is designed to cover a little bit less than the total size of the film being used for a given exam. The aperture diaphragm controls the beam such that an image on the radiograph is a little bit smaller than the film itself; usually it is about 1 centimeter smaller on all sides. That's why when a diaphragm is properly designed and used, you'll see an unexposed border on each edge of the radiograph.

Dedicated head units usually use this kind of beam restrictor. They generally have a standard SID and diaphragms of different sizes to match different film sizes. Aperture diaphragms are also commonly used in dental radiography.

It's important to put an aperture diaphragm into the head of the x-ray tube the right way. Its long axis should be parallel to the image receptor's long axis. If the two aren't lined up correctly, a large portion of the radiograph will end up being unexposed. This "diaphragm cutoff" will mean the exam will have to be repeated to get the diagnostic information required, and that will result in more radiation to the patient.

SLIDE 5-12/CD 5-10 Unsharpness
Aperture diaphragms are inexpensive and easy to use, and they do limit the beam, but they aren't perfect. The problem is that although we talk about x-ray photons emerging from a focal spot, there really isn't one exact spot. X-ray photons come from several points in the focal spot and travel in varying directions.

One problem with the aperture diaphragm, as you can see in this illustration, is that because it's placed close to the tube port, it causes some penumbra, or unsharpness, to show up around the edges of the radiograph. Moving it away from the port can cut down on this.

Another disadvantage of being close to the tube port is that an aperture diaphragm can also allow more off-focus, or stem radiation, to reach the film. This kind of radiation originates in the x-ray tube from areas other than the focal spot. It can produce shadowy images of the part being radiographed, which show up outside the boundaries of the primary exposure field.

MORE INFO LEADS TO THIS AUDIO RESPONSE: Although aperture diaphragms are rather inexpensive and simple to use, you won't see them much in modern radiography suites except with dedicated units, like those used for chest x-rays. That's because unlike the more sophisticated beam limiting device, the collimator, which you'll learn about shortly, aperture diaphragms don't provide any light to guide you as you try to line up the patient with the equipment.

SLIDE 5-13/CD 5-11 Cylinder
Modify the shape of an aperture diaphragm just a little bit and you get a cone or cylinder. Both of these circular metal parts serve essentially the same purpose as a diaphragm: they limit the useful beam to a particular size, in this case to a round shape. Cones are smaller at the upper part closest to the tube port and flare out as they extend. Cylinders maintain a consistent shape, equal in diameter at the top and bottom, as shown here.

Like diaphragms, cones and cylinders have fixed openings so they can't be used for every kind of examination. Once very popular because they're inexpensive and easy to manipulate, they're now used mainly for head, spine, and gallbladder examinations and in dentistry.

SLIDE 5-14/CD 5-12 Effect of cone
Which of these two radiographs do you think has the most diagnostic value? The one on the left, in which no cone was used, shows the entire skull. In the one on the right, a cone was used to restrict the x-ray beam to a particular portion of the skull. As you can see, this one exhibits better detail because limiting the field size limits the amount of scatter contributing to the image.

Although cones and cylinders are useful, one of the problems in using them is aligning them properly with the x-ray tube and film. If all three aren't on the same axis, the edge of the cone or cylinder can get in the way of the x-ray beam and underexpose one side of the radiograph. That's called cone cutting.

SLIDE 5-15/CD 5-13 Lead blocker

Besides aperture diaphragms, cones and cylinders, and the collimators you'll learn about next, there are other ways of restricting the x-ray beam. Ancillary devices like lead blockers and masks are used for specific kinds of examinations because they can restrict the beam to a specific shape.

A lead blocker is a sheet that can be cut to any shape and placed on the radiographic table. In this illustration, for example, a lead blocker is used for an examination of the lower spine. It will help to absorb some of the scatter radiation that is produced in the tissues of the patient's back. That means less scatter will reach the film to degrade the contrast on the radiograph. Lead masks can be cut to specific sizes placed over the end of the collimator for the same reason.

SLIDE 5-16/CD 5-14 Introduction to collimators

You've begun the topic of collimators. This subject builds on information covered in the preceding topic of beam limiting devices. If you have not worked through the earlier topic yet, you may want to quit this section now and return later after going through the earlier topic.

Now let's talk about another method of beam limitation. What has replaced the aperture diaphragm, cone, and cylinder as the most efficient beam restrictor used today? The collimator, which incorporates the best of the earlier beam restrictors and does an even better job of limiting the beam to cut down on scatter radiation.

Variable-aperture collimators, referred to simply as collimators, are permanently attached to the tube housing and have several advantages over the early models. They do a better job of protecting the patient from primary radiation, thereby reducing scatter production. They have a light to help you see as you try to position the central ray over the body part to be examined. And they're also easier and quicker for radiographers to use.

SLIDE 5-17/CD 5-15 Collimator compared to cone

The term collimator really isn't used precisely because, strictly speaking, the word collimate means to line up or make parallel. In radiography, the job of a collimator is to limit the x-ray beam to the desired field size.

A well-designed collimator will do a much better job of restricting the x-ray beam than earlier devices such as cones, as you can see here. When a cone was used, it produced a larger area of unwanted radiation.

SLIDE 5-18/CD 5-16 Collimator shutters

The specific design of collimators may vary by manufacturer and model, but all of them have three basic parts. These are the light source, a mirror, and shutters.

The first shutters, usually made of lead, are really more like a collar that forms an aperture right at the x-ray tube housing. These are called the entrance shutters. They control any off-focus radiation. Off-focus radiation, you'll recall, is radiation that is produced in the x-ray tube from areas other than the focal spot.

SLIDE 5-19/CD 5-17 Second set of shutters

The second set of shutters, or second stage shutters, consist of two pairs positioned at right angles to one another. Both are made of lead. These are located toward the bottom of the tube housing and thus reduce the unsharpness along the edge of the x-ray beam.

The two pairs of shutters in a collimator can be controlled independently to create different field sizes.

SLIDE 5-20/CD 5-18 Collimator control panel

A collimator makes it easier for you to limit the x-ray beam than earlier devices did because many of the settings are predetermined. Some collimator panels provide a scale of usual field sizes at various SIDs.

You can also attach cylinders and cones on many collimators if you want to restrict the beam further.

SLIDE 5-21/CD 5-19 Light localizer in collimator

Another major feature of collimators is the light localizer, a system that works with a light bulb and mirror. This is a big help to you as you position the tube, the central ray, and the patient. It projects a light field that matches the invisible radiation field coming from the x-ray tube. Both fields should be the same size; adjustments can be made in the equipment to be sure they are.

The light field is created by a mirror placed at a 45 degree angle to the path of the x-ray beam. The source of light is opposite the mirror. When the light hits the mirror, the mirror projects it into the collimator.

SLIDE 5-22/CD 5-20 Collimator cross-hairs

The center of the beam is indicated by the cross-hairs projected through the collimator. The central ray is at the center point where the cross-hair lines intersect. You use this guide to center the beam on the body part to be examined. This illustration shows how the cross-hairs are projected in the light coming through the collimator.

SLIDE 5-23/CD 5-21 Beam limitation device

After 1974 all fixed radiographic equipment has incorporated a positive beam limitation device, or PBL. This device automatically limits the size of the radiation field to the film size.

It works this way. When you put a cassette in a Bucky tray, sensors automatically gauge the size of the cassette and where it's placed. That activates an electric motor that puts the shutters into the right position. There should be a small unexposed border on all sides of the exposed film.

MORE INFO LEADS TO THIS AUDIO RESPONSE: It's your job as a radiographer to make sure the collimator is working properly. Remember that the exposure field should never be larger than the image receptor. The PBL should guarantee this, but you must make sure to limit the field to only the part being examined. That will reduce the amount of scatter radiation, which will produce a better image and also decrease the amount of radiation the patient is exposed to.

SLIDE 5-24/CD 5-22 Review: beam limiting devices

Now let's stop for a moment to review beam limiting devices. We've seen how they've evolved from diaphragms, cones and cylinders to the most common type used today, the collimator. Think for a minute about how the collimator's system of shutters, light, and mirror works to limit the size of the x-ray beam and lessen the amount of scatter radiation that is produced. What are the advantages of the collimator over the earlier devices?

a. Better patient protection
b. Light localizer
c. Ease of use
d. All of the above

There are several advantages. One is that a collimator reduces the amount of primary radiation that reaches the patient, thereby reducing the amount of scatter radiation. Another is the light localizer that lets you center the central ray. And a third is that, in general, a collimator is easier to use.

PRESENT THIS AUDIO IF ANSWER WAS d: Yes, you're right. There are several advantages. One is that a collimator reduces the amount of primary radiation that reaches the patient, thereby reducing the amount of scatter radiation. Another is the light localizer that lets you center the central ray. And a third is that, in general, a collimator is easier to use.

PRESENT THIS AUDIO IF ANSWER WAS a, b, or c: Well, you're partly right. But there are several advantages. One is that a collimator reduces the amount of primary radiation that reaches the patient, thereby reducing the amount of scatter radiation. Another is the light localizer that lets you center the central ray. And a third is that, in general, a collimator is easier to use. Maybe you should take a few minutes to go back over this material.

SLIDE 5-25/CD 5-23 Conclusion: collimation
This concludes the section on the collimator. You've seen its advantages over earlier types in cutting down on scatter radiation. The purpose of all of these devices is to reduce the radiation dose to the patient and to reduce scatter in order to produce a better quality radiograph.

SLIDE 5-26/CD 5-24 Introduction: beam filtration
You have begun the topic of beam filtration. In this section you'll learn the purpose of filtration, and how it affects patient dose, density, and contrast.

Filtration in radiography is like any other kind of filtration: the purpose is to strain material to remove parts you don't want. Just look to your kitchen for some good examples.

You may use a paper filter in your coffee pot to separate the coffee grounds from the water passing through the pot. Enough of the grounds cling to the water to make coffee, but the filter prevents the grounds themselves from passing whole into your morning cup of coffee.

Or think of using a metal strainer when you want to get rid of the cooking water but keep the carrots you've been simmering on the stove. The strainer holds the carrots in but lets the water you no longer want pass through.

SLIDE 5-27/CD 5-25 Beam hardening
In radiography, it's desirable to filter some of the x-ray photons that come from the tube. These are low-energy photons that probably would not reach the film and are of little diagnostic value. These photons would merely be absorbed in the patient, thus increasing the dose.

You may hear filtration referred to as hardening the x-ray beam. That term is used because as filtration removes the soft (or low-energy) photons, the average energy level of the remaining photons is higher.

In addition to the low-energy filtration used for patient protection, filters are used to compensate for the uneven rates at which different body parts absorb x-rays. Compensating filters come in many different sizes and shapes. As shown in this illustration, a wedge-shaped filter absorbs more of the primary radiation on one side than on the other.

MORE INFO LEADS TO THIS AUDIO RESPONSE: You'll never be able to get rid of all the low energy photons by filtering the beam, but by removing some, you'll have a better quality beam left.

SLIDE 5-28/CD 5-26 Inherent filtration

There are three types of filtration that you need to know about. They are inherent, added, and total filtration. When you combine inherent and added filtration, you get total filtration.

Let's begin with inherent filtration. When something is inherent to a thing or a place, it's a part of it. In radiography, the x-ray tube itself acts as a kind of filter for the beam that comes from within it. The beam passes through a thin glass "window" on the tube, and this window and the cooling oil layer around it become the first filter that filters some low-energy photons from the beam. The window and the oil comprise the inherent filtration.

SLIDE 5-29/CD 5-27 Aluminum equivalency

Inherent filtration is kept quite low on purpose. You measure it in terms of its relative thickness in comparison with the thickness of a piece of aluminum that would do the same job of filtering. The thickness, or the aluminum equivalency, as it's called, is abbreviated Al/Eq.

A general purpose x-ray tube has an inherent filtration capacity of about 0.5 mm Al/Eq. The mirror, plastic, and the attachments of a collimator also measures about the same Al/Eq.

MORE INFO LEADS TO THIS AUDIO RESPONSE: Although most filters are made of aluminum because it's inexpensive and available, other materials can also do the job. Beryllium, glass, oil, copper, and tin are some. Tubes used in mammography equipment, for example, are made to produce lower energy photons because of the soft tissue in the breast. Special windows made of beryllium can reduce filtration to 0.1 mm Al/Eq.

SLIDE 5-30/CD 5-28 Added filtration

Some photons are filtered after the x-ray beam exits from the tube housing and before it strikes the image receptor. This extra filtering system is called added filtration. It usually consists of thin sheets of aluminum positioned between the tube housing and the collimator.

Added filtration is measured in terms of aluminum equivalency or in terms of half-value layer, or HVL. This describes how thick the aluminum must be to cut the intensity of the original beam in half. Half-value layers are usually shown in terms of aluminum filtration equivalency. For example, HVL = 2.0 mm Al/Eq.

When a filter removes the low-energy photons, the x-ray beam becomes hardened, or attains a higher effective overall energy level. It becomes more highly penetrating and useful.

CD 5-28A Filtration related to kVp

The National Council on Radiation Protection (NCRP) sets the standards for the amount of filtration based on the kilovoltage being used. It recommends these minimum levels of total filtration:
0.5 mm Al/Eq for less than 50 kVp
1.5 mm Al/Eq for 50-70 kVp
2.5 mm Al/Eq for kVp over 70

SLIDE 5-31/CD 5-29 Added filtration

In a collimator there are two sources of added filtration: an aluminum filter and the collimator itself. Together these sources total from 2 to 3 mm Al/Eq. About 1 mm Al/Eq of that comes from the silver on the mirror of the collimator.

MORE INFO LEADS TO THIS AUDIO RESPONSE: Mammography units usually don't use collimators because they add another layer of filtration. That would absorb more low-energy photons, the best ones to use for imaging soft tissues like the breast.

SLIDE 5-32/CD 5-30 Compensating filters

There are other kinds of filters to use when you're examining body parts or tissues of various thicknesses and densities. These are called compensating filters. Their job is to filter radiation to compensate for the uneven rate at which different parts absorb x-rays. Doing this makes the primary beam penetrate more equally.

Compensating filters also prevent excess radiation from reaching the thinner, less dense parts of the anatomy being examined. Such filters can produce better diagnostic images because of the more uniform density and keep down the amount of radiation to which the patient is exposed.

CD 5-30A Varying density

It is difficult to get good images of a section of the body that has different thicknesses or whose tissue composition varies. In taking a chest radiograph, for example, one side could be radiopaque because it contains a lot of fluid or a mass. That side would show low density. But the other side, without fluid or a mass, would have a high density as shown at the left. Using a compensating filter will even this out.

SLIDE 5-33/CD 5-31 Wedge filter

Wedge and trough filters are the most common types of compensating filters. The wedge is shaped so that it's thick at one end and thinner at the other. (Think of a wooden doorstop that's shaped this way.) When you use a wedge filter, you put its thickest part over the thinner or less dense body parts.

You'll use a wedge filter when you're radiographing structures like the foot, which varies in thickness from toes to heel. In this case, you'd put the thickest part of the wedge so that it shadows the toes and the thinnest part toward the heel. Wedge filters can also be used to radiograph the thoracic spine and lower extremities during venography and angiography.

SLIDE 5-34/CD 5-32 Step filter

A variation of the wedge is the step-wedge filter, used sometimes when long sections of the body are radiographed using two or three films.

SLIDE 5-35/CD 5-33 Trough filter

Trough filters are used for radiographs of the spine and chest. For a chest radiograph, the filter is positioned such that the thicker end aligns with the lungs and the thinner portion aligns with the spine. This provides more uniform density on the radiograph.

CD 5-33A Conic filters

A bit less common than the wedge and the trough filters are "bow ties" and conic filters, which are shaped the way they sound. "Bow ties" compensate for the way the head or the whole body is unevenly shaped and are used with some CT equipment. Convex or concave cone-shaped filters are used in fluoroscopy with a round image receptor. Shown here are conic filters.

SLIDE 5-36/CD 5-34 Plexiglas filter

Lead-impregnated Plexiglas is a new material being developed to shape into compensating filters. An alternative to aluminum, Plexiglas is easy to mold into different shapes. It has another advantage too: it can use the light of the collimator to help position the patient and still partly attenuate the x-ray beam. Shown here is a Plexiglas bow tie filter.

SLIDE 5-37/CD 5-35 Quiz instructions

THIS AUDIO FOR SLIDE TAPE ONLY: This concludes the presentation section of this module. If you are not going to work through the self-assessment quiz that follows, you may stop the program at this point and turn off the equipment.

If your instructor has asked you to take this self-assessment quiz on the material you have learned in this module, you should have a piece of paper ready. There will be 10 questions with multiple-choice or short answers. After this self-assessment we will go back through these questions and briefly talk about the reasons for the correct answers. Ready?

THIS AUDIO IN CD ROM LECTURE MODE ONLY: You have reached the self-assessment quiz for this module. Here you will be asked 10 questions to help you assess how well you understand what you have learned in this module. The questions are multiple choice or have short answers. After this self-assessment we will go back through these questions and briefly talk about your answers and the reasons for the correct answers. Ready?

THIS AUDIO IN CD ROM STUDENT MODE ONLY: You have reached the self-assessment quiz for this module. Here you will be asked 10 questions to help you assess how well you understand what you have learned in this module. The questions are multiple choice or have short answers. For multiple-choice questions, click on the box next to your answer choice. For those questions that require a short answer, type in your answer at the keyboard and press enter.

After this self-assessment we will go back through these questions and briefly talk about your answers and the reasons for the correct answers.

SLIDE 5-38/CD 5-36 Quiz question 1

1. What factors affect the amount of scatter radiation produced in a radiograph?
   a. The thickness of the patient
   b. The kVp level
   c. The field size
   d. All of the above

SLIDE 5-39/CD 5-37 Quiz question 2

2. True or false: Compression devices even out the unequal thicknesses in certain areas of the body and cut down on scatter radiation.

SLIDE 5-40/CD 5-38 Quiz question 3

3. With a larger field size, what happens to the amount of scatter radiation?
   a. It is less.
   b. It is double.
   c. It is more.
   d. It is the same.

SLIDE 5-41/CD 5-39 Quiz question 4

4. When kVp is increased, which one of these things happens?
   a. More Compton scatter occurs.
   b. The radiation dose to the patient decreases.
   c. Scatter is totally eliminated.
   d. The mAs is automatically increased.

SLIDE 5-42/CD 5-40 Quiz question 5

5. Which of the following is true of the aperture diaphragm?
   a. It is made of aluminum.
   b. It is triangular in shape.
   c. It does not allow the primary beam to pass through to the patient.
   d. It limits the amount of radiation released at the tube port.

SLIDE 5-43/CD 5-41 Quiz question 6

6. Because the diaphragm is placed close to the tube port, it causes which of the following on the radiograph?
   a. Contrast
   b. Unsharpness
   c. Magnification
   d. Fog

SLIDE 5-44/CD 5-42 Quiz question 7

7. When are cones and cylinders typically used?
   a. For head and spine examinations
   b. For gallbladder examinations
   c. In dentistry
   d. For all of these

SLIDE 5-45/CD 5-43 Quiz question 8

8. True or false: There are two pairs of shutters in a collimator, and each pair can be controlled independently to change the field size.

SLIDE 5-46/CD 5-44 Quiz question 9

9. Which of the following is true of the light field and the radiation field in a collimator?
   a. They should be different sizes.
   b. They should be the same size.
   c. They have little relationship to one another.
   d. They are impossible for the radiographer to manipulate.

SLIDE 5-47/CD 5-45 Quiz question 10

10. Why are low-energy photons filtered out of the x-ray beam?
    a. Because they are otherwise absorbed by the film
    b. Because they scatter too much
    c. Because they are of little diagnostic use
    d. Because they make the image black

SLIDE 5-48/CD 5-46 Quiz review

That concludes the self-assessment quiz for Module 5: Beam Limitation and Filtration. Let's quickly go back through the questions and see how you did.

SLIDE 5-49/CD 5-47 Review question 1

Question 1 asked you what factors affect the amount of scatter radiation produced in a radiographic exam.

The correct answer is all of those listed. The thickness of the patient, the field size under examination, and the kVp level all affect the amount of scatter radiation that is produced.

CD 5-47A Review question 1

Question 1 asked you what factors affect the amount of scatter radiation produced in a radiographic exam.

PRESENT THIS AUDIO IF ANSWER WAS d: Congratulations on getting it right! The correct answer is d, because the thickness of the patient's body, the field size being examined, and the kVp level all affect the amount of scatter radiation produced.

PRESENT THIS AUDIO IF ANSWER WAS a, b, or c: You got only part of this right. In fact, the thickness of the patient's body, the field size being examined, and the kVp level all affect the amount of scatter radiation produced.

SLIDE 5-50/CD 5-48 Review question 2

Question 2 asked if it's true or false that compression devices even out the unequal thicknesses in certain areas of the body and cut down on scatter radiation.

The correct answer is true. If you remember, compression devices are used in mammography, for example, because breast tissue varies in thickness. Flattening it out somewhat makes it more equally thick. Such flattening also allows you to position the breast closer to the film cassette for improved detail.

CD 5-48A Review question 2

Question 2 asked you if it's true or false that compression devices even out the unequal thicknesses in certain areas of the body and cut down on scatter radiation.

PRESENT THIS AUDIO IF ANSWER WAS true: Congratulations on getting this right. It's true that compression devices even out the unequal thicknesses in certain areas of the body and cut down on scatter radiation. If you remember, compression devices are used in mammography, for example, because breast tissue varies in thickness. Flattening it out somewhat makes it more equally thick. Such flattening also allows you to position the breast closer to the film cassette for improved detail.

PRESENT THIS AUDIO IF ANSWER WAS false: No, you missed this one. It's true that compression devices even out the unequal thicknesses in certain areas of the body and cut down on scatter radiation. If you remember, compression devices are used in mammography, for example, because breast tissue varies in thickness. Flattening it out somewhat makes it more equally thick. Such flattening also allows you to position the breast closer to the film cassette for improved detail.

SLIDE 5-51/CD 5-49 Review question 3
Question 3 asked what happens to scatter radiation with a large field size.

The correct answer is that a larger field size produces more scatter radiation than a smaller one. That's because there is more body area for the photons to interact with.

CD 5-49A Review question 3
Question 3 asked what happens to scatter radiation with a large field size.

PRESENT THIS AUDIO IF ANSWER WAS a: Yes, you're correct in answering that the larger the field size, the more scatter radiation that is produced. That's because there is more body area for the photons to interact with.

PRESENT THIS AUDIO IF ANSWER WAS b: You incorrectly answered that less scatter radiation is produced. The correct answer is that more scatter is produced because there is more body area for the photons to interact with.

PRESENT THIS AUDIO IF ANSWER WAS c or d: Sorry, you missed this one. The correct answer is that the larger the field size, the more scatter radiation produced. That's because there is more body area for the photons to interact with.

SLIDE 5-52/CD 5-50 Review question 4
Question 4 asked what happens when the kVp is increased.

The correct answer is that the number of photons that go through Compton interaction increases. More high-energy photons are released, causing the interaction and more scatter.

CD 5-50A Review question 4
Question 4 asked what happens when the kVp is increased.

PRESENT THIS AUDIO IF ANSWER WAS a: You're right! More high-energy photons are released, causing the interaction and more scatter.

PRESENT THIS AUDIO IF ANSWER WAS b, c, or d: Sorry, you're answer is wrong. The correct answer is the number of photons that go through Compton interaction increases. More high-energy photons are released, causing interaction and more scatter.

SLIDE 5-53/CD 5-51 Review question 5
Question 5 asked which of several characteristics were typical of aperture diaphragms.

The correct answer is that the aperture diaphragm controls the amount of radiation that is released at the x-ray tube. This is one of the earliest devices invented to limit the x-ray beam.

CD 5-51A Review question 5
Question 5 asked which of several characteristics were typical of aperture diaphragms.

PRESENT THIS AUDIO IF ANSWER WAS d: You're right! The correct answer is that the aperture diaphragm controls the amount of radiation that is released at the x-ray tube. This is one of the earliest devices invented to limit the x-ray beam.

PRESENT THIS AUDIO IF ANSWER WAS a, b, or c: No, you missed this one. The purpose of a beam limiting device such as the aperture diaphragm is to limit the number of x-rays that reach the patient. The correct answer is that the aperture diaphragm controls the amount of radiation that is released at the x-ray tube. This is one of the earliest devices invented to limit the x-ray beam.

SLIDE 5-54/CD 5-52 Review question 6
Question 6 asked placing the diaphragm close to the tube port causes what effect on the radiograph.

The correct answer is that this placement causes some unsharpness to show up on the edges of the radiograph.

CD 5-52A Review question 6
Question 6 asked placing the diaphragm close to the tube port causes what effect on the radiograph.

PRESENT THIS AUDIO IF ANSWER WAS b: Yes, you got the correct answer, that this placement causes some unsharpness to show up on the edges of the radiograph.

PRESENT THIS AUDIO IF ANSWER WAS a, c, or d: Sorry, you missed this one. The correct answer is that this placement causes some unsharpness to show up on the edges of the radiograph.

SLIDE 5-55/CD 5-53 Review question 7
Question 7 asked what types of examinations usually use cones and cylinders.

The correct answer is d. Cones and cylinders are still generally used for head, spine, and gallbladder exams, as well as in dentistry.

CD 5-53A Review question 7
Question 7 asked what types of examinations usually use cones and cylinders.

PRESENT THIS AUDIO IF ANSWER WAS d: Yes, you were right. The answer is that cones and cylinders are generally still used for all of these purposes: head, spine, and gallbladder exams, as well as in dentistry.

PRESENT THIS AUDIO IF ANSWER WAS a, b, or c: No, you're only partially correct. The answer is that cones and cylinders are generally still used for all of these purposes: head, spine, and gallbladder exams, as well as in dentistry.

SLIDE 5-56/CD 5-54 Review question 8
Question 8 asked if it is true or false that the two pairs of shutters on a collimator can be controlled independently to create different field sizes.

The answer is true. The lateral and longitudinal shutters can be manipulated independently of each other to create different field sizes.

CD 5-54A Review question 8
Question 8 asked if it is true or false that the two pairs of shutters on a collimator can be controlled independently to create different field sizes.

PRESENT THIS AUDIO IF ANSWER WAS true: Yes, of course you're correct. The lateral and longitudinal shutters can be manipulated independently of each other to create different field sizes.

PRESENT THIS AUDIO IF ANSWER WAS false: No, you didn't get this one. The pairs of shutters don't always move in the same direction at the same time. They can be manipulated independently of each other to create different field sizes.

SLIDE 5-57/CD 5-55 Review question 9
Question 9 asked about the relationship of the light field and the radiation field in a collimator.

The correct answer is b. Both fields should be the same size in order to get the best quality radiograph.

CD 5-55A Review question 9
Question 9 asked about the relationship of the light field and the radiation field in a collimator.

PRESENT THIS AUDIO IF ANSWER WAS b: Yes, you're right. The correct answer is that both fields should match up and be the same size in order to get the best quality radiographs.

PRESENT THIS AUDIO IF ANSWER WAS a: Sorry, but you missed it. You answered that the fields should be of different sizes, but in fact, they must match and be the same size in order to get the best quality radiographs.

PRESENT THIS AUDIO IF ANSWER WAS c: Sorry, but you missed it. You answered that the size of the light and radiation fields don't have any relationship to one another, when in fact, they must be the same size to produce the best quality radiographs.

PRESENT THIS AUDIO IF ANSWER WAS d: Sorry, but when you said that the radiographer can't manipulate these fields, you were wrong. The correct answer is that both fields should match up and be the same size in order to get the best quality radiographs.

SLIDE 5-58/CD 5-56 Review question 10
Question 10 asked why low energy photons are filtered out of the x-ray beam.

The answer is c. Low energy beams are so weak they have no chance of reaching the film, so they have no diagnostic use. But they do reach the patient and expose him or her to more radiation than is necessary.

CD 5-56A Review question 10
Question 10 asked why low energy photons are filtered out of the x-ray beam.

PRESENT THIS AUDIO IF ANSWER WAS c: Yes, you're right. Low energy beams are so weak they have no chance of reaching the film, so they have no diagnostic use. But they do reach the patient and expose him or her to more radiation than is necessary.

PRESENT THIS AUDIO IF ANSWER WAS a, b, or d: Sorry, you missed it. The correct answer is c. Low energy beams are so weak they have no chance of reaching the film, so they have no diagnostic use. But they do reach the patient and expose him or her to more radiation than is necessary.

SLIDE 5-59/CD 5-57 Quiz conclusion
This concludes the self-assessment quiz. This was not intended as a test, so don't feel bad if you missed some. All that means is that you probably need to review this module or study your textbook more carefully.

CD 5-57A Quiz feedback

FOR SCORE OF 10, THIS AUDIO: You've done an excellent job here with a difficult subject. Clearly you are studying well, and you seem to have worked through the tutorial carefully.

FOR SCORE OF 9, THIS AUDIO: You've done well with a difficult subject. Clearly you are studying and paying attention to the subject. Maybe next time you'll get the perfect score!

FOR SCORE OF 7-8, THIS AUDIO: Your score is about average. I'd suggest you review this material in your textbook. You may also find it helpful, next time, to read the material in your book before coming to the computer to take the tutorial. And don't hesitate to talk to your instructor if you have trouble after both reading the textbook and working through the multimedia tutorial.

FOR SCORE OF 5-6, THIS AUDIO: Your score is below average. You need to review this material in your textbook, and perhaps you should come back and take this tutorial again afterwards. You may have just been unprepared this time, or if you are having trouble after both reading the textbook and working through the multimedia tutorial, be sure to talk to your instructor.

FOR SCORE OF 0-4, THIS AUDIO: Your score is rather low. Don't feel too bad; these are, after all, difficult concepts to grasp. If you tried your best here but are having this much difficulty with the material, you should first go to your textbook and see if you can understand the material there. If it still seems difficult, please ask your instructor for additional study aids.

SLIDE 5-60/CD 5-58 Exam instructions
In the next 7 or 8 minutes you will be presented with 15 multiple-choice questions. Select the one best answer choice. Get ready a blank sheet of paper numbered 1 to 15 down the left side. As you take the examination, write the letter corresponding to your answer choice next to the number for each question. Ready? You will not be asked to perform any complicated calculations.

CD 5-58A More exam instructions

In the next 7 or 8 minutes you will be presented with 15 multiple-choice questions. Select the one best answer choice. This examination covers the material you've been learning about in this tutorial over the last hour or so. It is designed to help you and your instructor determine how well you now grasp this material. You can use scratch paper during the exam if you want, but it shouldn't be necessary for any complicated calculations.

SLIDE 5-61/CD 5-59 Exam question 1

1. How does the positive beam limiting device (PBL) affect the size of the radiation field?
   a. It automatically limits it to the film size.
   b. It automatically doubles it as it cuts the field size in half.
   c. It automatically cuts it in half as it doubles the field size.

SLIDE 5-62/CD 5-60 Exam question 2

2. A general purpose x-ray tube has an inherent filtration of about how much?
   a. 0.3 mm Al/Eq
   b. 0.5 mm Al/Eq
   c. 1.0 mm Al/Eq
   d. 0.8 mm Al/Eq

SLIDE 5-63/CD 5-61 Exam question 3

3. A collimator acts as a kind of beam filter. About 1 mm Al/Eq comes from what part of the collimator?
   a. The shutters
   b. Cones
   c. Cylinders
   d. The mirror

SLIDE 5-64/CD 5-62 Exam question 4

4. When you use a wedge filter, what part of it do you place in such a way as to shadow the less dense body parts?
   a. Its thinnest part
   b. Positioning makes no difference
   c. Its thickest part
   d. Its longest part

SLIDE 5-65/CD 5-63 Exam question 5

5. How are the paths of scattered x-ray photons affected in relation to those that have not interacted with parts of the body?
   a. More angled
   b. Straighter
   c. Stronger
   d. More dangerous

SLIDE 5-66/CD 5-64 Exam question 6

6. Who will generate more scatter radiation, a 200-pound man or a 140-pound man?
   a. A 140-pound man
   b. A 200-pound man
   c. The amount of scatter produced will be the same.

SLIDE 5-67/CD 5-65 Exam question 7

7. What is the size of the aperture diaphragm in relation to the size of the film being used?
   a. A bit larger
   b. A bit smaller
   c. The same

SLIDE 5-68/CD 5-66 Exam question 8

8. A cone or cylinder that isn't properly aligned with the tube and the film can cause which of the following?
   a. Unsharpness
   b. Foreshortening
   c. Magnification
   d. Cone cutting

SLIDE 5-69/CD 5-67 Exam question 9

9. Which of the following is true of off-focus radiation?
   a. It is produced in the collimator shutters.
   b. It is produced from objects in the x-ray tube other than the focal spot.
   c. It is produced by hard x-ray beams.
   d. It is produced by the collimator mirror.

SLIDE 5-70/CD 5-68 Exam question 10

10. Which of the following is true of a state-of-the-art collimator?
    a. Many of the settings are precalculated.
    b. Many of the settings are difficult to read.
    c. Many of the settings are dependent on kVp.

SLIDE 5-71/CD 5-69 Exam question 11

11. A light-localizer on a collimator works with which of the following?:
    a. Shutters and mirror
    b. Shutters and a light bulb
    c. A light bulb and mirror
    d. The x-ray tube and mirror

SLIDE 5-72/CD 5-70 Exam question 12

12. What type of x-ray photons are filtered as they come from the tube port and travel toward the patient?
    a. High-energy photons
    b. Low-energy photons
    c. Neutral photons

SLIDE 5-73/CD 5-71 Exam question 13

13. Which of the following is true of inherent filtration?
    a. It is a variable part of the x-ray tube.
    b. It is not important to the efficiency of the x-ray tube.
    c. It is outside the path of beams emerging from the x-ray tube.
    d. It is a part of the x-ray tube.

SLIDE 5-74/CD 5-72 Exam question 14

14. Filtration is measured in terms of its relation to the thickness of which of the following?
    a. The collimator
    b. Aluminum
    c. Beryllium
    d. Plastic

SLIDE 5-75/CD 5-73 Exam question 15

15. How are compensating filters used?
    a. To compensate for poor equipment
    b. To compensate for inexperienced radiographers
    c. To compensate for unequal thickness levels of body parts or tissues
    d. To compensate for large field sizes

SLIDE 5-76/CD 5-74 Exam conclusion

INSTRUCTOR CD/SLIDE AUDIO: This concludes the examination section of Module 5 of Radiographic Imaging. Please follow your instructor's directions for your answer sheet to the questions.

STUDENT CD AUDIO: This concludes the examination section of Module 5 of Radiographic Imaging. Your score has been saved on the computer. Your instructor will report it to you later.

Answers to the Multimedia Examination

1. a	6. b	11. c
2. b	7. b	12. b
3. d	8. d	13. d
4. c	9. b	14. b
5. a	10. a	15. c

Technique Formation

6

Overview

Radiographic technique and exposure factors
- mA
- Exposure time
- kVp
- SID

Image quality
- Density
- Contrast
- Detail
- Distortion

Patient considerations
- Thickness
- Positioning
- Motion blur

Technique charts
- Variable-kVp charts
- Fixed-kVp charts
- High kVp charts
- Automatic exposure control system

This module focuses on radiographic technique and the use of technique charts in making exposure selections. So that students understand how technique charts are developed and why they are used, the module begins with a review of exposure factors and image quality factors.

From earlier modules students should already have an understanding of the meaning of kVp, mA, exposure time, and SID. The effect of each of these factors on the image is considered individually. These factors are balanced to obtain the best diagnostic image with adequate density and contrast and minimal patient dose.

Density, contrast, recorded detail, and distortion are reviewed to emphasize the importance of developing radiographic technique to provide the best contrast and detail with a minimum of distortion. Patient factors such as positioning and the thickness of the body area are explored as important complementary aspects of radiographic technique.

The reasons for using technique charts are explored, as well as the process of developing them. The most common types of technique charts are described, along with their advantages and disadvantages. The module ends with discussion of more recent developments related to technique: automatic exposure control systems and anatomically programmed radiography.

Learning Objectives

Upon completion of this module, the student should be able to do the following:

1. Define all the key terms in the module.
2. Describe how selecting each of the following exposure factors affects image quality:
   - mA
   - Exposure time
   - kVp
   - SID
3. Explain how each of the following image quality factors is affected by exposure variables:
   - Density
   - Contrast
   - Recorded detail
   - Distortion
4. Describe the importance of patient factors, including thickness of the body area, tissue density, and positioning, for radiographic technique.
5. For each of the following types of technique charts, describe how the chart is used and its advantages and disadvantages:
   - Variable-kVp technique
   - Fixed-kVp technique
   - High-kVp technique
   - Automatic exposure control systems
6. Successfully complete the activities and posttest in the Study Guide.

Key Terms

Automatic exposure control system
Automatically programmed radiography (APR)
Blur
Calipers
Central ray
Contrast
Density
Distortion
Elongation
Exposure guide
Exposure variables
Fifteen percent rule
Film contrast
Fixed kVp technique chart
Foreshortening
Grid
High kVp technique chart
Intensifying screen
Inverse square law
mA
Magnification
mAs
Object-to-image receptor distance (OID)
Pathology, pathological condition
Radiographic technique
Recorded detail
Shape distortion
Size distortion
Source-to-image receptor distance (SID)
Subject contrast
Technique chart
Unsharpness
Variable kVp technique chart

Instructional Outline

I. Radiographic technique refers to manipulating exposure factors to get the highest quality images.
   A. Quality images protect the patient by minimizing the patient dose that would be incurred with a repeat exam.
   B. mA controls the current flowing through the tube's filament.
      1. With a low mA, the kVp must be higher or the exposure time longer to achieve adequate density on the image.
      2. A higher mA allows for a shorter exposure time but may lead to loss of detail because of increased focal spot size.
   C. Exposure time determines how long the x-ray beam continues.
      1. Shorter exposure times are beneficial because there is less motion blur.
      2. Often a short exposure time with a high mA produces the most effective mAs.
      3. High-speed screen-film combinations allow for shorter exposure times.
   D. kVp is the most important exposure factor because of its many effects.
      1. kVp determines the velocity of the electrons striking the anode and thus the energy level of the x-rays produced in the beam.
      2. kVp must be high enough to penetrate the body sufficiently to produce enough density on the image; low-energy x-rays are absorbed in the body but do not contribute to the image.
      3. Increasing the kVp 15% doubles the density.
      4. Whereas increasing the mAs to produce more x-ray photons increases the patient dose, increasing the kVp decreases the dose because more x-rays penetrate the body to reach the image receptor rather than being absorbed by the body.
      5. Higher kVp causes more scatter to exit the patient; overall scatter may be reduced by collimation and when appropriate by use of a grid.
      6. Higher kVp also lowers the contrast on the image.
   E. SID is an important exposure factor because it determines the intensity of the x-ray beam.
      1. The inverse square law applies to SID, meaning that doubling the SID causes the intensity of the beam to be one-fourth.
      2. SID is usually standardized at an effective distance for most exams.

II. Image quality factors include density, contrast, recorded detail, and distortion.
   A. Density is the overall blackening on an image.
      1. A good radiograph shows a variation of densities to clearly distinguish the different tissues in the area examined.
   B. Contrast is a combination of subject and film contrast.
      1. Subject contrast is produced on the image by the variable absorption rates of the different tissues in the areas being imaged.
      2. Film contrast refers to the sensitivity of an x-ray film to show a range of different densities.
      3. Higher kVp settings produce more scatter, which causes fog on the image that lowers contrast.
   C. Recorded detail is the degree of sharpness of structures recorded in a radiograph.
      1. Patient motion causes blur that decreases detail.
      2. Visible detail depends on good density and contrast.
      3. Detail is better with a small OID, a smaller focal spot, a slower intensifying screen, and a longer SID.
   D. Distortion includes magnification and shape distortion.
      1. Magnification is less with a longer SID and a shorter OID.
      2. Shape distortion is minimized by aligning the x-ray beam, the body part being examined, and the image receptor.

III. Patient considerations in radiographic technique include the patient's size, the tissues being examined, the pathological condition, and positioning.
   A. Patient thickness affects how many x-rays are absorbed in the body.
      1. Either the kVp or mAs must be increased to compensate for thicker patient areas.
      2. Patient thickness is measured using calipers.
      3. Thicker patients and body parts produce more scatter radiation.
   B. kVp and mAs selections depend on the tissues being examined and the variations in tissue density in the body area.
   C. Correct patient positioning is necessary to minimize distortion.
IV. Technique charts establish suggested settings for exposure for a particular exam with the equipment used in the department.
   A. Technique charts are established by radiologists, radiographers, and medical physicists in the department, using the specific equipment present for specific types of standard exams.
   B. Radiologic technologists consult technique charts to determine the best exposure factors for a given patient for a standard exam.
   C. Technique charts protect the patient because they minimize the need for repeat exams.
   D. The technique chart states whether and when to use grids, different screen-film combinations, and the kVp and mAs selections for different patient thicknesses.
   E. There are four standard types of technique charts.
      1. The variable-kVp chart uses a standard mAs and a variable kVp setting based on the patient's thickness.
         a. Contrast may vary with a variable kVp chart.
         b. Exposure changes are easy to make to compensate for different body sizes.
         c. Calipers are used to accurately measure body thickness.
      2. The fixed kVp system uses one kVp setting and varies the mAs depending on the body thickness.
         a. Contrast and density are more consistent.
         b. Exposure time is shorter.
         c. More scatter is produced, lowering overall contrast.
      3. The high kVp technique keeps the kVp high (over 100 kVp) for all studies and is typically used for chest exams.
      4. The automatic exposure control system has an electronic timer that ends the exposure as soon as there is optimum density on the image.
   F. Anatomically programmed radiography uses a computerized system to guide exposure selections based on the desired projection and the patient's size.

Teaching Tips

Exposure Factors and Image Quality Factors

From earlier modules and course work, students should already be familiar with the physical principles involved in mA, exposure time, kVp, and SID—the factors covered in the beginning of this module. They should already understand the 15% rule for kVp and density, for example, as well as the general principle that higher kVp selections generally produce more scatter. What is important about how these factors are revisited in this module is that they are now placed in a larger perspective of radiographic technique in general, leading to a fuller understanding of what technique charts are and how they are used. Although each factor is again explored in some basic terms—such as mA determining the number of x-rays in the beam, while kVp determines the energy level of those x-rays—the real point is to understand how each exposure factor fits into an overall picture. Your students should come away from this material with a feel for how, rather than some simple perfect combination of selections, these variables are balanced against each other in complex ways, even in routine examinations.

It is important, of course, that students understand each factor individually before trying to build to this larger picture. In class discussions, an effective way to help students fully grasp the technique implications of each factor is to ask students questions that lead them to realize how there can be no completely perfect setting for each factor. Try to get them to use their imagination in a problem-solving way. For example, in a discussion of SID, ask what the "ideal" SID would be to eliminate magnification. The answer actually is an infinite SID, of course, or nearly so. But then what happens to the intensity of the x-ray required, because the inverse square law tells us how the intensity diminishes over distance? And how practical would it be to have the x-ray tube a long distance from the patient? Help students work through the problems in establishing a practical SID—and understand why this "compromise" is quite acceptable for the images that result.

Take students through the same process for each variable. With kVp, for example, ask students what kVp would be best to eliminate or reduce scatter radiation to prevent fog on the image and thereby to obtain the best image. Then introduce the issue that the x-ray beam must penetrate the body sufficiently for the image to have enough density—and is this "ideal" kVp the same as that needed to prevent scatter? Then introduce the issue of patient dose—what kVp selection will minimize patient dose?

Similar questions can be asked also about exposure time and mA. What exposure time is best to prevent motion blur if the patient moves? But with extremely short exposure times, how high must the mA be to have the same mAs—and what problem may result from very high mA selections? What mAs is best for patient dose? What mAs is best for penetrating the body sufficiently to obtain enough density in the image? And so on.

As you ask students these questions, some students will begin to reply, "That depends on ..." — such as the relationship between mAs and kVp. Ultimately, as each factor is explored, they will see how the selection of each influences the selection of all the others. Students will begin to see how complex this balancing act is.

Through this discussion you can also increasingly bring into the perspective the image quality factors described in this module: density, contrast, recorded detail, and distortion. These factors help students recall that the goal is not merely to produce the image but to provide the best possible image with diagnostic value. For example, if density was the only characteristic needed, the kVp selection would not be so complicated—but contrast is equally important. At this stage in the class discussion you might want to show students radiographs (or reproductions in a textbook) that are deficient because of poor contrast, low recorded detail, or distortion. Ask students what exposure factor might have been changed to obtain a better image. Again, there is always a balancing act; one selection may be "perfect" to improve contrast, but that selection may have some other drawback.

Finally, once students have a sense of how complex this balancing can be, introduce the patient as yet another variable. Even when all the exposure factors have been worked out as ideally as possible for an "average patient," something must change with a larger or smaller patient. Change the mAs or kVp?

What effect will that change then have on image quality? What about other patient issues, such as the difference between an area of little variation in tissue densities (such as the breast) and an area with much variation (bone and muscle)? Furthermore, what adjustment should be made for pathological conditions affecting tissue density, such as a large mass in the abdomen?

Technique Charts

The goal of the preceding discussion of the complexity of radiographic technique is not to confuse or overwhelm students. A sense that it all is somewhat overwhelming, however, may be beneficial. Indeed, if every radiological technologist did have to "reinvent the wheel" by figuring this all out before every exposure, it truly would be overwhelming. Fortunately, radiography builds on past success in determining exposure selections, so that the technologist can work from standardized settings that have proven effective for producing diagnostic images. The discussion therefore leads very naturally and easily to the topic of technique charts.

Once students understand the value of using technique charts to help determine exposure selections for a given patient and type of exam, there is a risk that some students may view them as the automatic "answer" to all that balancing complexity and lose sight of the active role the radiographic technologist still has in terms of technique. There still is no "ideal" combination of selections, and the patient always remains a major dimension in the exam. Measuring and positioning the patient correctly, as well as adjusting the exposure based on size and other factors, remain important skills even when technique charts are used. Students need to gain a balanced perspective of how technique charts do simplify the examination process but how their judgment and skills are still needed.

The module describes four common types of technique charts in terms of their advantages and disadvantages. That there is no one type of chart used everywhere is a fact related to the complexity of balancing exposure factors, as described earlier. However, the discussion of these different types of charts should move from a balanced view of the four types to a focus on the particular types of charts used in the students' clinical setting. Photocopies of charts used in that setting can be brought into the classroom so that students gain some familiarity working with them (given hypothetical situations) before encountering them in the radiography department.

Workbook Posttest Answers and Rationales

1. Using technique charts helps ensure which of the following?
   a. **Patients receive minimal radiation.** When the best possible image is obtained in this controlled manner, the exposure is minimal and the need for a repeat exam is avoided.
   b. Equipment receives routine maintenance.
   c. Chemicals are periodically changed in the developer.
   d. All of the above are true.
   e. None of the above is true.

2. Control panel selections allow determination of which of the following?
   a. How many x-rays reach the patient
   b. The energy level of the x-rays
   c. The length of time the x-ray beam is on
   d. All of the above—These three characteristics are controlled by the mA, the kVp, and the exposure time.
   e. None of the above

3. In general, which is better?
   a. A longer exposure time
   b. A shorter exposure time—A shorter exposure time minimizes the risk of motion blur.
   c. An exposure time standardized for all exams
   d. Any exposure time is fine

4. kVp affects which of the following?
   a. Contrast in the image
   b. The amount of scatter radiation produced
   c. Patient dose
   d. All of the above—Higher kVp increases scatter while decreasing contrast and patient dose.
   e. None of the above

5. Increasing the kVp by 15% does which of the following?
   a. Doubles the density on the film—This is known as the 15% rule.
   b. Halves the density on the film
   c. Has no effect on density but doubles the contrast
   d. None of the above

6. When high kVp technique is used, which of the following is true?
   a. Collimation is needed to reduce scatter.
   b. A grid may be needed to absorb some of the scatter.
   c. Contrast is reduced.
   d. All of the above are true. Because scatter is produced (which lowers contrast), collimation and use of a grid may be important.
   e. None of the above is true.

7. The radiologic technologist applies the inverse square law to which of the following?
   a. Distance from cathode to anode
   b. Object to image receptor distance
   c. Source to image receptor distance—This is important because the x-ray beam becomes significantly less intense as the image receptor is moved further away from the x-ray tube.
   d. All of the above
   e. None of the above

8. Image quality factors include which of the following?
   a. Density
   b. Contrast
   c. Detail
   d. All of the above—All three of these are essential aspects of the quality of the image.
   e. None of the above

9. A high-contrast film is generally used for which of the following?
   a. Larger patients
   b. Smaller patients
   c. Body areas with large variations in absorption rates
   d. Body areas with small variations in absorption rates—Because of the slight differences in absorption, high-contrast film is needed to differentiate between subtle differences in the tissues.

10. For the best result, the central ray should be which of the following?
    a. Perpendicular to the image receptor
    b. Perpendicular to the part being imaged
    c. Positioned in the center of the area being imaged
    d. All of the above—This alignment produces the least shape distortion as well as the best view of the area being imaged.
    e. None of the above

11. Technique charts are established based on which of the following?
    a. Small patients
    b. Large patients
    c. Specific x-ray equipment—Each piece of equipment should have its own technique charts (based on patients of average size, with different settings for thicker or thinner patients).
    d. An average of all the equipment in the department

12. Technique charts take into account which of the following?
    a. kVp
    b. The x-ray equipment
    c. Screen-film combinations
    d. All of the above—These are key factors that determine the settings given on the technique chart, along with mAs and use of grids.
    e. None of the above

13. Why do technique charts help reduce patient dose?
    a. Because kVp is always kept low
    b. Because mAs is always kept low
    c. The need for repeated exams is minimal. Standardized settings usually give better results (the kVp or mAs selections may be changed).
    d. Because faster screen-film combinations are used

14. Technique charts are created by which of the following?
   a. The equipment manufacturer
   b. **Radiologists and technologists in the department**—Although manufacturers do provide much information, the specific uses of the equipment in the department usually results in the technique charts being made there by radiologists and others in the department, including medical physicists.
   c. The authors of radiographic textbooks
   d. Darkroom technicians

15. With a variable kVp chart, the kVp for a particular exam is selected based on which of the following?
   a. **The patient's thickness**—Thickness determines the kVp needed to penetrate the body well for an image, all other factors being equal.
   b. The patient's ability to hold still
   c. The patient's age
   d. The varying mAs setting

Testbank Questions

1. Which goal best reflects the primary reason for using technique charts?
   a. To make exams easier to perform
   b. To obtain the best image the first time
   c. To ensure the exam is most comfortable for the patient
   d. To standardize exams so that only one kind of film is needed in the department

2. Exposure variables include which of the following?
   a. kVp
   b. mA
   c. Exposure time
   d. All of the above
   e. None of the above

3. mA is a measure of which of the following?
   a. The energy level of electrons flowing from cathode to anode
   b. The current through the filament in the x-ray tube
   c. The potential difference between cathode and anode
   d. The power supply to the x-ray machine

4. A shorter exposure time in general is desirable to do which of the following?
   a. Reduce the risk of motion blur
   b. Allow use of lower kVp
   c. Allow use of lower mA
   d. Shorten the SID

5. A high-speed screen-film combination allows using which of the following?
   a. Higher kVp
   b. Higher mA
   c. Shorter exposure time
   d. All of the above
   e. None of the above

6. Higher kVp levels are needed for which of the following?
   a. Reducing scatter
   b. Imagining thin body areas
   c. Eliminating shape distortion
   d. Obtaining a broader range of densities in the image

7. The "15% rule" refers to increasing what factor in order to double the density?
   a. kVp
   b. mA
   c. mAs
   d. SID

8. If the kVp is set too low, what may result?
   a. The patient absorbs too many of the x-rays.
   b. The film absorbs too many of the x-rays.
   c. Too much scatter is produced.
   d. Density is good but contrast is poor.

9. Doubling the SID causes the radiation intensity to become which of the following?
   a. Twice what it was
   b. Half of what it was
   c. Four times what it was
   d. One-fourth of what it was

10. Which of the following exposure factors is most important because its selection affects density, scatter, and patient dose?
    a. mA
    b. kVp
    c. SID
    d. OID

11. A high-quality radiograph is characterized by which of the following?
    a. A variation in densities
    b. Little density
    c. A great amount of density
    d. None of the above

12. Radiographic contrast involves which of the following?
    a. X-ray tube focal spot and film contrast
    b. Film contrast and subject contrast
    c. Film-screen combinations and grid contrast
    d. Patient thickness and film speed

13. Patient motion blur can be minimized by which of the following?
    a. Shorter exposure times
    b. Higher kVp
    c. Use of a collimator
    d. Grids

14. As the SID is increased, which of the following is true?
    a. Magnification increases.
    b. Magnification decreases.
    c. The OID decreases.
    d. The OID increases.

15. Even when automated systems determine much of the technique used, the radiologic technologist must still consider which of the following?
    a. Patient size
    b. Patient positioning
    c. Individual patient factors such as pathology
    d. All of the above
    e. None of the above

16. Technique charts generally specify the settings for which of the following?
    a. kVp
    b. mAs
    c. Varying patient thicknesses
    d. All of the above
    e. None of the above

17. A variable kVp technique chart has which of the following?
    a. Constant mAs
    b. Constant kVp
    c. Constant patient thickness
    d. All of the above
    e. None of the above

18. Using a fixed kVp technique chart, the mAs is variable depending on which of the following?
    a. Patient age
    b. Body thickness
    c. OID
    d. All of the above
    e. None of the above

19. What is a possible disadvantage of fixed kVp technique?
    a. More production of scatter
    b. High patient doses
    c. Long exposure times
    d. All of the above
    e. None of the above

20. Anatomically programmed radiography uses which of the following?
    a. A computerized system for making exposure selections for various exams
    b. A moving examination table for automatic field positions
    c. A video camera system to guide patient position
    d. All of the above
    e. None of the above

Answers to Testbank Questions

1. b	6. d	11. a	16. d
2. d	7. a	12. b	17. a
3. b	8. a	13. a	18. b
4. a	9. d	14. b	19. a
5. c	10. b	15. d	20. a

Audiovisual Script

SLIDE 6-1/CD 6-i Welcome
Welcome to Mosby's Radiographic Instructional Series.

SLIDE 6-2/CD 6-ii Technique formation
The module you are about to experience is the sixth of eight in the Radiographic Imaging program: Technique Formation.

This module will help you understand exposure techniques that affect radiographs, the factors that affect the quality of the image, patient considerations in technique formation, and technique charts and processing.

SLIDE 6-3/CD 6-1 Introduction
When photographers talk about technique, they consider things like the amount of light available, the composition of the photo they want to take, film speed, and different camera settings. Skilled photographers understand these variables very well, and they know how to manipulate them to come up with the particular images and special effects they want.

Radiographers don't have quite the creative range that photographers do. There's just one ultimate reason for taking a radiograph, and that is to provide an accurate image of the body so that radiologists and other physicians can use it to make informed diagnoses of illness or injury.

SLIDE 6-4/CD 6-2 Density differences
But being limited in purpose doesn't mean you can ignore technique, or that it isn't important. In radiography, the word just has a different emphasis.

Radiographic technique refers to the way you manipulate exposure factors on the radiographic equipment control panel to get the best quality images possible. Technique is influenced by the type of exam being performed, the patient's body habits, and the type of image receptor. Like the photographer, the radiographer needs a good understanding of how these variables affect technique.

As you can see in these radiographs, the one on the left has an excellent level of density, as opposed to the one on the right, which doesn't. The radiographer chose the right settings to get the good results.

We'll begin this module by taking a look at the three categories of technique elements.

SLIDE 6-5/CD 6-3 Technique chart
Understanding the interrelationships among the factors that influence radiographic technique isn't as daunting as it sounds. With experience, you'll learn how to make the right adjustments for the exam you're doing. And you'll get help in the imaging department, where standards have been established to guide you toward getting high-quality images.

Technique charts are present in most imaging departments, although they vary among different facilities. They establish suggested settings for exposure for a particular exam with the equipment being used in that department. When equipment is calibrated properly and maintained well, that ensures a certain level of consistency in the resulting radiographs, no matter who operates the equipment.

With the help of technique charts and with experience, you'll begin to understand how the influencing factors affect technique selection. Your goal will be to select factors that will produce the best image on the first exposure.

CD 6-3A Patient exposure
The reason for striving for high-quality images is to protect the patient. Every time you repeat an exam, you expose the patient to more radiation. You want to do everything you can to prevent that.

Over time, equipment may need to be adjusted for exposure, collimation, or other errors. The chemicals in the processor also need to be checked and adjusted. These factors can affect the quality of images. You also need to be aware of what type of screen-film combinations and grid ratios you are using.

Usually, however, those kinds of cumulative effects are less of a problem than errors in technique. The things you can influence as the radiographer are more likely to make a difference in image quality.

SLIDE 6-6/CD 6-4 Three elements of technique
Let's break down the technique elements into three different categories to make them easier to understand. They are exposure factors, the image quality, and the patient.

In a previous module in this series, you studied the exposure variables that affect the quality of the radiograph produced. They are kilovoltage (kVp), milliamperage (mA), source-to-image receptor distance (SID), and exposure time. We'll talk more about them and how you can alter them for particular purposes as we go along.

You've also learned about detail, density, contrast, and distortion. They determine the quality of the image that's produced on the radiograph, and we'll talk more about these also.

And we'll also discuss patients and how their body size and the way you position them during an exam influences the result of the image you take.

SLIDE 6-7/CD 6-5 Review: technique elements

Now let's take a minute to digest what you've just heard. What are the three categories of factors at work in radiographic technique, the ones that make a difference in whether you get good or poor quality images?

If you are thinking of exposure factors, the patient, and the things that affect image quality (such as density, contrast, distortion, and detail) you're right. Now we'll build on those concepts so you'll understand each one and how they work together. Let's start with exposure factors.

SLIDE 6-8/CD 6-6 The control panel

The essential elements under your control as you get ready to perform a radiographic examination are the quantity, quality, and intensity of the x-rays that are produced. How many x-rays reach the patient, the energy of those x-rays, and the length of time the x-ray beam is on are decisions you must make. You adjust settings on the control panel to achieve the results you want.

SLIDE 6-9/CD 6-7 Exposure technique factors

There are four exposure factors you need to consider to get the best possible image. The first is milliamperage (mA). mA controls the current that flows through the filament in the x-ray tube, which in turn controls the number of x-rays produced during a given exposure.

A low mA means fewer x-rays are produced during the exposure. A lower mA setting requires a longer exposure time or a higher kVp setting in order to produce an image with adequate density.

A higher mA setting will allow you to use a shorter exposure time, which can be beneficial. There is a potential problem with higher mA settings, however. It can lead to "focal bloom," which means that the effective focal spot size will be increased during the exposure. This will result in lower detail in the image.

CD 6-7A Origin of x-rays

Recall what you've already learned about how x-rays are produced. In simple terms, x-rays are produced when high-speed electrons collide with the metal of the anode inside the tube, creating x-ray photons. The x-ray tube is designed to allow the x-rays to escape the tube in a controlled beam. As the radiographer, you have the ability to select the energy and number of x-rays in the beam by adjusting settings on the control panel.

SLIDE 6-10/CD 6-8 Exposure time

The second factor, which goes hand-in-hand with mA, is exposure time, or how long an exposure takes. Usually, it's better to have a shorter exposure time because that leaves less opportunity for the patient to move, voluntarily or involuntarily, during the exam. The patient's motion can cause blur on the image.

A short exposure time combined with a high mA will maintain adequate density and also minimize the possibility of patient motion adversely affecting the radiograph. This is particularly useful in studies such as chest radiography, angiography, and pediatric imaging.

You'll set the exposure time on some kinds of equipment, while others have automatic exposure controls.

CD 6-8A Involuntary motion
Many exams are not affected by involuntary motion, but short exposure times should always be used. Sedation may be used for some exams to lessen the possibility of patient motion.

A high-speed screen film combination will also allow you to use shorter exposure times for all exams.

SLIDE 6-11/CD 6-9 kVp levels
A third factor in this mix, and probably the most significant, is kilovoltage, the kVp level. kVp affects several things: radiographic contrast, the penetrating ability of the x-ray beam, scatter radiation, and patient dose.

For there to be enough radiographic density to produce a readable image, the part of the body being examined has to be well penetrated by the x-ray beam. At a higher kVp, the quality of the beam is higher, and more x-rays penetrate the body. That results in a broader range of densities, which is the same as lower contrast.

SLIDE 6-12/CD 6-10 kVp doubling
Do you remember the 15% rule? Experience has proven that increasing the kVp by 15% doubles the density on the film. The converse is also true: cutting the kVp by 15% cuts the density in half.

Cutting kVp by 15% has the same effect as reducing mAs by half, while increasing it by the same amount is like doubling the mAs.

CD 6-10A kVp density
Kilovoltage is the force that drives the electrons from the cathode to the anode in the x-ray tube to create x-ray photons. The kVp setting you choose affects the velocity of those electrons. More high-energy photons are produced when the electrons strike the target from a higher kVp setting.

Remember that within the x-ray tube, there's a negative charge at the cathode and a positive charge at the anode. Electrons always flow from the cathode to the anode.

Keep this distinction in mind. Boosting the kVp doesn't produce more x-rays that in turn create more density on the film. What it does is increases the energy of the x-ray photons, which lets more x-rays penetrate the body. That results in more density.

SLIDE 6-13/CD 6-11 kVp and mA relationship
In some situations you'll have to decide whether to alter the mAs or the kVp in order to achieve the desired density.

Large body parts or large patients pose a particular problem because they absorb more of the x-ray photons. Increasing mAs may not be sufficient to increase density because this does not increase the overall effective energy of the x-ray beam. You may need to increase kVp to adequately penetrate the part and reach an adequate density on the film.

Using a higher mAs will produce more x-ray photons, but that means a higher dose of radiation to the patient. Increasing the kVp will accomplish the same result but will decrease patient dose. But as we already discussed, changing the kVp will also change the resultant contrast.

Collimators will decrease the amount of scatter produced. Grids absorb much of the scatter that is produced. Therefore both of these are important with high kVp techniques.

CD 6-11A kVp and contrast levels
Experience will help you judge which kVp is sufficient for a particular exam. The right amount will produce a high amount of contrast as thicker body parts absorb low-energy photons and the x-ray beam penetrates less dense parts. If the kVp is too low, the patient, rather than the film, will absorb most of the x-rays. If it's too high, there's a more even absorption of photons, which results in less contrast.

CD 6-11B Protection from scatter
Increasing the kVp also increases the amount of scatter radiation, which can travel away from the body in several different directions. The patient becomes a source of radiation, which is why you must be shielded from him or her when you make the exposure. When you stand behind a wall or glass that contains lead, you're protected from the scatter radiation because the lead absorbs it.

A lower kVp lowers the amount of scatter radiation produced.

Do you see what might go wrong in this photograph? The technologist seems about to make the exposure with the door still open! The lead-lined door with leaded glass is part of the protection from the scatter radiation. The technologist must have the door closed between her and the patient.

SLIDE 6-14/CD 6-12 SID and image quality
The last factor in this group is source-to-image receptor distance, or SID. The SID will determine how intense the x-ray beam will be when it hits the image receptor, and that, of course, affects the quality of the image.

The inverse square law is the principle at work here. That principle, you'll recall, is that the intensity of x-rays or light diminishes as it travels away from its source. Think, for example, of how well you can read a magazine when you're sitting close to a 100-watt bulb, but how different your ability to see the print becomes if you move the magazine several feet from the light bulb. The same holds true with radiation coming from an x-ray tube.

SLIDE 6-15/CD 6-13 Inverse square law
The inverse square law simply states that the amount of radiation that reaches a certain point is inversely proportional to the square of the distance between the point and the source of radiation.

Here are a couple of examples of how this works. When the distance from the source to the receptor is doubled, the radiation intensity is one-fourth. On the other hand, when the distance is cut in half, the intensity increases fourfold.

SLIDE 6-16/CD 6-14 Review: Control elements
Now let's pause for a quick review. What are the three major elements that you control and that make the difference between producing high-quality and low-quality radiographic images?

If your answer is the quantity, quality, and intensity of the x-rays that are produced, you're right. What's important are how many x-rays reach the patient, the energy of those x-rays, and how long they are allowed to flow to the patient. You adjust settings for those variables on the control panel.

SLIDE 6-17/CD 6-15 Review: importance of kVp

Now here's another question for you. Of the four exposure factors you need to think about to get high-quality images, which is considered the most important?

Type in your answer now.

The correct answer is kVp. Kilovoltage is so significant because it affects so many things: contrast, the x-ray beam's penetrating ability, the amount of scatter radiation produced, and the radiation dose to the patient.

PRESENT THIS AUDIO IF ANSWER WAS kilovoltage or kVp: You're right. Kilovoltage is so significant because it affects so many things: contrast, the x-ray beam's penetrating ability, the amount of scatter radiation produced, and the radiation dose to the patient.

PRESENT THIS AUDIO IF ANSWER WAS anything else: No, you might want to go back over this material. Kilovoltage, or kVp, is the right answer. It's so significant because it affects so many things: contrast, the x-ray beam's penetrating ability, the amount of scatter radiation produced, and the radiation dose to the patient.

SLIDE 6-18/CD 6-16 Conclusion of exposure techniques

This concludes the section on the exposure techniques that affect the quality of radiographs.

SLIDE 6-19/CD 6-17 Introduction: quality factors

You have begun the topic of image quality factors and patient considerations. This topic builds on the preceding topic of exposure techniques. If you haven't yet worked through the earlier topic, you may want to quit this section now and return later after going through it.

Now let's talk about image quality factors.

SLIDE 6-20/CD 6-18 Density and contrast

The second category of principles that affect the quality of radiographs is image quality factors. Like exposure techniques, these factors are linked closely together. They are density, contrast, detail, and distortion.

You have studied these in some depth in an earlier module in this series and touched on them here because they're intertwined with technique factors. But it's important to take another look at them to understand what difference they make to image quality.

Shown here are high-quality radiographs with the right amount of contrast and density to make them useful to a radiologist. The radiographer knew how to select the correct exposure settings to get these results.

Let's begin with a review of these four factors and then move on to the adjustments you can make to affect them.

SLIDE 6-21/CD 6-19 Density

Density, you remember, is the overall blackening visible on a radiograph. Actually, there can be a range of density from almost all black (many photons reach the film) to almost clear (no photons reach the film). At higher mAs settings, there is more density on the film, as you see here.

A good radiograph shows a variation of densities, particularly between areas close to each other, because the differences in darkness clearly distinguish the body part under examination. That clear distinction should be your aim.

SLIDE 6-22/CD 6-20 Contrast and density

Radiographic contrast, a combination of subject and film contrast, you'll recall, is produced when there are different densities (or shades of gray) on a radiograph. How well you can see a body part on a radiograph depends on the variations in density of that part as well as how it's set apart from areas around it.

Without differences in densities, everything would look the same and it would be difficult to distinguish different patient anatomy. You can see in this illustration how different the same thing can look with differing degrees of contrast. Think of a room where the walls, ceiling, woodwork, and other details are all painted the same shade of blue. You have to look hard to see architectural features, curves, or cracks because everything is the same color and no details stand out. If those details were painted black, they'd be much more obvious.

Subject contrast refers to the amount of x-radiation that has been absorbed by different parts of the body in the path of the x-ray beam. The more pronounced that absorption is, the greater the contrast.

SLIDE 6-23/CD 6-21 Film contrast

Film contrast is different. It refers to how sensitive a particular x-ray film is to photons that strike it, a sensitivity that's built into the film itself. You can regulate contrast by choosing from different films depending on what kind of examination you're performing. This illustration shows that different films absorb photons at different rates.

The area in and around the chest, for example, has tissue that absorbs x-rays at different rates, so it has high subject contrast. If you used a high contrast film for this area, you'll likely get too much contrast on the image. Breast tissue, on the other hand, doesn't have much absorption difference, so if you used a high-contrast film you'd end up with a better image with enough contrast.

CD 6-21A Film processing

Choosing the right film alone doesn't guarantee a perfect image. Much depends on the chemical reactions that occur in processing, as well as other variables like the temperature of the developing solution. We'll talk more about processing later. Just keep in mind that it's also an important factor in contrast.

Remember, too, that kVp has a definite effect on contrast. As kVp increases, more photons are transmitted through the body, and more of the image is produced by scatter radiation. This means lower contrast.

SLIDE 6-24/CD 6-22 Detail and unsharpness

Detail is the term used to describe how well the structural lines of a body part are recorded on a radiograph. It may sound contradictory, but there may be excellent detail even if you can't see it because it can be obscured by poor levels of density or contrast. A radiograph that has too much unsharpness or blurring around the edges has a poor level of detail.

When a patient moves, that also causes blur on the radiograph, so you should always instruct the patient to stay as still as possible. There are other changes you can make to get sharper detail, but you have to be careful because they may also increase radiation exposure to the patient.

These changes include reducing the object-to-image receptor distance (OID); reducing the focal spot size; reducing the speed of intensifying screens; and increasing the source-to-image receptor distance (SID).

SLIDE 6-25/CD 6-23 Distortion

Distortion, the fourth factor that affects the image quality, occurs when the size or the shape of the body part being examined is misrepresented. Either it shows up as too large, or it's stretched out or shortened and does not reflect the actual shape.

Body structures are always magnified on a radiograph, which makes them look as though they're larger than they really are. Reducing the magnification increases detail, and you can achieve that by increasing the SID and decreasing the OID.

Magnification decreases as the SID is increased. A common SID in many radiographic exams is 40 inches (100 cm), although some exams may require a shorter or longer SID.

Magnification also decreases as the OID decreases. Your goal should be to try for the shortest OID possible. That depends on the body part being examined, the size of the patient, and the way you position the patient for the exam.

SLIDE 6-26/CD 6-24 Elongation/foreshortening

Distortion also refers to the way the shape of an object appears on an image. When it's elongated, it looks longer than it really is. When it's foreshortened, is looks shorter.

An object appears to be elongated if the x-ray tube or the image receptor is not aligned properly. When the body part is not in alignment, foreshortening occurs.

To refresh your memory, the central ray, the body part, and the image receptor must be carefully positioned in order to get an undistorted image. That means making sure the central ray is perpendicular to the part and to the image receptor. (This also means the part and image receptor have to be parallel.)

CD 6-24A Density, contrast, and detail

Now it's time for a quick review. You've just learned about the four factors that influence image quality: density, contrast, detail, and distortion. Think for a moment about how these factors all intertwine to produce what you see on a radiograph.

These are the factors that affect the overall quality of the radiograph. The radiologist is concerned with the degree of density, the contrast level, the overall detail, and any distortion present on the image. These can all affect the eventual diagnosis.

SLIDE 6-27/CD 6-25 Patient size

The patient is the final consideration in radiographic technique. The size of the person being examined, the tissue composition of the body part being examined, and how you position that person make a difference in the quality of the radiograph that results.

One of the first things you have to do in preparing for an exam is consider the body thickness of the patient, because it takes more radiation to properly expose a large body than a small one. Depending on the kind of equipment you're using, you can change the mAs or the kVp to accommodate differences in body sizes.

But body thickness by itself isn't the only determining factor. You'll recall that different parts of the body absorb radiation at different rates, so you must keep that in mind. As a general rule, if you're imaging just soft tissue, use a low kVp and a high mAs technique.

If you're examining a thin body part such as a hand or foot, use a slightly higher kVp technique to penetrate the bone. With a chest radiograph, a high kVp technique may be used because more penetration is needed for a thicker body part.

SLIDE 6-28/CD 6-26 kVp and scatter

As you learned earlier, the kVp setting you choose affects the amount of scatter radiation produced and the amount of radiation the patient absorbs. While a higher kVp results in more scatter, it also means more radiation will leave the patient and get to the film.

Keep in mind, then, that a higher kVp reduces the amount of radiation the patient absorbs.

SLIDE 6-29/CD 6-27 Automated control panel

You'll discover as we move on that new advances in technology are leading to more automation in technique factor selection. But even so, it will always be important for radiographers to position patients correctly and consider factors such as patient size that may affect the image.

SLIDE 6-30/CD 6-28 Conclusion: exposure techniques

This concludes the section on the exposure techniques and patient considerations that affect the quality of radiographs.

SLIDE 6-31/CD 6-29 Introduction: technique charts

You have begun the topic of technique charts and the different types that are used in radiography. You'll also learn how processing affects image quality. This topic builds on the preceding topic of exposure techniques and patient considerations. If you haven't yet worked through the earlier topic, you may want to quit this section now and return later after going through it.

Now let's begin by talking about a term you've heard referred to in this module, the technique chart. You may also hear it called an exposure guide. The technique chart is common in examination rooms and is unique to the kind of equipment and the types of examinations performed in that department. Wherever you work, you'll learn to rely on it to help you choose the proper settings for examinations.

A technique chart for a particular room is geared toward the average-sized patient and the generator and x-ray tube in that room. Consulting it won't eliminate having to make adjustments for specific exams, but it will go a long way in guiding you toward getting the best images and in maintaining consistency within the department.

SLIDE 6-32/CD 6-30 Use of technique charts

The technique chart should be posted in a prominent spot on the wall or kept in a notebook in the radiography room so you can easily refer to it. Its purpose is to guide you toward the standard settings for that equipment that will yield the proper levels of contrast and density for the radiograph. Without those predetermined standards, you'd have to estimate the correct technical factors each time you performed an examination.

Radiographic equipment continues to become more and more computerized, and the technology does more and more of the work in choosing the appropriate settings for examinations. Radiographers still need to understand the variables that affect the image because each patient is different in body type, tissue composition, water content, and pathologic conditions, and each examination is different.

That's why technique charts are so important. There are four kinds: variable kilovoltage, fixed kilovoltage, high kilovoltage, and automatic exposure control. Radiologists and radiographers work together to create charts based on the equipment, screen-film combinations used, and accessories at hand in their departments.

CD 6-30A Technique chart

Technique charts are an important consideration for patient protection. Calculated properly and evaluated regularly, they help keep the radiation dose to the patient as low as possible because using them increases the chances for producing good-quality radiographs with the first attempt.

SLIDE 6-33/CD 6-31 Development of technique charts

The purpose of technique charts is to limit the number of variable factors, so it makes sense that before the charts are developed, a lot of work has to be done to evaluate the equipment and the accessories available.

The first step is for radiologists and radiographers to come to an agreement on what they consider to be acceptable quality in a radiograph. From there, they can establish the exposure factor settings to achieve the level of density and contrast they agree is satisfactory and which will also keep the patient's exposure to radiation at a minimum.

As you begin your work in this field, you'll rely on technique charts, but not be expected to create them. However it's helpful for you to understand the steps that responsible professionals take as they develop these important charts.

Once the needed image quality is determined, the next step is for a medical physicist to test and calibrate the equipment. That involves checking the mA, timer, and kVp controls, and total filtration to make sure they're working within acceptable limits. Collimators and grids are checked at this stage as well, and any piece of equipment that isn't functioning within acceptable parameters must be adjusted.

SLIDE 6-34/CD 6-32 Photograph of calipers

Next, tube rating charts (usually supplied by the equipment's manufacturer) must be reviewed to make sure that exposure settings conform to the recommended limits of the equipment. The heating and cooling capacity of the equipment must be evaluated, too.

Standards have to be set for the processing system. This is also the time to set up a schedule for regular testing to make sure the system is working as it should.

What might seem like a piece of old fashioned equipment, calipers, can't escape this initial review. They're used to measure the body mass of patients and should be present in every radiographic room.

SLIDE 6-35/CD 6-33 Photograph of grid
Grids are devices that improve contrast on the image. These should be checked as well to make sure they are not damaged in any way. The technique chart should specify which exams require a grid.

The same is true for film-screen combinations, which are usually standardized within the department.

SLIDE 6-36/CD 6-34 Variable kVp technique chart
Now let's move on to the four types of technique charts and discuss the differences among them. The first we'll consider is one of the most common, and also the first to be developed in the 1920s, the variable-kVp chart.

This kind of chart is based on a kVp setting that changes depending on the thickness of the part of the body being examined and pairs it with the mAs setting that stays the same. The kVp increases by two for each centimeter of thickness, so accurate measurement of the patient is important.

Using this type of chart as a guide usually produces a short scale of contrast, which means a fairly small number of density ranges on the image, and a higher radiation dose to the patient.

SLIDE 6-37/CD 6-35 Exposure adjustments
One advantage to this kind of system over others is that it allows you to make small exposure changes if you need to compensate for body size.

There's a possible disadvantage related to the kind of image you get when you change kVp, that is increasing it reduces contrast. If the kVp is too high, it can obscure the detail the radiologist needs to interpret the image because of low contrast.

SLIDE 6-38/CD 6-36 Patient measurement
This is where the importance of measuring the patient comes in. You need to know the thickness of the patient and of the particular body part you're examining so you can properly set the kVp. If there's a fairly low kVp, you must be sure that enough x-rays will penetrate the body. The density on the image will be affected if that doesn't happen, and you may need to take more exposures, which increases the radiation dose to the patient.

The people who developed the chart use phantom models of different body parts and use average figures to come up with the settings on the chart. Of course, there's no such thing as an "average" patient, so you must use the settings as a base and do your own measuring.

CD 6-36A Where to measure patient
With calipers, you measure either at the central ray entrance and exit points, or at the thickest part of the body part. The technique chart for a particular radiography department must say which method is used, and every radiographer must measure in exactly the same way to maintain a level of consistency.

In this illustration, you can see that the caliper measurement is made at point B, where the x-ray beam enters and leaves the body. When you measure a body part, always look for the thickest section of the area you're radiographing.

SLIDE 6-39/CD 6-37 Fixed kVp technique chart

The fixed kVp system came along during World War II and has become more popular than the variable kVp chart with many radiographers. The system calls for setting the kVp at a certain rate and changing the mAs in relation to body thickness to get the right density. Usually it calls for a higher kVp than other techniques to make sure the body part is thoroughly penetrated.

There are a number of advantages to the fixed kVp system. It allows you to lower the mAs to compensate, which usually means a lower radiation dose to the patient; it produces better consistency in density and contrast; it offers more diagnostic information on the image; and it calls for a shorter exposure time.

SLIDE 6-40/CD 6-38 Fixed kVp technique

There are some disadvantages to a fixed kVp system. Although it does produce better consistency in density and contrast, a fixed kVp system produces more scatter radiation and therefore lower overall contrast. In some systems it may also be harder to make small changes in exposure for different body thickness because the mAs setting is less flexible.

It isn't as crucial to measure the body part with a fixed kVp. In fact, body size is categorized as small, medium, or large, which is specific enough.

CD 6-38A Body part thicknesses

People who develop technique charts categorize body parts by looking at the range of thickness in various parts. Take the abdomen as an example. Small could be considered from 14 to 20 cm, medium from 21 to 25 cm, and large from 26 to 31 cm.

As a general rule, mAs is decreased by up to 50% for a small anatomy and increased by the same amount for an anatomy considered large. For a part of the body that's swollen by trauma you might have to increase the mAs even more.

SLIDE 6-41/CD 6-39 Good density

The high kVp chart does just what it says: it sets a high kVp for all studies. High means a kVp setting greater than 100 kVp. Routine chest exams can be done at a kVp of 100 to 120 kVp because the many tissue densities present in the chest area show up well at that setting.

A high kVp is also useful in barium studies because it guarantees the x-rays will penetrate the barium-filled body part under examination and produce a good image.

SLIDE 6-42/CD 6-40 Automatic exposure system

The growth of computer-assisted technology has given birth to the last type of technique chart, the automatic exposure control system. Actually there are several different types of automated exposure systems, but they have similar characteristics. Most of them have standard kVp and mA settings and a set time for each exposure. While that helps guide you, it doesn't mean that just anyone can operate automatic exposure control systems. As always, you have to know much more than how to simply recognize correct settings to perform a radiographic exam.

The main feature of this kind of system is that it has an electronic timer that ends the exposure as soon as there is optimum density on the image. As a safety feature, there is usually a backup timer that you must set in case the automatic timer fails.

SLIDE 6-43/CD 6-41 Measuring patient

Although automatic exposure control systems take a lot of the calculations out of radiography, with some you may still have to make decisions about density settings. Because these settings are shown on a number scale to take different body thicknesses into consideration, you should measure the patient before you begin.

Positioning the patient properly is crucial when you're using an automatic exposure control system. To make sure you get the correct exposure, you must place the body part being examined exactly over the timing device. If the placement isn't perfect, there may be too little or too much density, and the patient may be exposed to more radiation than necessary.

CD 6-41A Mobile equipment

Automated exposure control systems used in mobile equipment are becoming more common. Often, a sensor is placed under the film cassette with a cable linking it to the mobile unit.

SLIDE 6-44/CD 6-42 APR

Radiologic technology is changing all the time, and exciting new developments are taking place. Anatomically programmed radiography, or APR, the latest in computer-aided technique charts, uses graphics like those you see on a personal computer to guide you in choosing the right settings for particular exams.

Let's say you're getting ready to examine a patient's lumbar spine. You can push a button to bring up either a written description or a graphic of a lumbar spine on the screen and actually see a variety of projections. The one you choose will automatically set the right exposure factors and you'll get excellent quality images if you position the patient correctly. You can adjust the exposure factors if your patient's particular body size or pathological condition is not average.

CD 6-42A Review: technique charts

Time for a quick review. Radiologists and radiographers develop technique charts for a facility and make them unique to the equipment and types of examinations conducted in that facility. Is it accurate to say that you, as a radiographer, can rely totally on a technique chart and not have to worry about making any decisions about exposure factors and patient positioning? Yes or No

Click on your answer.

PRESENT THIS AUDIO IF ANSWER WAS no: You're right to understand that you can't turn all your decision-making over to the guides established on the technique chart. Depending on the kind of chart used where you're working, you'll still have to understand how all the factors work together and how changing one affects another. And no matter how computer-aided the technology is, it's still important to measure the patient and take each patient's size and possible pathologic condition into account.

PRESENT THIS AUDIO IF ANSWER WAS yes: No, you're making a big mistake if you think you can hand all your decision-making over to the guides established on the technique chart. Depending on the kind of chart used where you're working, you still have to understand how all the factors work together and how changing one affects another. And no matter how computer aided the technology is, it's still important to measure the patient and take each patient's size and possible pathological condition into account.

SLIDE 6-45/CD 6-43 Film processing
We mentioned earlier that processing has an affect on image quality. In fact, the whole issue of film processing is a module in itself in this series that you'll be exploring later.

For now, keep in mind that processing, like all of the other technical factors we've discussed here, is another factor in producing an image that a radiologist can study and interpret. Like technique and image quality factors and patient positioning, it's another of the variables that makes radiography as much an art as a science.

The technologist is the expert when it comes to producing the best image possible. From that solid basis, the radiologist can analyze the image.

SLIDE 6-46/CD 6-44 Quiz instructions
THIS AUDIO FOR SLIDE/TAPE ONLY: This concludes the presentation section of this module. If you are not going to work through the self-assessment quiz that follows, you may stop the program at this point and turn off the equipment.

If your instructor has asked you to take this self-assessment quiz on the material you have learned in this module, you should have a piece of paper ready. There will be 10 questions with multiple-choice or short answers. After this self-assessment we will go back through these questions and briefly talk about the reasons for the correct answers. Ready?

THIS AUDIO IN CD ROM LECTURE MODE ONLY: You have reached the self-assessment quiz for this module. Here you will be asked 10 questions to help you assess how well you understand what you have learned in this module. The questions are multiple choice or have short answers. After this self-assessment we will go back through these questions and briefly talk about your answers and the reasons for the correct answers. Ready?

THIS AUDIO IN CD ROM STUDENT MODE ONLY: You have reached the self-assessment quiz for this module. Here you will be asked 10 questions to help you assess how well you understand what you have learned in this module. The questions are multiple choice or have short answers. For multiple-choice questions, click on the box next to your answer choice. For those questions that require a short answer, type in your answer at the keyboard and press enter.

After this self-assessment we will go back through these questions and briefly talk about your answers and the reasons for the correct answers.

SLIDE 6-47/CD 6-45 Quiz question 1

1. Radiographic technique refers to the way several variables are adjusted to produce the best possible image. Which of the following is not one of those variables?
    a. The patient
    b. Exposure settings on the control panel of the x-ray machine
    c. Position of the x-ray tube and image receptor
    d. Type of technique chart used

SLIDE 6-48/CD 6-46 Quiz question 2

2. As a radiographer, what are the important technique factors you control?
   a. Patient position
   b. Image quality
   c. Exposure factors
   d. All of the above

SLIDE 6-49/CD 6-47 Quiz question 3

3. There are several exposure factors that you must understand so you can alter the exposure when one or more variables are changed. Which is considered to be the most important?
   a. Kilovolts peak (kVp)
   b. Milliamperes (mA)
   c. Exposure time
   d. Source-to-image receptor distance (SID)

SLIDE 6-50/CD 6-48 Quiz question 4

4. Four image quality factors affect the quality of radiographs: density, contrast, detail, and distortion. What is the relationship among these factors?
   a. They are independent of one another.
   b. They are loosely related to one another.
   c. They are closely intertwined with each other.

SLIDE 6-51/CD 6-49 Quiz question 5

5. True or false: You can help regulate contrast on a radiograph by choosing a particular type of film for a specific examination.
   a. True
   b. False

SLIDE 6-52/CD 6-50 Quiz question 6

6. Blur is often caused by patient movement, resulting in a poor level of detail on a radiograph. Which of the following changes can help to get sharper detail?
   a. Increase the focal spot size
   b. Reduce the source-to-image receptor distance
   c. Reduce exposure time
   d. Increase the speed of screens

SLIDE 6-53/CD 6-51 Quiz question 7

7. The patient is an important factor in choosing the appropriate exposure and image quality techniques. What are the things you must consider as you get ready to radiograph a patient?
   a. The patient's body size
   b. The x-ray absorption rate of the area to be studied
   c. The position of the patient on the examining table
   d. All of the above

SLIDE 6-54/CD 6-52 Quiz question 8

8. True or false: Every technique chart developed is unique to the facility where it will be used by radiographers; it sets the standards for quality and consistency for that department.
   a. True
   b. False

SLIDE 6-55/CD 6-53 Quiz question 9

9. The variable kVp technique chart calls for which of the following?
   a. Choosing as high a kVp as possible
   b. Slightly increasing mAs as kVp changes
   c. Changing kVp depending on the patient's body thickness
   d. Slightly decreasing kVp depending on body size

SLIDE 6-56/CD 6-54 Quiz question 10

10. Which of the following is not one of the several advantages of the fixed kVp system?
    a. It usually lowers radiation dose to the patient.
    b. It produces better consistency in contrast and density.
    c. It shortens exposure time.
    d. It eliminates the need to consider patient thickness.

SLIDE 6-57/CD 6-55 Quiz review

That concludes the self-assessment quiz for Module 6: Technique Formation. Let's quickly go back through the questions and see how you did.

SLIDE 6-58/CD 6-56 Review question 1

Question 1 stated that radiographic technique refers to the way several variables are adjusted to get the best possible image. It asked which was not one of those variables.

The correct answer is d, the type of technique chart used. Congratulate yourself if you got it right! The patient, the exposure settings (kVp, mA) on the control panel, and where the x-ray tube and the image receptor are placed in relation to each other are all variables the radiographer can adjust to get the best possible image.

CD 6-56A Review question 1

Question 1 stated that radiographic technique refers to the way several variables are manipulated to get the best possible image. It asked which was not one of those variables.

PRESENT THIS AUDIO IF ANSWER WAS d: Yes, you're right. The correct answer is the type of technique chart used. The patient, the exposure settings (kVp, mA) on the control panel of the equipment, and where the x-ray tube and the image receptor are placed in relation to each other are all variables the radiographer can adjust to get the best possible image.

PRESENT THIS AUDIO IF ANSWER WAS a, b, or c: No, sorry, your answer is incorrect. The correct answer is d, the type of technique chart used. The patient, the exposure settings (kVp, mA) on the control panel of the equipment, and where the x-ray tube and the image receptor are placed in relation to each other are all variables the radiographer can adjust to get the best possible image.

SLIDE 6-59/CD 6-57 Review question 2
Question 2 asked what are the important technique elements that are under the radiographer's control.

CD 6-57A Review question 2
Question 2 asked you what are the important technique elements that are under the radiographer's control.

PRESENT THIS AUDIO IF ANSWER WAS d: Yes, you correctly answered that you must position the patient correctly and measure the patient for body thickness, make sure the exposure settings will ensure that enough penetrating x-rays will reach the patient at the lowest possible radiation dose, and determine how to influence image quality factors to produce high-quality radiographs.

PRESENT THIS AUDIO IF ANSWER WAS a, b, or c: Sorry, you incorrectly answered this one. The right answer is d, that you must position the patient correctly and measure the patient for body thickness, make sure the exposure settings will ensure that enough penetrating x-rays will reach the patient at the lowest possible radiation dose, and determine how to influence image quality factors to produce high-quality radiographs.

SLIDE 6-60/CD 6-58 Review question 3
Question 3 asked about the several exposure factors that you must understand so that you can alter the exposure when one or more variables are changed, and asked which is considered to be the most important.

The correct answer is A, kilovolts peak (kVp). That's because it affects so many things: the amount of contrast on the radiograph; the x-ray beam's intensity; the amount of scatter radiation created; and the radiation dose to the patient. You must adjust it in conjunction with mAs.

CD 6-58A Review question 3
Question 3 asked about the several exposure factors that you must understand so that you can alter the exposure when one or more variables are changed, and asked which is considered to be the most important.

PRESENT THIS AUDIO IF ANSWER WAS a: Yes, you're correct in answering a, kilovolts peak (kVp). That's because it affects so many things: the amount of contrast on the radiograph; the x-ray beam's intensity; the amount of scatter radiation created; and the radiation dose to the patient. You must adjust it in conjunction with mAs.

PRESENT THIS AUDIO IF ANSWER WAS b, c, or d: Sorry you incorrectly answered this one. The right answer is a, kilovolts peak (kVp). That's because it affects so many things: the amount of contrast on the radiograph; the x-ray beam's intensity; the amount of scatter radiation created; and the radiation dose to the patient. You must adjust it in conjunction with mAs.

SLIDE 6-61/CD 6-59 Review question 4
Question 4 asked about the relationship among the four image quality factors (density, detail, distortion, and contrast) that affect the quality of radiographs.

The correct answer is c. It's impossible to look at these factors independently because they are very closely intertwined with each other. Changing technique settings and making choices in film and accessories will have an impact on all of these factors in different ways.

CD 6-59A Review question 4

Question 4 asked about the relationship among the four image quality factors (density, detail, distortion, and contrast) that affect the quality of radiographs.

PRESENT THIS AUDIO IF ANSWER WAS c: You're right! It's impossible to look at these independently because they are very closely intertwined with each other. Changing technique settings and making choices in film and accessories will have an impact on all of these factors in different ways.

PRESENT THIS AUDIO IF ANSWER WAS a, b, or d: Sorry, your answer is wrong. It's impossible to look at these independently because they are very closely intertwined with each other. Changing technique settings and making choices in film and accessories will have an impact on all of these factors in different ways.

SLIDE 6-62/CD 6-60 Review question 5

Question 5 asked if it is true or false that you can regulate contrast on a radiograph by choosing a particular type of film for a specific examination.

The correct answer is true. You remember that different parts of the body absorb x-rays at different rates. X-ray film is manufactured with different sensitivities to the photons that strike it. Depending on the kind of examination you're performing, you can choose film that will produce the level of contrast you want.

CD 6-60A Review question 5

Question 5 asked if it is true or false that you can regulate contrast on a radiograph by choosing a particular type of film for a specific examination.

PRESENT THIS AUDIO IF ANSWER WAS true: You're right! The correct answer is true. You remember that different parts of the body absorb x-rays at different rates. X-ray film is manufactured with different sensitivities to the photons that strike it. Depending on the kind of examination you're performing, you can choose film that will produce the level of contrast you want.

PRESENT THIS AUDIO IF ANSWER WAS false: Sorry, you missed this one. The answer is true. Different parts of the body absorb x-rays at different rates. X-ray film is manufactured with different sensitivities to the photons that strike it. Depending on the kind of examination you're performing, you can choose film that will produce the level of contrast you want.

SLIDE 6-63/CD 6-61 Review question 6

Question 6 stated that blur is often caused by patient movement, resulting in a poor level of detail on a radiograph. It asked which change could be made to help get a sharper detail.

The correct answer is c, reduce the exposure time. You could also improve detail by reducing the focal spot and by increasing the SID.

CD 6-61A Review question 6

Question 6 stated that blur is often caused by patient movement, resulting in a poor level of detail on a radiograph. It asked which change could be made to help get a sharper detail.

PRESENT THIS AUDIO IF ANSWER WAS c: Yes, you got the correct answer, reduce the exposure time. You could also improve detail by reducing the focal spot and by increasing the SID.

PRESENT THIS AUDIO IF ANSWER WAS a, b, or d: Sorry, you missed it. The correct answer is c, reduce the exposure time. You could also improve detail by reducing the focal spot and by increasing the SID.

SLIDE 6-64/CD 6-62 Review question 7

Question 7 stated that the patient is an important factor in choosing the appropriate exposure and image quality techniques. It asked which things you must consider as you get ready to radiograph a patient.

The correct answer is d, all of the points listed. You have to consider the size of the patient, how well the area to be studied absorbs x-rays, and the patient's position on the examining table.

CD 6-62A Review question 7

Question 7 stated that the patient is an important factor in choosing the appropriate exposure and image quality techniques. It asked which things you must consider as you get ready to radiograph a patient.

PRESENT THIS AUDIO IF ANSWER WAS d: Yes, you were right, the answer is all of the points listed. You have to consider the size of the patient, how well the area to be studied absorbs x-rays, and the patient's position on the examining table.

PRESENT THIS AUDIO IF ANSWER WAS a, b, or c: No, you missed it. The correct answer is all of the points listed. You have to consider the size of the patient, how well the area to be studied absorbs x-rays, and the patient's position on the examining table.

SLIDE 6-65/CD 6-63 Review question 8

Question 8 asked whether the following statement is true or false: Every technique chart developed is unique to the facility where it will be used by radiographers. It sets the standards for quality and consistency for that department.

The answer is true. Each technique chart is developed specifically for use in a particular imaging department and is based on the equipment being used and the kinds of examinations being performed in that department. The technique chart is designed to guide radiographers in choosing the settings that will yield a diagnostic level of contrast and density on images.

CD 6-63A Review question 8

Question 8 asked whether the following statement is true or false: Every technique chart developed is unique to the facility where it will be used by radiographers. It sets the standards for quality and consistency for that department.

PRESENT THIS AUDIO IF ANSWER WAS true: Yes, of course you're correct. The answer is true. Each technique chart is developed specifically for use in a particular imaging department and is based on the equipment being used and the kinds of examinations being performed in that department. The technique chart is designed to guide radiographers in choosing the settings that will yield a diagnostic level of contrast and density on images.

PRESENT THIS AUDIO IF ANSWER WAS false: Nope, you missed this one. The answer is true. Each technique chart is developed specifically for use in a particular imaging department and is based on the equipment being used and the kinds of examinations being performed in that department. The technique chart is designed to guide radiographers in choosing the settings that will yield a diagnostic level of contrast and density on images.

SLIDE 6-66/CD 6-64 Review question 9

Question 9 asked what the distinguishing factor of the variable kVp technique chart is, or what it calls for.

The correct answer is c, changing kVp depending on the patient's body thickness. As the kVp changes, the mAs setting stays the same. The kVp increases by two for each centimeter of body thickness.

CD 6-64A Review question 9

Question 9 asked what the distinguishing factor of the variable kVp technique chart is, or what it calls for.

PRESENT THIS AUDIO IF ANSWER WAS c: Yes, you're right. The correct answer is that this kind of chart calls for changing kVp depending on the patient's body thickness. As the kVp changes, the mAs setting stays the same. The kVp increases by two for each centimeter of body thickness.

PRESENT THIS AUDIO IF ANSWER WAS a, b, or d: Sorry, but you missed it. The correct answer is c, that this kind of chart calls for changing kVp depending on the patient's body thickness. As the kVp changes, the mAs setting stays the same. The kVp increases by two for each centimeter of body thickness.

SLIDE 6-67/CD 6-65 Review question 10

Question 10 asked which of the listed items is not one of the several advantages of the fixed kVp system.

The correct answer is d, that it eliminates the need to consider patient thickness. Unlike other systems, in the fixed kVp system body size is precategorized as small, medium, or large, and that is specific enough.

CD 6-65A Review question 10

Question 10 asked which of the listed items is not one of the several advantages of the fixed kVp system.

PRESENT THIS AUDIO IF ANSWER WAS d: Well, you're right. It eliminates the need to consider patient thickness. Unlike other systems, in the fixed kVp system body size is precategorized as small, medium, or large, and that is specific enough.

PRESENT THIS AUDIO IF ANSWER WAS a, b, or c: Sorry, you missed it. The correct answer is d, it eliminates the need to consider patient thickness. Unlike other systems, in the fixed kVp system body size is precategorized as small, medium, or large, and that is specific enough.

SLIDE 6-68/CD 6-66 Quiz conclusion

This concludes the self-assessment quiz. This was not intended as a test, so don't feel bad if you missed some. All that means is that you probably need to review this module or study your textbook more carefully.

CD 6-66A Quiz feedback

FOR SCORE OF 10, THIS AUDIO: You've done an excellent job here with a difficult subject. Clearly you are studying well, and you seem to have worked through the tutorial carefully.

FOR SCORE OF 9, THIS AUDIO: You've done well with a difficult subject. Clearly you are studying and paying attention to the subject. Maybe next time you'll get the perfect score!

FOR SCORE OF 7-8, THIS AUDIO: Your score is about average. I'd suggest you review this material in your textbook. You may also find it helpful, next time, to read the material in your book before coming to the computer to take the tutorial. And don't hesitate to talk to your instructor if you have trouble after both reading the textbook and working through the multimedia tutorial.

FOR SCORE OF 5-6, THIS AUDIO: Your score is below average. You need to review this material in your textbook, and perhaps you should come back and take this tutorial again afterwards. You may have just been unprepared this time, or if you are having trouble after both reading the textbook and working through the multimedia tutorial, be sure to talk to your instructor.

FOR SCORE OF 0-4, THIS AUDIO: Your score is rather low. Don't feel too bad; these are, after all, difficult concepts to grasp. If you tried your best here but are having this much difficulty with the material, you should first go to your textbook and see if you can understand the material there. If it still seems difficult, please ask you instructor for additional study aids.

SLIDE 6-69/CD 6-67 Exam instructions

In the next 7 or 8 minutes you will be presented with 15 multiple-choice questions. Select the one best answer choice. Get ready a blank sheet of paper, numbered 1 to 15 down the left side. As you take the examination, write the letter corresponding to your answer choice next to the number for each question.
Ready? You will not be asked to perform any complicated calculations.

CD 6-67A More exam instructions

In the next 7 or 8 minutes you will be presented with 15 multiple-choice questions. Select the one best answer choice. This examination covers the material you've been learning about in this tutorial over the last hour or so. It is designed to help you and your instructor determine how well you now grasp this material. You can use scratch paper during the exam if you want, but it shouldn't be necessary for any complicated calculations.

SLIDE 6-70/CD 6-68 Exam question 1

1. Technique charts are posted either on the wall of every radiography suite or in a notebook in a prominent place. A technique chart is unique to the suite it was developed for. In addition to establishing suggested settings for exposure, what else does it do?
   a. Eliminates the need to think about the size of the patient
   b. Means just about anyone can follow the guide without having to make any decisions at all
   c. Establishes suggested settings for x-ray penetration for the equipment being used
   d. Restricts the kinds of film that can be used to just a few

SLIDE 6-71/CD 6-69 Exam question 2

2. As a general rule, it's always better to have which of the following?
   a. A long exposure time
   b. A short exposure time
   c. A medium exposure time
   d. A non-timed exposure time

SLIDE 6-72/CD 6-70 Exam question 3

3. The 15% rule means that increasing kVp by 15% results in which of the following?
   a. Cuts contrast by half
   b. Cuts by 15% the amount of blackening on the film
   c. Increases density by 15%
   d. Doubles the amount of overall blackening on the film

SLIDE 6-73/CD 6-71 Exam question 4

4. Generally, a high kVp exposure will get better results than a low kVp exposure. If kVp is too low, which of the following will absorb most of the x-rays?
   a. The film
   b. The patient
   c. The grid
   d. The intensifying screen

SLIDE 6-74/CD 6-72 Exam question 5

5. A higher kVp usually does which of the following?
   a. Produces a lower quality x-ray beam
   b. Raises the contrast
   c. Increases the amount of scatter radiation produced
   d. Exposes the patient to excessive radiation

SLIDE 6-75/CD 6-73 Exam question 6

6. Which of the following is an image quality factor?
   a. Density
   b. Contrast
   c. Detail
   d. Distortion
   e. All of the above
   f. None of the above

SLIDE 6-76/CD 6-74 Exam question 7

7. Why is it important to know the thickness of the patient being examined?
   a. It takes less radiation to penetrate a large body than a small one.
   b. It takes more radiation to penetrate a large body than a small one.
   c. You have to adjust the height of the examining table depending on body size.
   d. It takes longer to examine a large patient.

SLIDE 6-77/CD 6-75 Exam question 8

8. Which of the following is not a kind of technique chart?
   a. Variable kilovoltage
   b. Fixed kilovoltage
   c. Low kilovoltage
   d. High kilovoltage
   e. Automatic exposure control

SLIDE 6-78/CD 6-76 Exam question 9

9. What is the most common technique chart that also was developed first?
   a. Variable kVp
   b. Automatic exposure control
   c. High kVp
   d. Fixed kVp

SLIDE 6-79/CD 6-77 Exam question 10

10. Which of the technique charts is generally the most popular these days?
   a. High kVp
   b. Fixed kVp
   c. Automatic exposure control
   d. Variable kVp

SLIDE 6-80/CD 6-78 Exam question 11

11. Because the many tissue densities present in the chest area show up well at this setting, routine chest exams are done at which of the following?
   a. A low kVp
   b. A medium kVp
   c. A high kVp

SLIDE 6-81/CD 6-79 Exam question 12

12. What is the main feature of the automatic exposure control system?
   a. It's the easiest to use.
   b. It has an electronic timer that stops exposure when there is optimum density on the image.
   c. It makes exposure times the same for all examinations.
   d. It means even nontrained people can easily choose the right exposure settings.

SLIDE 6-82/CD 6-80 Exam question 13

13. In an automatic exposure control system, which of these variables is crucial?
   a. Selecting the mAs
   b. Selecting the kVp
   c. Setting exposure time
   d. Positioning the patient properly over the timing device

SLIDE 6-83/CD 6-81 Exam question 14

14. Which of these factors do you control as you prepare to perform a radiographic examination?
    a. The quantity of x-rays that reach the patient
    b. The penetrating ability of the x-rays
    c. The length of time the x-ray beam is on
    d. All of the above
    e. None of the above

SLIDE 6-84/CD 6-82 Exam question 15

15. Which of the following is true of increasing kVp?
    a. It produces more x-rays.
    b. It increases the energy of the x-rays.
    c. It lowers mAs.
    d. It keeps exposure time the same.

SLIDE 6-85/CD 6-83 Exam conclusion

INSTRUCTOR CD/SLIDE AUDIO: This concludes the examination section of Module 6 of Radiographic Imaging. Please follow your instructor's directions for your answer sheet to the questions.

STUDENT CD AUDIO: This concludes the examination section of Module 6 of Radiographic Imaging. Please follow your instructor's directions for your answer sheet to the questions.

Answers to the Multimedia Examination

1. c	6. e	11. c
2. b	7. b	12. b
3. d	8. c	13. d
4. b	9. a	14. e
5. c	10. b	15. b

Exposure Selection

7

Overview

Primary technique factors
- kVp
- mAs

Secondary factors
- SID
- OID
- Focal spot
- Grid
- Intensifying screen

Filtration
- Inherent
- Added
- Compensating

Generators
- Falling load generator
- Ripple factor

This module brings together many of the subjects students have learned individually in order to show their interrelationships when exposure factors are selected. With greater understanding of the meaning of each variable, students can better make adjustments as needed in situations not covered well by technique chart guidelines.

The primary technique factors are covered first: kVp and mAs. The effect of kVp on density in the image is explored, along with the problem of scatter with higher kVp selections. The balance of kVp with mAs is considered, along with the direct relationship between density and mAs.

Secondary factors discussed include SID, OID, focal spot size, grids, and intensifying screens. SID is considered in terms of the inverse square law, magnification, loss of detail because of unsharpness, and the need to alter primary exposure factors when the SID is changed. OID is considered in terms of magnification and loss of detail to unsharpness. Focal spot size is an issue of better detail from smaller focal spots balanced against the problem of overheating the tube. The advantage of using a grid in absorbing scatter and improving contrast is balanced against the higher patient dose resulting from the more intense exposure needed when a grid is used.

The effects of inherent, added, and compensating filtration are considered in terms of reducing the patient dose and evening out density when needed in a radiograph. Finally, the effect of different types of generators is briefly considered.

Learning Objectives

Upon completion of this module, the student should be able to do the following:

1. Define all the key terms in the module.
2. Explain the impact of kVp selection on density, patient dose, and scatter.
3. Explain how mAs selection relates to balance with kVp, density, SID, and motion blur.
4. State the inverse square law and describe how it relates to SID.
5. Describe the advantage and disadvantage of using a grid.
6. Explain why added filtration is used generally and why compensating filters are used in some circumstances.
7. Describe what is different about falling load generators.
8. Successfully complete the activities and posttest in the Study Guide.

Key Terms

Added filtration
Aluminum equivalency
Collimator
Compensating filter
Contrast
Contrast medium
Contrast improvement factor
Density
Filter
Focal spot
Generator
Grid
Grid ratio
Hardening
Inherent filtration
Intensifying screen
Inverse square law
kVp
mA
mAs
Magnification
Object-to-image receptor distance (OID)
Quality
Quantity
Recorded detail
Ripple factor
Scatter radiation
Source-to-image receptor distance (SID)
Technique chart
Unsharpness

Instructional Outline

I. Primary technique factors—kVp and mAs—affect exposure selection and determine levels of density and contrast.
   A. High-density indicates more x-rays exiting the patient; low-density areas indicate fewer x-rays exiting the patient.
   B. The perfect balance of high and low densities, or contrast, depends on the right combination of exposure factors.

1. Technique charts guide exposures but do not replace the need for knowledge of the effects of all variables and judgments about how the variables interact.

C. The kVp determines the quality, or energy level, of the x-ray beam.
   1. At higher kVp levels, there is more penetration of the patient, resulting in higher density.
   2. Higher kVp levels reduce patient exposure caused by the absorption of lower-energy x-rays.
   3. Higher kVp levels cause more scatter radiation, however, reducing contrast.
   4. Selection of the appropriate kVp involves considerations of the thickness of the part being examined, the use of a grid to reduce scatter, the screen-film combination, and the use of any contrast media.

D. The mAs determines the quantity of photons in the x-ray beam.
   1. The number of x-ray photons produced is directly proportional to the filament current, measured in mA.
   2. mAs, or the mA multiplied by the exposure time, determines the total number of x-ray photons during an exposure.
   3. The exposure time is usually kept as short as possible to minimize the chance of motion blur.
   4. With some radiographic equipment you can select the mA and the exposure time separately, whereas with falling load generators you may be able to select only the mAs, and the equipment will determine the precise mA and time factors.
   5. Density in the radiograph is directly proportional to the mAs; doubling the mAs doubles the density.

II. Secondary factors also affect exposure selection.

A. SID is an important consideration because the x-ray beam spreads out as it travels from the tube.
   1. Following the inverse square law, doubling the SID produces one-fourth as much density on the radiograph.
   2. SID is standardized, usually at 40 or 72 inches, to balance practicality with good detail and acceptable levels of magnification.
   3. SID is determined by the technique chart; when SID is increased, increase the mAs to compensate.
   4. SID might be altered because of other equipment in place around a patient or because an extremely large patient needs more penetrating energy.

B. OID is usually kept as short as possible because a larger OID increases magnification and unsharpness, reducing the amount of detail.

C. Choice of focal spot size is another important determination.
   1. Smaller focal spots result in less unsharpness and produce greater detail, but more heat is produced in the anode and therefore higher energy levels are limited.
   2. Larger focal spots result in more unsharpness and thus less detail but can be used with higher-energy technique.
   3. Small focal spots are generally used for examining thinner parts of the body, and larger focal spots for more dense or thicker areas or when very high technique factors are required.

D. A grid may be used with higher kVp selections to absorb up to 90% of the scatter.
   1. The grid is made of strips of radiopaque material such as lead separated by radiolucent material that lets x-rays pass through only when they are in a straight line from the tube to the image receptor.
   2. The contrast improvement factor measures how much better contrast is in the image when a grid is used.
   3. The disadvantage of grids is that the exposure must be increased to penetrate the grid, resulting in an increased patient exposure.

E. Intensifying screens are used in combination with the film in most radiographic procedures because the fluorescent light produced by the screen helps expose the film, allowing for a lower radiation dose to the patient.

III. Filtration also affects exposure selection.
   A. Filtration includes inherent filtration and added filtration.
   B. The benefit of added filtration is the absorption of low-energy x-rays that could add nothing to the image but would be absorbed in the body, increasing the patient dose.
   C. Compensating filters are used to even out density when wide differences in body tissues or density would cause too much variation in density on the finished radiograph.

IV. The radiographic equipment's generator is a final factor affecting exposure.
   A. A falling load generator allows for selecting only mAs, and the equipment selects the optimal mA and time exposure.
   B. Ripple factor, the difference between the maximum voltage and the lowest level to which it falls, causes fluctuation in the x-ray beam.
   C. Three-phase power generators produce a more consistent beam than the original single-phase generators, but modern high-frequency generators are still better and provide a ripple factor less than 1%.

Teaching Tips

This module is in many ways a review of several topics students have learned about already in other contexts. Therefore the subjects covered here are generally already familiar to students, and introduction to new material is not needed.

What is more important is helping students understand how all these factors interrelate when it comes to making exposure selections for a given examination of a particular patient. Ideal situations are generally covered by a department's technique charts and other standardized approaches. Students need to understand when it becomes necessary to use their own judgment to vary from the technique chart's guidelines.

An effective way to help students understand how each factor affects exposure selection and make the appropriate variation from the standard exam is to work through a series of hypothetical situations. First, obtain copies of a number of technique charts from the department where your students gain their clinical experience. Make copies for all the students.

Then create a number of scenarios in which students must make a variation from the standard technique. Not all hypothetical situations are likely or possible using the specific types of equipment available in that radiology department, so it is important that you construct hypotheticals that are realistic in the students' setting.

Students can work through these hypotheticals individually or in small groups. Give them the written scenario, stating all needed technical information, along with a copy of the appropriate technique chart, and have them work out the appropriate exposure selections for the different situations. Then discuss these with the whole class, perhaps having each group or individual report on how and why they made the technique adjustments that they did.

You might base some of your scenario on situations similar to the following:

- For an extremity exam, the technique chart says use a small focal spot with specified kVp and mAs. The patient is a weight lifter with a very thick upper arm, off the scale for thickness. Should the focal spot change? What adjustment is needed in the exposure factors?
- The patient is in traction and cannot be moved. Equipment over the bed will not allow you to use your desired 40 inch SID, but a 30 inch SID is possible. Adjust the exposure factors appropriately.
- The technique chart for a particular exam states to use a grid and gives the appropriate exposure factors. Because the patient has had significant occupational radiation exposure in the past, the patient's doctor wants the lowest possible exposure dose, so you will not be using the grid. Adjust the exposure factors appropriately.
- A repeat exam is necessary because the density on a radiograph was only a third of what was desired. Adjust the exposure factors accordingly.
- Because of equipment surrounding the patient, the OID must be longer than usual. Is there anything that can be done to help minimize the effects of the increased magnification?

Workbook Posttest Answers and Rationales

1. What does kVp selection determine?
   a. The quantity of x-rays in the beam
   b. The quality of x-rays in the beam—Quality is the energy level of the x-rays in the beam, which is determined by the kVp.
   c. The exposure time
   d. All of the above
   e. None of the above

2. Factors that affect the kVp selection may include which of the following?
   a. Tissue thickness
   b. Use of a grid
   c. Use of contrast media
   d. All of the above—All of these factors influence the energy level of the x-rays needed to ensure adequate penetration to provide good density in the image.
   e. None of the above

3. The more electrons that pass from the cathode to the anode,
   a. The more x-rays are produced
   b. The higher the mAs setting
   c. The higher the quantity of the x-ray beam
   d. All of the above—The number of incident electrons, which is determined by the mAs, determines how many x-rays are produced, which is the definition of beam quantity.
   e. None of the above

4. Reducing the exposure time also helps reduce which of the following?
   a. Patient exposure
   b. Motion blur
   c. **Both of the above**—Assuming the mA setting is not increased, using a shorter exposure time reduces patient exposure, and the shorter time also means there is less likelihood of blur caused by patient motion.
   d. Neither of the above

5. Because of the inverse square law, how is density on a radiography affected if the SID is doubled?
   a. Density is doubled.
   b. Density is halved.
   c. Density is four times as much.
   d. **Density is one-fourth as much.** Because of the inverse square law, the strength of the beam is one fourth at twice the distance, resulting in one-fourth the density.

6. If you are using a longer SID than that listed in the technique chart, what should you do to maintain good density?
   a. Decrease the kVp
   b. Increase the OID
   c. Use a grid
   d. **Increase the mAs**—Because of the inverse square law, the beam's intensity diminishes with a greater SID, and therefore the mAs must be increased to compensate.

7. If you double the SID from that listed in the technique chart, how much should you change the mAs to have the same level of density?
   a. Set the mAs twice as high
   b. **Set the mAs four times as high**—Again, because of the inverse square law, the mAs must be set four times as high to compensate for the beam being one-fourth as intense at twice the distance.
   c. Set the mAs half as high
   d. Set the mAs one-fourth as high

8. In what situation might you have to use an SID shorter than that given in the technique chart?
   a. With a very thin patient
   b. **When equipment interferes with positioning**—At such times the tube might have to be positioned closer to the patient.
   c. When the x-ray tube is overheating
   d. When children are fidgety

9. A larger OID has what effect on unsharpness?
   a. **Increased unsharpness**—This is a geometric principle resulting from the beam coming from an area rather than a single point source.
   b. Decreased unsharpness
   c. No effect on unsharpness
   d. Effect depends on kVp

10. What is the main reason small focal spots cannot always be used?
   a. The generator could not consistently supply enough power.
   b. Patient exposure would be too great in some circumstances.
   c. Grids cannot be used with small focal spots.
   d. **The x-ray tube would overheat.** Heat is produced where the incident electrons strike the anode (the focal spot), and the smaller this area, the hotter the tube becomes, limiting the use of small focal spots to lower-energy exams.

11. Grids are used to do which of the following?
   a. Improve density
   b. Reduce magnification
   c. **Reduce scatter**—They do this by allowing only those x-rays traveling in a straight line to pass through.
   d. Lower patient exposure

12. Which x-rays can pass through a grid?
   a. **Those traveling in a straight line**—X-rays traveling at an angle (as results with scatter) are absorbed in the lead strips of the grid.
   b. Those deflected in the patient's body
   c. Those scattered inside the patient
   d. Those absorbed inside the patient

13. A contrast improvement factor of 2 means that using a grid does which of the following?
   a. **Doubles the amount of contrast on an image**—This is the basic definition of the contrast improvement factor.
   b. Halves the amount of contrast on an image
   c. Doubles the density with out changing the contrast
   d. Halves the density without changing the contrast

14. Inherent filtration includes which of the following?
   a. **The x-ray tube glass envelope**—Inherent filtration is filtration that occurs naturally by part of the tube and collimator, as opposed to intentionally added filtration.
   b. Aluminum filters mounted in the tube port
   c. Intensifying screens
   d. Grids

15. Why do federal regulations require minimum filtration levels?
   a. To standardize image quality
   b. To protect radiographers
   c. **To minimize patient dose**—Filtration removes low-energy x-rays that are typically absorbed in the patient and add nothing to the diagnostic image.
   d. To guard against x-ray tube malfunctions

Testbank Questions

1. One kilovolt equals which of the following?
   a. 1/1000 of 1 volt
   b. 100 volts
   c. 1000 volts
   d. None of the above

2. The higher the kVp,
   a. The more x-rays are produced
   b. The fewer x-rays are produced
   c. The more high-energy x-rays are produced
   d. The more low-energy x-rays are produced

3. Which factor has the greatest effect on contrast in a radiograph?
   a. kVp
   b. SID
   c. Focal point size
   d. All have equal effect

4. If the mA is 400 and the mAs is 80, how long is the exposure time?
   a. 0.02 seconds
   b. 0.2 seconds
   c. 2 seconds
   d. 20 seconds

5. When using a radiographic unit with a falling load generator, you usually cannot select which of the following?
   a. mAs
   b. mA
   c. kVp
   d. All of the above
   e. None of the above

6. If the kVp is high enough that the beam penetrates the part, the density on the radiograph is directly proportional to which of the following?
   a. kVp
   b. contrast
   c. SID
   d. mAs

7. An SID of 72 inches is typically used for which of the following?
   a. Chest exams
   b. Extremity exams
   c. Contrast exams
   d. All of the above
   e. None of the above

8. The technique chart says to use an mAs of 100 and an SID of 72 inches; instead, you need to use an SID of 36 inches. What should the mAs be?
   a. 25 mAs
   b. 50 mAs
   c. 100 mAs
   d. 200 mAs

9. OID is generally kept as small as possible to minimize which of the following?
   a. Motion blur
   b. Magnification
   c. Scatter
   d. Patient exposure

10. A smaller focal spot does which of the following?
    a. Reduces unsharpness and requires lower mAs settings
    b. Reduces unsharpness and allows higher mAs settings
    c. Increases unsharpness and requires lower mAs settings
    d. Increases unsharpness and allows higher mAs settings

11. A grid can absorb up to how much of scatter radiation?
    a. 10%
    b. 50%
    c. 90%
    d. 100%

12. Where is the grid positioned?
    a. Between the x-ray tube and the patient
    b. Between the patient and the image receptor
    c. On the back side of the film cassette
    d. Any of the above
    e. None of the above

13. Which of the following is a common grid ratio?
    a. 1:1
    b. 8:1
    c. 40:1
    d. 100:1

14. Intensifying screens are used primarily because they provide which of the following?
    a. Greater contrast
    b. More recorded detail
    c. Lower patient doses
    d. All of the above
    e. None of the above

15. For an exam of the toes, would a larger or smaller focal spot produce a better image?
    a. Smaller focal spot
    b. Larger focal spot
    c. Makes no difference
    d. Depends on other factors

16. Filtering the x-ray beam is said to do which of the following?
    a. Soften it
    b. Harden it
    c. Liquefy it
    d. Solidify it

17. Use of added filtration is usually guided by which of the following?
    a. The radiologist's orders
    b. The department's technique charts
    c. The equipment manufacturer's recommendations
    d. All of the above
    e. None of the above

18. Which of the following is an example of a compensating filter?
    a. Wedge filter
    b. Trough filter
    c. Step filter
    d. All of the above
    e. None of the above

19. What is the problem with ripple in the high-voltage power generated for x-ray equipment?
    a. The voltage is too high, causing too much patient exposure.
    b. The voltage is too low, causing too little density in the image.
    c. The voltage produces an alternating current that overheats the rectifiers.
    d. The voltage fluctuates and produces a pulsating x-ray beam.

20. Three-phase power in the high-voltage generator is better than single-phase power because three-phase power has which of the following?
    a. Lower ripple
    b. Higher ripple
    c. Higher voltage
    d. Lower voltage

Answers to Testbank Questions

1. c	6. d	11. c	16. b
2. c	7. a	12. b	17. b
3. a	8. a	13. b	18. d
4. b	9. b	14. c	19. d
5. b	10. a	15. a	20. a

Audiovisual Script

SLIDE 7-1/CD 7-i Welcome
Welcome to Mosby's Radiographic Instructional Series

SLIDE 7-2/CD 7-ii Exposure selection
The module you are about to experience is the seventh of eight in the Radiographic Imaging program: Exposure Selection.

This module will help you understand the relationships of technique factors and their effects on exposure selection. You will learn how factors, such as mAs and kVp, affect radiographic qualities such as density and contrast so that you can make selections that will produce the best images possible.

SLIDE 7-3/CD 7-1 Introduction
Let's begin this module on exposure selection by repeating that what you've already learned is the very essence of medical radiography. It's the science surrounding the transmission of x-rays through parts of the body to create images that can be used for diagnosis and treatment of illness.

You'll recall that as x-rays pass through the body, they interact in different ways. The kind of interaction depends on the intensity of the x-rays and the size and tissue density of the part of the body being examined. These variables produce different degrees of density, or film blackening. Recall that contrast is the variation of density in adjacent areas on the finished radiograph. Contrast makes the detail visible. Density and contrast are the properties that show the structural details on a radiograph.

Areas of high density appear dark on the radiograph, indicating more x-rays exiting from the patient. Low density appears whiter on the radiograph, indicating fewer x-rays exiting the patient. A good quality radiograph shows a balance of lighter and darker densities, making diagnosis easier.

SLIDE 7-4/CD 7-2 Density
That perfect balance of high to low densities doesn't just happen. To achieve it, you need to know how to select the right combination of exposure factors for each radiographic procedure you do.

And in order to be able to make those kinds of judgments on a routine basis, you have to thoroughly understand each of these exposure factors and how they relate to one another. That knowledge builds on what you know about anatomy, patient positioning, and pathological conditions. When all of those factors come together, you'll get the excellent results you want in every examination you perform.

CD 7-2A Exposure settings
As you've learned in earlier modules, technological advances are producing radiographic equipment that is more and more sophisticated. Technique charts, if followed closely, can help guide the use of this equipment and produce consistent results on the finished radiographs.

Still, there are lots of variables you have to control and decisions you need to make. Automation takes some of the guesswork out of radiography, but it doesn't eliminate the need for sound knowledge and the ability to make technical decisions specific to each exam. As the radiographer, you're still the human, and the most important player.

SLIDE 7-5/CD 7-3 mAs and kVp

Your biggest responsibility is to decide, for each procedure, how many and what energy level x-rays to direct through the patient to get the results you want. You've already learned quite a bit about kilovoltage peak (kVp), and milliampere seconds (mAs), the two factors that control x-ray quality and quantity. Those are the most important factors under your control and are closely linked.

Other factors come into play too, as we'll discuss as we go along. They are variables like the size of the focal spot, distance, filtration, and so on. On newer equipment, those factors are often standardized, or there may be fewer options to choose from.

CD 7-3A Kilovoltage

You've heard over and over again the term kilovoltage. It means the amount of energy that's needed to produce usable x-rays. But you also know that when you're talking about the energy required to power a hair dryer or your CD player, you talk about volts. Why the difference?

The prefix "kilo," or thousand, is always attached to the word "volts" in radiography, and is expressed as kilovolts because a high energy is needed to produce x-rays capable of penetrating the body. It's just easier to refer to 70 kV (or kVp, the peak energy level), than saying 70,000 volts.

SLIDE 7-6/CD 7-4 High and low kVp settings

Let's first discuss kVp and the ways to manipulate it as you select exposure factors. What you must remember is that kVp is the most important influence on the quality of the x-ray beam and, therefore, the beam's ability to penetrate the body. How thoroughly the beam penetrates the body determines the density level and how wide a scale of contrast there will be on the radiograph.

The higher the kVp, the more high-energy x-rays are produced, making the x-ray beam more penetrating and lowering the dose to the patient. These are reasons why most radiography departments prefer to use high kVp techniques. However, as you may remember, high kVp increases the amount of scatter radiation reaching the film, thus decreasing contrast.

SLIDE 7-7/CD 7-5 Body part thickness

The first step in selecting the appropriate kVp is to assess the thickness and tissue type of the body part you are examining. The goal is to have sufficient penetration to produce a radiograph with adequate contrast and density.

Other factors may affect your choice of kVp. They include the use of a grid, use of beam-restricting devices, the radiologists' preferred density and contrast levels, screen-film combinations used, and use of any contrast media.

Most radiography departments don't use the minimum kVp settings. Consult your technique chart to find out what the recommended kVp is for the particular exam you're about to perform, and use it as a starting point for choosing the correct kVp.

CD 7-5A High kVp technique

Use of high kVp allows you to use lower mAs. This results in lower contrast while maintaining adequate density. It may, however, result in a slightly decreased visibility of detail on the finished radiograph.

SLIDE 7-8/CD 7-6 Milliamperage

You should be rather confident by now in your understanding of how kilovoltage controls the quality of the x-ray beam being produced in the tube. Now let's talk about milliamperage, which, on the other hand, controls how many x-rays are produced.

When you choose the mA setting on the control panel of an x-ray machine, you are choosing the quantity of electrons that will be released to strike the anode and create the x-ray beam. The more electrons traveling through the tube, the more x-rays there will be produced.

The relationship between the number of electrons and the number of x-rays produced is directly proportional. That means if you change the mA setting from 200 to 400, for example, you are doubling the number of electrons passing through the tube. This doesn't affect the quality of the x-rays: quality remains the same. Remember that quality refers to the energy level of the x-rays, while quantity refers to how many x-rays are produced.

SLIDE 7-9/CD 7-7 Milliamperage seconds

You'll notice that the terms mA and mAs seem to be used interchangeably. But make sure you know the difference between the two, even though the consoles on much newer radiographic equipment have only one setting, mAs.

The ampere (A) is one unit of electric current and is equal to one coulomb (C) traveling through a conductor each second.

A milliampere (mA) is one thousandth (1/1,000) of an ampere. When you multiply the quantity of electricity in milliamperes by the time in seconds you get mAs.

CD 7-7A Review: kVp and mA

Let's take a moment to review. kVp and mAs are the two primary factors to consider when making your exposure selection. kVp determines the quality of the x-ray beam and the beam's ability to penetrate the body to produce a visible image. What property of radiographs does kVp influence?

a. Density
b. Contrast
c. Fog
d. Distortion

Click on your answer now.

PRESENT THIS AUDIO IF ANSWER WAS b: Yes, of course you're right. When x-rays have a high energy level and penetrate the body part well, the image will show differences between adjacent shades of density. This is called contrast.

PRESENT THIS AUDIO IF ANSWER WAS a, c, or d: No, you missed this one. It's easy to get a bit confused when you talk about contrast and density. But when the kVp is at a high enough setting to produce x-rays that penetrate the body part well, the image will show differences between adjacent shades of density. This is called contrast.

SLIDE 7-10/CD 7-8 Maximum equipment capacity

Radiographic equipment is commonly labeled by how much electricity the tube uses. Those intended to be used in a relatively limited way, such as those in physicians' offices, generally have a high capacity of 600 mA and a low setting of 50 mA.

More sophisticated equipment (which is usually more expensive, too) is designed to be used in modern radiography suites for a variety of procedures. It has a higher mA capacity, usually a top of 1200 mA.

SLIDE 7-11/CD 7-9 mA and second relationships

Just as kVp controls contrast on the radiograph, mAs controls optical density. These two exposure factors work closely together. To determine the mAs, you multiply the milliamperage by the exposure time, which is usually kept as short as possible.

It's always important to keep the exposure as low as possible to reduce the amount of radiation the patient is exposed to. But in fact, a short exposure time also reduces patient motion. Patient motion, you may remember, causes blur on the image.

So let's say the technique chart in your department calls for a milliamperage rate (mA) of 400 and an exposure time of 200 milliseconds (ms) for a particular examination. You can see in this illustration that 1000 ms is equal to 1 second. How do you calculate the correct mAs?

If you said multiply 400 mA by 0.2 seconds for an mAs of 80, you're right.

CD 7-9A Review: milliampere-seconds

Let's take a moment to review here to make sure you understand the relationship between mA and exposure time. Assume you must perform a procedure that calls for an mA of 300 and an exposure time of 500 milliseconds. What is the mAs?

a. 200
b. 100
c. 150
d. 80

Click on your answer now.

PRESENT THIS AUDIO IF ANSWER WAS c: Yes, you calculated correctly. The mAs is 150, which means you're thinking straight. To get that number, you multiply 300 by 0.5 seconds.

PRESENT THIS AUDIO IF ANSWER WAS a, b, or d: No, you missed this one. The mAs is 150. To get that number, you multiply 300 by 0.5 seconds.

SLIDE 7-12/CD 7-10 mA and seconds combinations

There isn't one magic combination of numbers that will achieve the right mAs. You can get a consistent result by manipulating mA and time in different ways to get the mAs you want. Remember that mA is inversely proportional to exposure time.

Look, for example, at this chart to see the different mixes of time and milliamperes that result in the same mAs of 10. When you know the mAs you want for a procedure, you have enough flexibility to change the settings in various ways to reach that mAs.

Not all equipment will allow you this flexibility, though. In more up-to-date and expensive units with a falling-load generator, the only choice you can make is the mAs. The exposure factors have already been set at the highest mA and the shortest exposure time the generator can accommodate. We'll talk more about generators later on in this module.

SLIDE 7-13/CD 7-11 mA and number of x-rays

Increasing the mAs increases the number of projectile electrons, thus increasing the number of x-rays produced. When the kVp is set at a particular level, the electrons going from cathode to anode will have varying energy levels. The x-ray beam will be made of x-ray photons with varying energies.

There's another principle to remember. When the kVp is set high enough that the beam penetrates the part, the density on the resulting radiograph is directly proportional to the mAs.

For example, the kVp might be high enough to penetrate the part, but there may not be enough density on the image to see it clearly. You can double the density by doubling the mAs.

SLIDE 7-14/CD 7-12 Image quality and kVp and mA

This concludes this section on kVp and mAs, the primary technique factors that influence density and contrast. You've seen how closely related kVp and mAs are, and how changing one will frequently require a compensating change of the other.

SLIDE 7-15/CD 7-13 Technique factors

You have begun the topic of secondary technique factors and how they affect exposure selection. This topic builds on the preceding topic of the primary factors affecting exposure selection and how they influence radiographic qualities such as density and contrast. If you haven't yet worked through the earlier topic, you may want to quit this section now and return later after going through it.

kVp and mAs are the first variables to think about as you select exposure factors, but there are several other considerations to keep in mind that will also make a difference in the kind of image you produce. Let's turn our attention now to distance, focal spots, grids, and intensifying screens.

SLIDE 7-16/CD 7-14 Effects of SID

We'll begin with distance, specifically the distance between the source of the x-rays and the image receptor. This is called the SID, for source-to-image receptor distance. This distance can influence the sharpness of the radiographic image. As a general rule, there is more magnification as the SID decreases.

An x-ray beam, like other electromagnetic radiation, is strongest at its point of origin and decreases as the beam spreads out. The quality of the x-rays doesn't change, but the beam fans out as it spreads over a larger distance, and its intensity is decreased the farther it goes. Exposure factors must be changed to maintain the intensity of the beam when the distance is changed.

SLIDE 7-17/CD 7-15 Beam intensity and SID

You can calculate the difference in intensity of the x-ray beam by using the inverse square law, which you may remember from an earlier module. It states that the amount of radiation reaching an object is inversely proportional to the square of the distance between the object and the source.

Doubling the SID will reduce the beam's intensity and the resultant density to one quarter. Or, conversely, cutting the SID in half will make the intensity of the beam and the density as they reach the film four times as great.

MORE INFO LEADS TO THIS AUDIO RESPONSE: To repeat, the inverse square law goes like this: the amount of light or radiation reaching an object from a source is inversely proportional to the square of the distance between the object and the source.

Think of it this way in radiography. A patient positioned 1 meter from the x-ray tube is exposed to four times as much radiation as that patient would be if positioned 2 meters away. The reason for this decrease in intensity at the longer distance is because the total amount of radiation is spread over a larger area.

SLIDE 7-18/CD 7-16 Technique chart and SID

Every radiology department has its own SID standards for examinations of different parts of the body. The SID is usually set at a standard of 40 inches for most routine procedures. That ensures an acceptable level of detail and magnification. The standard SID for a chest radiograph is 72 inches in most institutions.

It is not common to use an SID longer than 72 inches. Anything over that does provide better detail, but it's impractical with most equipment.

The standard SID depends on a number of exposure variables. The most important considerations are achieving a balance of resolution and acceptable patient dose. Increasing the SID decreases magnification of the image if the OID remains constant. Effective technique charts will list the SID for each exam.

SLIDE 7-19/CD 7-17 SID and mA

If a radiologist asks for a different SID or if exposure conditions exist that warrant changing it, you'll also have to change other factors to maintain an acceptable level of density. A longer SID will produce more sharpness on the image.

To get a specific level of density on an image, you have to change the mAs. The general rule is that if the SID is greater than the one listed on the technique chart, increase the mAs. If the SID is less, decrease the mAs.

SLIDE 7-20/CD 7-18 Formula: mA and SID changes

But increase or decrease the mAs by how much? Calculations can be done in different ways, but probably the easiest is the one you see in this illustration.

Here's what the numbers mean: mAs 1 equals the value from the technique chart; mAs 2 equals the value to be calculated; D1 equals the SID from the technique chart; and D2 equals the SID to be used.

CD 7-18A Exercise: mA and SID formula

Now let's try putting the formula to work. Let's say the technique for a particular procedure calls for an mAs of 100 and an SID of 72 inches. If the new SID is to become 36 inches, what should the new mAs be?

a. 150
b. 125
c. 75
d. 50
e. 25

Click on your answer now.

PRESENT THIS AUDIO IF ANSWER WAS e: You're right. The new mAs is 25. You can see that when the SID is cut in half, the new mAs is a quarter of the original setting.

PRESENT THIS AUDIO IF ANSWER WAS a, b, c, or d: No, take a minute to think this one through again. The new mAs is 25. What's happened here is that when the SID is cut in half, the new mAs is a quarter of the original setting.

SLIDE 7-21/CD 7-19 SID and inverse square law

As you study this illustration, you can better understand why this rule applies. Remember that mAs controls the quantity of x-rays produced. They move out in a cone shape from the x-ray tube and spread out, so that fewer reach the body area being examined as the distance is increased.

In this illustration, we've superimposed one x-ray path over another, showing what happens as the x-rays exit the tube and head towards the patient. The SID is set at 36 inches for the first patient in line, but is doubled to 72 inches for the second patient. Four times as many x-rays reach the first patient's chest as reach the second's. At a SID of 72 inches, the number of x-rays is only a quarter of what it was originally.

Do you see how the inverse square law works here?

SLIDE 7-22/CD 7-20 Short SID uses

There are some situations that might require changing the SID. If you're having difficulty penetrating an extremely large patient and have reached maximum tube potential, you might have to decrease the SID in order to get a diagnostic exposure.

You may also have difficulty positioning the equipment in some cases to maintain the standard SID. For example, traction beds can pose a challenge when trying to position portable equipment over the patient. Operating rooms may also have other equipment present that interferes with positioning. Using different SIDs in such cases will require that you adjust the technique.

SLIDE 7-23/CD 7-21 OID and magnification

The object-to-image receptor distance (OID) is another factor to consider. As it increases, there is more magnification on the image, so it should always be kept as short as possible. Magnification decreases the radiographic detail. The radiograph you see here shows magnification.

SLIDE 7-24/CD 7-22 OID and unsharpness

On the other hand, when the OID is increased, that increases the amount of penumbra, or radiographic unsharpness, in the image. You can see that in this illustration. And unsharpness, of course, means the radiographic detail is not as good.

CD 7-22A Review: standard SIDs

Let's pause a moment to review. As you've just learned, most routine radiography examinations are performed at an SID of 40 inches or 72 inches. Why are these the standards for the source-to-image receptor distance?

The reason why a 40 inch SID is standard is that it provides an acceptable balance between magnification and detail as well as being a practical tube-over-table height. A 72 inch SID is used for chest radiographs in order to reduce magnification of the heart.

SLIDE 7-25/CD 7-23 Focal spot and unsharpness

Now let's move on to focal spot size and see how this makes a difference when you're selecting exposure factors. If there were one tiny point that x-rays emerged from, there would never be any unsharpness or poorly defined edges on the radiograph. But in reality, the x-ray tube emits x-rays from a wider area of the anode, so there is always some unsharpness.

The large focal spot has a higher technique capacity than the small one. Most tubes have focal spots ranging from 0.6 mm to 1.2 mm. The size of the focal spot chosen depends on the body part thickness to be examined.

Using a small focal spot will produce higher detail on the radiograph, but a larger focal spot may be necessary so that you can select a mAs setting high enough to produce the exposure you need.

SLIDE 7-26/CD 7-24 Unsharpness and detail

The reason there's less detail on a radiograph when a large focal spot has been used is that x-rays are emitted from a wider area of the anode. That creates more unsharpness on the image. A high mA, usually over 200, frequently necessitates use of a large focal spot.

The best detail and the least amount of unsharpness will occur with a small focal spot, a long SID, and a short OID. This illustration shows two different sized focal spots and how they affect the amount of unsharpness created on the image.

CD 7-24A Focal spot size and mA

The reason a small focal spot cannot be used with high mA techniques is that the small area will not produce enough x-ray photons without overheating. Most tubes are designed to indicate to the user when a technique using a small focal spot is not possible.

Small focal spots are good for examining thin parts of the body when a large number of x-rays is not needed to expose dense areas.

SLIDE 7-27/CD 7-25 Grid

Besides changing exposure settings, you have accessories that can be used to help obtain a quality image. A grid is an accessory used with an x-ray machine to lower the amount of scatter radiation reaching the film and thereby improve contrast. Decisions about when to use a grid and what kind to use are part of the overall decision-making process.

The grid is related most directly to kVp. When you choose a high kVp setting to make sure the intensity of the x-ray beam will penetrate the part you want to examine, a side effect is that more scatter radiation is produced. Too much scatter radiation reduces contrast, and you can end up with a gray film that isn't particularly useful for diagnostic purposes.

Using a grid to absorb some of the scatter radiation will increase the contrast. A grid is said to have good "cleanup" when it's able to absorb a large percentage (up to 90%) of scattered radiation.

CD 7-25A Composition of grids

A grid is composed of strips of radiopaque material such as lead, which doesn't let radiation through, separated by radiolucent material such as aluminum or plastic, which lets radiation pass through. The purpose of the grid is to allow only x-rays traveling in a direct line from the tube to pass through the radiolucent material to reach the film. The lead strips absorb scattered x-rays traveling at an angle. The grid is placed between the patient and the image receptor.

SLIDE 7-28/CD 7-26 Grids absorb scatter

Contrast in the image is better when scatter radiation is absorbed by a grid. How much better is measured by what's called the contrast improvement factor, which is usually measured at a baseline of 100 kVp.

The contrast improvement factor is the ratio of contrast on the image taken with a grid to contrast on the image taken without a grid. It's constant at 1: anything over that, such as 1.5 to 2.5, is proof the grid is doing it's job. A contrast improvement factor of 2, for example, means the level of contrast is doubled by using the grid.

SLIDE 7-29/CD 7-27 Grid ratio

The grid ratio is the ratio between the height of the lead strips in a grid and the width of the interspace material between them. You can see the lead strips in this illustration. There are lots of different grid ratios available.

You'll see the grid ratio expressed in two numbers representing lead-strip height and interspace width. Common ratios, for example, include 5:1, 6:1, 8:1, 12:1, and 16:1.

Grid ratios of 5:1 and 6:1 are used in mobile radiography and work efficiently at kVp levels of up to 80. A ratio of 8:1 works well at up to 100 kVp. Exposures above 100 kVp usually use a grid ratio of 12:1 and 16:1.

Mammography uses lower grid ratios, those of 2:1 to 4:1.

SLIDE 7-30/CD 7-28 Grid ratio and kVp and mA

The disadvantage of using a grid is that the exposure must be increased in order to penetrate the grid, and that increases the dose of radiation to the patient. Still, with dedicated equipment, the dose is offset by the benefit of the image quality.

SLIDE 7-31/CD 7-29 Intensifying screens

You should recall learning about intensifying screens in an earlier module. These screens, used along with the film and classified by their speed, are sheets coated with phosphors that give off light when they're struck by x-rays. The fluorescing light creates most of the density on the film.

Intensifying screens react to exposures differently depending on the kVp setting. They respond less and create less fluorescent light at lower settings than at higher ones. Exposures that use intensifying screens produce shorter contrast scales than those that don't use them. Almost all radiographic procedures done today use intensifying screens.

SLIDE 7-32/CD 7-30 Film cassettes

Some film cassette screens contain a dye in the phosphor that helps absorb some scattered light photons that contribute to density but provide no useful image information.

CD 7-30A Review: focal spot sizes

Let's pause to review before we move on. You've learned there are small and large focal spots, and the size you choose has an impact on the image that's created. A larger focal spot is used with thicker body parts that require higher exposure settings for adequate penetration. If you were performing an examination of a hand, would you choose a small or a large focal spot? Click on your answer.

PRESENT THIS AUDIO IF ANSWER WAS small: Yes, you're right. A hand is a relatively thin part of the body and doesn't require an intense x-ray beam to penetrate it. That holds true also with other parts of the body that are not too dense.

PRESENT THIS AUDIO IF ANSWER WAS large: No, you missed this one. Performing a radiographic examination of the hand can be accomplished with a small focal spot. A hand is a relatively thin part of the body and doesn't require an intense x-ray beam to penetrate it. That holds true also with other parts of the body that are not too dense.

SLIDE 7-33/CD 7-31 Radiographs comparing detail

This concludes this section on the secondary technique factors that influence exposure selection and the way they impact density and contrast. As you've seen, the choices you make about distance, focal spot, grids, and intensifying screens make a difference in the kind of image quality you'll get.

SLIDE 7-34/CD 7-32 Introduction to filtration

You have begun the topic of filtration and generation of x-rays and how they affect exposure selection. This topic builds on the preceding topic of the secondary factors affecting exposure selection. If you haven't yet worked through the earlier topic, you may want to quit this section now and return later after going through it.

So far, we've been dealing with settings that often you can change on the operating console of the x-ray equipment. Two other factors, filtration and generation of x-rays, also affect exposure selection, but you have less ability to control them. Let's turn our attention now to the different kinds of filtration and the generation of x-rays and what relationship they have to exposure selection.

SLIDE 7-35/CD 7-33 Filtration removes photons

Filtration involves a substance passing through a material that stops or "catches" some of the substance trying to pass through. Think of water mixing with coffee grounds and being filtered so that only the coffee drips into the pot, not the coffee grounds.

In radiography, filtration means removing some x-ray photons from the x-ray beam, somewhat like removing coffee grounds from the coffee. Certain types of materials are put in the path of the beam to filter it. The beam generated inside the tube is first filtered by the glass envelope of the x-ray tube as the x-rays pass out of the tube. That's called inherent filtration because the glass tube is part of the equipment and naturally filters some of the photons.

SLIDE 7-36/CD 7-34 Inherent and added filtration

The standard rate of inherent filtration for common x-ray tubes is 0.5 to 1.0 mm Al equivalent. The reflective surface of the collimator mirror in the x-ray machine adds another 0.5 to 0.1 mm Al equivalent. Federal regulations call for 2.5 mm Al equivalent with a tube potential greater than 70 kVp, so equipment manufacturers add another layer of filtration between the x-ray tube housing and the collimator.

The benefit of filtration is that it hardens the beam, or increases its energy, by filtering out low-energy x-ray photons.

MORE INFO LEADS TO THIS AUDIO RESPONSE: Let's recall the meaning of the term Al equivalent. When the rate of filtration is being measured, it's compared to the same amount of filtration in the same amount of aluminum. For example, an x-ray tube whose inherent filtration is 1 mm has the same amount of filtration capacity as 1 mm thickness of aluminum.

SLIDE 7-37/CD 7-35 Inherent filtration
Inherent filtration that's contained inside the equipment is, obviously, beyond your control. But you may use equipment that has filtration added to it, and you can make adjustments to that. The technique chart in your department will guide you towards making the proper setting. Usually, the level of added filtration is fairly low and is standardized.

SLIDE 7-38/CD 7-36 Compensating filters
You can also use filters to even out the density on the image. That's often done for examinations of parts of the body that have significant differences in tissue density or thickness. Wedge and trough filters, which you learned about in an earlier module, are examples of this kind of compensating filter.

Using these types of filters usually means you have to adjust settings on the control panel to get the density the radiologist wants. But a higher kVp, for example, might result in such a loss of contrast that the image isn't helpful in diagnosis. The imaging department, therefore, has standards for the degree of density and contrast.

MORE INFO LEADS TO THIS AUDIO RESPONSE: All kinds of filtration make an impact on density and contrast. Filtration increases the average photon energy of the beam, thus decreasing contrast. To maintain the same level of contrast, you would need to lower the kVp.

SLIDE 7-39/CD 7-37 Electric generators
The x-ray generator is a combination of circuits and electrical components that supplies power to the x-ray tube. Although you can't choose the type of generator available to you, you do make decisions about other settings influenced by the generator. It's helpful to know a little about how generators work and how to consider them when selecting exposure factors.

You can see the basic elements of an electric generator with an alternating current (AC) in this illustration. There's a coil of wire between two magnetic poles, N and S. Some form of mechanical energy rotates the coil, producing a current in it. Since the current flows in different directions, it produces an alternating current and is not constant.

SLIDE 7-40/CD 7-38 Control panel for falling-load generator
Some x-ray equipment is powered by a high-voltage generator called a falling-load generator. The control panel has a setting for mAs, not two separate settings for mA and exposure time. The mAs is set automatically at optimal settings for the best image production.

SLIDE 7-41/CD 7-39 Single-phase waveform
As you work in radiography you'll become familiar with different types of high-voltage generators in use. These include single-phase (which you see in this illustration), three-phase, and high frequency. The type of generator used affects how many and what kind of x-rays are produced in the x-ray tube.

One way generators are rated is by the ripple factor, expressed as a percentage. Remember that kVp measures the peak amount of kilovoltage. The ripple factor is the amount the voltage drops from the maximum. Single-phase power, for example, has a 100% ripple, which means the voltage goes from 100% to 0, causing a pulsating x-ray beam. The x-rays produced when the waveform has a value of zero or little more than that aren't of much diagnostic use because they are too weak to penetrate the body.

SLIDE 7-42/CD 7-40 Three-phase waveform

Three-phase power is a big improvement on single-phase. Waveforms are at a consistently high voltage, so the x-rays have a higher average photon energy level and are of more diagnostic use.

SLIDE 7-43/CD 7-41 High-frequency waveform

More recently developed, the high-frequency generator delivers high voltage to the x-ray tube and results in a waveform with less than 1% ripple.

SLIDE 7-44/CD 7-42 Quiz instructions

THIS AUDIO FOR SLIDE/TAPE ONLY: This concludes the presentation section of this module. If you are not going to work through the self-assessment quiz that now follows, you may stop the program at this point and turn off the equipment. If your instructor has asked you to take this self-assessment quiz on the material you have learned in this module, you should have a piece of paper ready. There will be 10 questions with multiple-choice or short answers. After this self-assessment we will go back through these questions and briefly talk about the reasons for the correct answers. Ready?

THIS AUDIO IN CD ROM LECTURE MODE ONLY: You have reached the self-assessment quiz for this module. Here you will be asked 10 questions to help you assess how well you understand what you have learned in this module. The questions are multiple-choice or have short answers. After this self-assessment we'll go back through these questions and briefly talk about your answers and the reasons for the correct answers. Ready?

THIS AUDIO IN CD ROM STUDENT MODE ONLY: You have reached the self-assessment quiz for this module. Here you will be asked 10 questions to help you assess how well you understand what you have learned in this module. The questions are multiple-choice or have short answers. For multiple-choice questions, click on the box next to your answer choice. For those questions that require a short answer, type in your answer at the keyboard and press Enter. After this self-assessment we'll go back through these questions and briefly talk about your answers and the reasons for the correct answers.

SLIDE 7-45/CD 7-43 Quiz question 1

1. As you prepare the exposure settings for each examination you perform, what is your biggest responsibility?
   a. To select patient dose
   b. To select length of the exposure
   c. To select quality and quantity of the x-rays produced
   d. To select the distance from the source of x-rays to the film

SLIDE 7-46/CD 7-44 Quiz question 2

2. The quality of the x-ray beam, or its penetrating ability, depends on which of the following?
   a. mAs
   b. kVp
   c. The amount of scatter radiation present
   d. The length of the exposure

SLIDE 7-47/CD 7-45 Quiz question 3

3. As a general rule, most radiology departments prefer which of these kVp settings?
   a. High
   b. Low

SLIDE 7-48/CD 7-46 Quiz question 4

4. Which one of these factors does mAs control?
   a. Optical density on the radiograph
   b. Contrast on the radiograph
   c. The amount of scatter radiation produced
   d. The penetrating ability of the x-ray beam

SLIDE 7-49/CD 7-47 Quiz question 5

5. mAs is calculated by multiplying milliamperage by exposure time measured in seconds. Can you mix different time and milliamperages to produce the same mAs?
   a. No
   b. Yes

SLIDE 7-50/CD 7-48 Quiz question 6

6. What is the standard SID setting for most routine radiography procedures?
   a. 60 inches
   b. 40 inches
   c. 56 inches
   d. 72 inches

SLIDE 7-51/CD 7-49 Quiz question 7

7. The use of a grid and how it affects the radiograph is linked most closely to the kVp setting used. Which of the following does a grid affect most?
   a. Detail
   b. Unsharpness
   c. Magnification
   d. Contrast

SLIDE 7-52/CD 7-50 Quiz question 8

8. True or false: A disadvantage to using a grid is that it increases the radiation dose to the patient.
   a. True
   b. False

SLIDE 7-53/CD 7-51 Quiz question 9

9. The advantage of filtration is that it increases the energy of the x-ray beam, making it harder and more able to penetrate the body. How does it do this?
   a. By deflecting scatter radiation
   b. By slowing down the x-ray flow
   c. By increasing the number of x-rays produced
   d. By removing low-energy photons

SLIDE 7-54/CD 7-52 Quiz question 10

10. True or false: Exposures using intensifying screens produce shorter contrast scales than those that don't use them.
   a. False
   b. True

SLIDE 7-55/CD 7-53 Quiz review

This concludes the self-assessment quiz for Module 7: Exposure Selection. Let's quickly go back through the questions and see how you did.

SLIDE 7-56/CD 7-54 Review question 1

Question 1 asked you what your biggest responsibility is as you get ready to select the exposure.

The correct answer is c, the quality and quantity of the x-ray beams produced. kVp determines the quality of the beam, and mAs controls how many x-rays there are in the beam. This is important because various parts of the body absorb x-rays at different rates. How many x-rays you direct to the part being examined, and how penetrating they are, are what determine the quality of the image that is produced.

CD 7-54A Review question 1

Question 1 asked you what your biggest responsibility is as you get ready to select exposure.

PRESENT THIS AUDIO IF ANSWER WAS c: Yes, you're right. The correct answer is c, the quality and quantity of the x-ray beams produced. kVp determines the quality of the beam, and mAs controls how many x-rays there are in the beam. This is important because various parts of the body absorb x-rays at different rates. How many x-rays you direct to the part being examined, and how penetrating they are, are what determine the quality of the image that is produced.

PRESENT THIS AUDIO IF ANSWER WAS a, b, or d: No, sorry, your answer is incorrect. The correct answer is c, the quality and quantity of the x-ray beams produced. kVp determines the quality of the beam, and mAs controls how many x-rays there are in the beam. This is important because various parts of the body absorb x-rays at different rates. How many x-rays you direct to the part being examined, and how penetrating they are, are what determine the quality of the image that is produced.

SLIDE 7-57/CD 7-55 Review question 2

Question 2 asked what the quality of the x-ray beam, or its penetrating ability, depends on.

The correct answer is b, kVp. The higher you set the kVp, the more high-energy x-rays are produced and the better their ability to penetrate the body part being examined. The drawback to a high kVp is that it also produces more scatter radiation, so you must compensate for that by using grids and tight collimation.

CD 7-55A Review question 2
Question 2 asked you what the quality of the x-ray beam, or its penetrating ability, depends on.

PRESENT THIS AUDIO IF ANSWER WAS b: Yes, you correctly answered this one, which is kVp. The higher you set the kVp, the more high-energy x-rays are produced, and the better their ability to penetrate the body part being examined. The drawback to a high kVp is that it also produces more scatter radiation, so you must compensate for that by using grids and tight collimation.

PRESENT THIS AUDIO IF ANSWER WAS a, c, d: No, you incorrectly answered this one. The right answer is b, kVp. The higher you set the kVp, the more high energy x-rays are produced, and the better their ability to penetrate the body part being examined. The drawback to high kVp is that it also produces more scatter radiation, so you must compensate for that by using grids and tight collimation.

SLIDE 7-58/CD 7-56 Review question 3
Question 3 asked, as a general rule, which kVp setting most radiology departments prefer.

The correct answer is a high kVp setting. A higher kVp produces x-rays that better penetrate the body. That's most useful to the radiologist. But as you've learned, a by-product of high kVp is more scatter radiation, so you must make adjustments for that.

CD 7-56A Review question 3
Question 3 asked if whether, as a general rule, which kVp setting most radiology departments prefer.

PRESENT THIS AUDIO IF ANSWER WAS a: Yes, you're correct in answering a high kVp setting. A higher kVp produces x-rays that better penetrate the body. That's most useful to the radiologist. But as you've learned, a by-product of high kVp is more scatter radiation, so you must make adjustments for that.

PRESENT THIS AUDIO IF ANSWER WAS b: Your answer was incorrect. The right answer is a high kVp setting. A higher kVp produces x-rays that better penetrate the body. That's most useful to the radiologist. But as you've learned, a by-product of high kVp is more scatter radiation, so you must make adjustments for that.

SLIDE 7-59/CD 7-57 Review question 4
Question 4 asked what mAs controls.

The correct answer is a, optical density on the radiograph. But the mAs setting is closely related to kVp in affecting the image. To calculate the mAs, multiply the milliamperage by the exposure time as measured in seconds. The exposure time should always be as short as possible.

CD 7-57A Review question 4
Question 4 asked what mAs controls.

PRESENT THIS AUDIO IF ANSWER WAS a: You're right! mAs controls optical density on the radiograph. But the mAs setting is closely related to kVp in affecting the image. To calculate the mAs, multiply the milliamperage by the exposure time as measured in seconds. The exposure time should always be as short as possible.

PRESENT THIS AUDIO IF ANSWER WAS b, c, or d: Sorry, your answer is wrong. mAs controls optical density on the radiograph. But the mAs setting is closely related to kVp in affecting the image. To calculate the mAs, multiply the milliamperage by the exposure time as measured in seconds. The exposure time should always be as short as possible.

SLIDE 7-60/CD 7-58 Review question 5

Question 5 stated that mAs is calculated by multiplying milliamperage by exposure time in seconds. It asked if you can mix different time and milliamperages to produce the same mAs.

The correct answer is b. Yes, it's true there isn't just one combination of numbers that will produce the correct mAs. mA is inversely proportional to exposure time: you can manipulate different milliamperages and exposure times in different ways to get the mAs you want.

CD 7-58A Review question 5

Question 5 stated that mAs is calculated by multiplying milliamperage by exposure time in seconds. It asked if you can mix different time and milliamperages to produce the same mAs.

PRESENT THIS AUDIO IF ANSWER WAS b: You're right! The correct answer is b, yes, it's true there isn't just one combination of numbers that will produce the correct mAs. mA is inversely proportional to exposure time: you can manipulate different milliamperages and exposure times in different ways to get the mAs you want.

PRESENT THIS AUDIO IF ANSWER WAS anything else: Your answer was incorrect. The correct answer is b, yes, it's true there isn't just one combination of numbers that will produce the correct mAs. mA is inversely proportional to exposure time: you can manipulate different milliamperages and exposure times in different ways to get the mAs you want.

SLIDE 7-61/CD 7-59 Review question 6

Question 6 asked what the standard SID setting is for most routine radiography procedures.

The correct answer is b, 40 inches. The SID can range up to 72 inches, which is common for chest x-rays. But most routine procedures are done at 40 inches.

CD 7-59A Review question 6

Question 6 asked what the standard SID setting is for most routine radiography procedures.

PRESENT THIS AUDIO IF ANSWER WAS b: You got the correct answer, b. The SID can range up to 72 inches, which is common for chest x-rays. But most routine procedures are done at 40 inches.

PRESENT THIS AUDIO IF ANSWER WAS a, c, or d: Sorry, you missed it. The right answer is b. The SID can range up to 72 inches, which is common for chest x-rays. But most routine procedures are done at 40 inches.

SLIDE 7-62/CD 7-60 Review question 7
Question 7 stated that the grid is most closely linked to kVp. It asked which of the four factors listed it affected most strongly.

The correct answer is d, contrast. A high kVp setting creates more penetrating x-ray beams, but it also produces more scatter radiation. Using a grid will help to absorb some of that scatter radiation and thereby increase the contrast.

CD 7-60A Review question 7
Question 7 stated that the grid is most closely linked to kVp. It asked which of the four factors listed it affected most strongly.

PRESENT THIS AUDIO IF ANSWER WAS d: Yes, you were right, the answer is d, contrast. A high kVp setting creates more penetrating x-ray beams, but it also produces more scatter radiation. Using a grid will help to absorb some of that scatter radiation and thereby increase the contrast.

PRESENT THIS AUDIO IF ANSWER WAS a, b, or c: No, you missed it. The correct answer is d, contrast. A high kVp setting creates more penetrating x-ray beams, but it also produces more scatter radiation. Using a grid will help to absorb some of that scatter radiation and thereby increase the contrast.

SLIDE 7-63/CD 7-61 Review question 8
Question 8 stated that one disadvantage of the grid is that it increases radiation dose to the patient and asked whether this is true or false.

The answer is a, true. A grid will increase the radiation exposure to the patient.

CD 7-61A Review question 8
Question 8 stated that one disadvantage of the grid is that it increases radiation dose to the patient and asked whether this is true or false.

PRESENT THIS AUDIO FOR ANSWER a: Yes, of course you're correct. The answer is a, true. A grid will increase the radiation exposure to the patient.

PRESENT THIS AUDIO IF ANSWER WAS b: No, you missed this one. The answer is a, true. A grid will increase the radiation exposure to the patient.

SLIDE 7-64/CD 7-62 Review question 9
Question 9 asked how filtration increases the energy of the x-ray beam, making it more able to penetrate the body.

The correct answer is d, by removing low-energy photons. These photons are filtered out. That raises the average energy level of the remaining photons.

CD 7-62A Review question 9
Question 9 asked how filtration increases the energy of the x-ray beam, making it more able to penetrate the body.

PRESENT THIS AUDIO IF ANSWER WAS d: Yes, you're right. The correct answer is d, by removing low-energy photons. These photons are filtered out. That raises the average energy level of the remaining photons.

PRESENT THIS AUDIO IF ANSWER WAS a, b, or c: Sorry, but you missed it. The correct answer is d, by removing low-energy photons. These photons are filtered out. That raises the average energy level of the remaining photons.

SLIDE 7-65/CD 7-63 Review question 10
Question 10 asked if it is true or false that exposures using intensifying screens produce shorter contrast scales than those that don't use them.

The correct answer is b, true. Intensifying screens react less and produce less fluorescent light at lower kVp settings than at higher ones. When intensifying screens are used with high kVp settings, they produce shorter contrast scales than procedures where no intensifying screen is used.

CD 7-63A Review question 10
Question 10 asked if it is true or false that exposures using intensifying screens produce shorter contrast scales than those that don't use them.

PRESENT THIS AUDIO IF ANSWER WAS b: Yes, you're right. It's true. Intensifying screens react less and create less fluorescent light at lower kVp settings than at higher ones. When intensifying screens are used with high kVp settings, they produce shorter contrast scales than procedures where no intensifying screen is used.

PRESENT THIS AUDIO IF ANSWER WAS a: Sorry, you missed it. The correct answer is b, true. Intensifying screens react less and create less fluorescent light at lower kVp settings than at higher ones. When intensifying screens are used with high kVp settings, they produce shorter contrast scales than procedures where no intensifying screen is used.

SLIDE 7-66/CD 7-64 Quiz conclusion
This concludes the self-assessment quiz. This was not intended as a test, so don't feel bad if you missed some. All that means is that you probably need to review this module or study your textbook more carefully.

CD 7-64A Quiz feedback
FOR SCORE OF 10, THIS AUDIO: You've done an excellent job here with a difficult subject. Clearly you are studying well, and you seem to have worked through the tutorial carefully.

FOR SCORE OF 9, THIS AUDIO: You've done well with a difficult subject. Clearly you are studying and paying attention to the subject. Maybe next time you'll get the perfect score!

FOR SCORE OF 7-8, THIS AUDIO: Your score is about average. I'd suggest you review this material in your textbook. You may also find it helpful, next time, to read the material in your book before coming to the computer to take the tutorial. And don't hesitate to talk to your instructor if you have trouble after both reading the textbook and working through the multimedia tutorial.

FOR SCORE OF 5-6, THIS AUDIO: Your score is below average. You need to review this material in your textbook, and perhaps you should come back and take this tutorial again afterwards. You may have just been unprepared this time, or if you are having trouble after both reading the textbook and working through the multimedia tutorial, be sure to talk to your instructor.

FOR SCORE OF 0-4, THIS AUDIO: Your score is rather low. Don't feel too bad; these are, after all, difficult concepts to grasp. If you tried your best here but are having this much difficulty with the material, you should first go to your textbook and see if you can understand the material there. If it still seems difficult, please ask your instructor for additional study aids.

SLIDE 7-67/CD 7-65 Exam instructions

In the next 7 or 8 minutes you will be presented with 15 multiple-choice questions. Select the one best answer choice. Get ready a blank sheet of paper, numbered 1 to 15 down the left side. As you take the examination, write the letter corresponding to your answer choice next to the number for each question. Ready? You will not be asked to perform any complicated calculations.

CD 7-65A More exam instructions

In the next 7 or 8 minutes you will be presented with 15 multiple-choice questions. Select the one best answer choice. This examination covers the material you've been learning about in this tutorial over the last hour or so. It is designed to help you and your instructor determine how well you now grasp this material. You can use scratch paper during the exam if you want, but it shouldn't be necessary for any complicated calculations.

SLIDE 7-68/CD 7-66 Exam question 1

1. Two main factors control the image quality of the radiograph. What are these two factors that you must consider as you select exposure?
   a. mAs and SID
   b. kVp and exposure time
   c. mAs and patient thickness
   d. kVp and mAs

SLIDE 7-69/CD 7-67 Exam question 2

2. True or false: The use of higher kVp requires the radiographer to reduce the mAs to avoid excessive density, and this results in shortened exposure times.
   a. True
   b. False

SLIDE 7-70/CD 7-68 Exam question 3

3. A high kVp setting increases the amount of scatter radiation and density produced. To compensate, which of these exposure factors would you choose?
   a. Higher mAs
   b. Lower mAs
   c. Longer exposure time
   d. Shorter SID

SLIDE 7-71/CD 7-69 Exam question 4

4. What is the top mA setting in up-to-date radiographic equipment designed to be used for a variety of procedures in a busy radiographic suite?
   a. 1,000
   b. 800
   c. 1,200
   d. 900

SLIDE 7-72/CD 7-70 Exam question 5

5. For a particular procedure, a technique chart calls for the mA to be 800 and the exposure time to be 200 milliseconds. What is the correct mAs?
   a. 80
   b. 120
   c. 160
   d. 40

SLIDE 7-73/CD 7-71 Exam question 6

6. True or false: With a high kVp, density is directly proportional to the mAs.
   a. True
   b. False

SLIDE 7-74/CD 7-72 Exam question 7

7. What happens to the degree of magnification on a radiograph when you increase the SID?
   a. It stays the same.
   b. It increases.
   c. It decreases.
   d. It disappears.

SLIDE 7-75/CD 7-73 Exam question 8

8. According to the inverse square law, if you double the distance between the x-ray tube and the film, what happens to the intensity?
   a. It is reduced to 25% of the original.
   b. It is increased by 25% of the original.
   c. It is not affected.
   d. It is doubled.

SLIDE 7-76/CD 7-74 Exam question 9

9. What happens as the OID increases?
   a. Magnification decreases
   b. More scatter radiation is produced
   c. Detail increases
   d. Magnification increases

SLIDE 7-77/CD 7-75 Exam question 10

10. Which of the following is true of a large focal spot?
    a. It may be required with large body parts.
    b. It provides less detail on the image.
    c. It allows you to reduce exposure time.
    d. All of the above are true.

SLIDE 7-78/CD 7-76 Exam question 11

11. Which of the following is a benefit of a small focal spot?
    a. More detail
    b. Less contrast
    c. Less detail
    d. More magnification

SLIDE 7-79/CD 7-77 Exam question 12

12. Which of these procedures typically uses a low-ratio grid?
    a. Chest x-ray
    b. Mammography
    c. Abdominal x-ray
    d. Foot x-ray

SLIDE 7-80/CD 7-78 Exam question 13

13. Which of the following is true?
    a. The more filtration, the less magnification
    b. The more filtration, the less contrast
    c. The more filtration, the less radiation dose to the patient
    d. The more filtration, the less distortion

SLIDE 7-81/CD 7-79 Exam question 14

14. True or false: Using a filter can even out density on a radiograph.
    a. False
    b. True

SLIDE 7-82/CD 7-80 Exam question 15

15. What is the relationship between the number of electrons and the number of x-rays produced in the x-ray tube?
    a. Directly proportional
    b. Inversely proportional
    c. Nonexistent
    d. Difficult to determine

SLIDE 7-83/CD 7-81 Exam conclusion

INSTRUCTOR CD/SLIDE AUDIO: This concludes the examination section of Module 7 of Radiographic Imaging. Please follow your instructor's directions for your answer sheet to the questions.

STUDENT CD AUDIO: This concludes the examination section of Module 7 of Radiographic Imaging. Your score has been saved on the computer. Your instructor will report it to you later.

Answers to the Multimedia Examination

1. d
2. a
3. b
4. c
5. c
6. a
7. c
8. a
9. d
10. d
11. a
12. b
13. c
14. b
15. a

Film Processing

8

Overview

- Film Composition
  - Base
  - Emulsion
  - Supercoat
- Film characteristics
  - Speed
  - Contrast
  - Latitude
  - Recorded detail
- Film storage and handling
  - Temperature
  - Humidity
  - Light
  - Radiation
  - Shelf life
  - Handling
- Intensifying screens
  - Screen composition
  - Screen film contact
  - Cassettes
- Film processing
  - Daylight processing units
  - Automatic processing
  - Developer
  - Fixer
  - Bath
- Darkrooms
- Film Artifacts
- Silver Recovery

The module opens with a discussion of the composition of film, leading into an exploration of how film characteristics originate in differences in the silver halide crystals in the film. The process of x-ray photons interacting with the crystals to produce atomic silver is reviewed. Film speed and contrast are related to the size and evenness of crystals in the emulsion. The concept of graininess is discussed in terms of film speed as well as recorded detail.

Film storage and handling are important concepts because students need to understand how careful they must be when working with film. The effects of many variables are described, including temperature, humidity, light, radiation, shelf life, and physical handling.

Intensifying screens are first considered in terms of their composition, and screen speed and resolution are related to the size of the phosphor crystals. Students see how the size of the screen's crystals has a greater impact on resolution in the image than the film's crystals. The importance of continuous direct contact of the screen with the film is discussed, leading into exploration of problems that may result with a warped, scratched, or broken cassette or film holder.

The process of film developing is then described. Students learn what happens inside an automatic processor, both in terms of the mechanics of processing and the atomic level changes in the film. This discussion leads into practical issues of how a darkroom is set up and used.

The module ends with a review of the causes of artifacts and a description of silver recovery units and the importance of recycling silver from the development chemicals as well as films.

Learning Objectives

Upon completion of this module, the student should be able to do the following:

1. Define all the key terms in the module.
2. Describe what happens in the film emulsion from exposure to the x-ray beam through to development and production of the radiograph.
3. Explain the basis in the film for each of the four fundamental film characteristics: film speed, contrast, latitude, and recorded detail.
4. Give examples of why different films are used for different types of examinations.
5. Explain the basic principles for safe film handling and storage and the potential effects of temperature, humidity, or exposure to light or radiation.
6. Describe how intensifying screens function and how artifacts may result from problems with film cassettes or holders.
7. Explain the importance of silver recovery.
8. Successfully complete the activities and posttest in the Study Guide.

Key Terms

Artifact
Atomic silver
Automatic processor
Base
Cassettes
Clearing agent
Contrast
Darkroom
Daylight film processing unit
Density
Double-emulsion film
Emulsion
Film characteristics
Fixer
Fluorescence
Grain
Intensifying screen
Latent image
Latitude
Luminescence
Manifest image
Phosphor
Phosphorescence
Recorded detail
Reduction
Replenisher reservoir
Safelight
Sensitivity specks
Shelf life
Silver recovery
Speed
Supercoat

Instructional Outline

I. Film characteristics vary among different kinds of film for different purposes.
   A. Most films are composed of a base, an emulsion on one or both sides of the base, and covered with a supercoat.
      1. Silver halide crystals are suspended in a gelatin in the emulsion.
      2. The latent image is formed when x-ray photons interact with the emulsion.
         a. Electrons are freed, which migrate to sensitivity specks in the crystals.
         b. Positively-charged silver ions are attracted to the negatively-charged sensitivity specks, creating atomic silver.
         c. The chemical processing converts the atomic silver into grains of black silver.
   B. Specialty films include mammography film, cine film, and duplicating film.
   C. Film characteristics include speed, contrast, latitude, and recorded detail.
      1. Film speed refers to how much blackening occurs as a result of a set exposure.
         a. The size of the crystals in the emulsion is the primary determinant of film speed.
         b. Larger crystals lead to a faster film speed but less resolution because of the larger film grain.
      2. Contrast is the difference in densities on a radiographic image.
         a. High-contrast films have a relatively even grain size, and low-contrast films have more varying crystal sizes.
         b. The choice of a high- or low-contrast film depends on the body areas being imaged and other factors.
      3. Film latitude refers to the range of exposures that can be performed with a film to obtain diagnostically useful densities.
         a. The wider the latitude, the lower contrast.
         b. A film with narrow latitude differentiates more clearly subtle differences in tissue densities.
      4. Recorded detail refers to the extent that small structures can be recorded on a film with sharpness, or high resolution.
         a. The smaller the grain of a film the better the resolution and recorded detail.
         b. Most modern films have such small grain that differences can be seen only if the radiograph is magnified.

II. To prevent problems with radiographs, careful film handling is necessary.
   A. High temperatures can cause fogging on stored film; some departments refrigerate film that will not be used for a while.
   B. High humidity can cause fogging, whereas very low humidity can cause static electricity and potential artifacts.
   C. Any light exposure can cause artifacts or fogging; film should be opened and handled only under a safelight.
   D. Film is very sensitive to radiation, even to scatter from the patient or personnel.
   E. Shelf life is important, and film should not be used beyond its expiration date.
   F. Physical handling must be careful to avoid creasing or bending the film or getting any hand cream or lotion on it.

III. Understanding intensifying screens and film holders is important to obtain good images and prevent artifacts.
   A. The screen is composed of a base layer, a phosphor layer, a reflective layer, and a protective coating.
   B. Fluorescence is the property of phosphor that creates light photons from an interaction with x-ray photons; old screens must be replaced to avoid phosphorescence, which is a delayed light emission.

C. The phosphor crystals are larger than the film crystals and thus reduce image sharpness somewhat; faster screens give off more light photons per x-ray photon.
D. The screen must be in direct, continuous contact with the film; loss of contact causes artifacts in the image.
E. Screens and film holders must be handled carefully, as any damage or warping can cause artifacts.

IV. Film processing involves a number of steps to create the finished radiograph.
A. Daylight film processing units eliminate the need for a darkroom, as the unit loads and unloads film to and from the cassette automatically.
B. Automatic processors carry the film through the cycle of developer, fixer, washing, and drying.
1. A roller transport system moves the film in and out of the baths.
2. Chemicals in the baths are automatically kept at the correct temperature and replenished from separate tanks as needed.
C. The development process makes a manifest image from the latent image.
1. In the developing step, the reducing agent neutralizes the positively-charged silver ions, and visible black specks of silver are converted from the atomic silver.
2. The clearing agent in the fixer removes unexposed silver halide crystals, leaving the manifest image.
3. The wash step dissolves any residual chemicals.
4. The dryer completes the process.
D. Darkrooms are used to load film into cassettes, remove film from cassettes, and load film into the automatic processor.
E. Darkrooms have light-protected entrances and pass boxes for films, using safelights for personnel working inside.

V. Film artifacts may occur from poor film storage conditions, mishandling of film, damaged cassettes or film holders, or problems with the developing process.

VI. Silver recovery is the process of reclaiming silver from processing chemicals and unneeded films to be recycled.
A. The three types of silver recovery systems are metallic replacement units, electrolytic units, and chemical precipitation units.
B. Unneeded films themselves are stored for recycling.

Teaching Tips

This unit, the last of eight on imaging techniques, presents an opportunity for students to firmly join theory and practicality in their understanding of film and film development. Most of the general principles explored in this unit, from choice of a specific film for a particularly examination to safe handling of film and cassettes, can be related directly to the physics of what happens during the processes of film exposure and film development. Unifying all the different topics in this unit—film characteristics, storage and handling, use of intensifying screens, and film developing—in terms of these processes make it easier for students to grasp the rationales for everyday practices and procedures in the radiology department.

Film Characteristics

An effective teaching approach, therefore, can begin with a review of silver halide crystals and what happens through exposure to x-ray photons and later development: the creation of the latent and then the manifest image. Help students visualize the atomic processes by using a large diagram of silver halide crystals in the emulsion. Work through the steps of exposure: the interaction with an x-ray photon, the migration of free electrons to the sensitivity speck, the attraction of positive silver ions to the negatively-charged sensitivity speck, and so on. Make sure students can visualize exactly what is happening. Then move on to the development process using the same diagram, leading to the formation of black metallic silver grains.

From this point you can move up a level from single crystals and grains to show how separate grains comprise the final image. Build on the original diagram to show several crystals in a pattern forming grains. From this more complex diagram students can easily visualize and understand the concepts of graininess and resolution. Continue building on these concepts with film speed and latitude. Another diagram can be added beside the first to illustrate a different film with fewer or more crystals in the same area, to show differences in speed and the consequent level of recorded detail. Add a third diagram showing a wider variety of crystal sizes to illustrate differences in contrast.

If you are so equipped, show students films magnified at different levels. Magnification, under a low-power microscope or by other means, will show the actual grain in a manner students can obviously relate to the atomic principles by which the latent and manifest images are formed.

Film Storage and Handling

Using the same diagrams of film crystals, demonstrate how exposing the film to light, radiation, heat, or humidity can affect areas of the film. Even one random light photon or an x-ray photon scattered from a patient in the next examining room can interact with a film crystal. Show how a smudge of hand lotion can cover an area of film when it is immersed in the developer chemicals, such that some atomic silver is not converted into black metallic silver. Each cause of artifacts can be illustrated on this same molecular level.

Intensifying Screens

Continue the same use of illustrations as you move to a discussion of intensifying screens, first with the composition of phosphor crystals and the parallel characteristic of screen speed. Most importantly, illustrate visually how x-ray photons reach the phosphor crystals to produce light photons, and how the light photons move from the screen to the film. From a diagram showing those principles it is easy to show why the film must be in direct contact with the screen and what will happen if it is not. You can modify your diagram, for example, to show an area where the screen is bent back away from the film; show the light photons spreading more widely before they reach the film, causing a larger area of interaction in the film and the blur that results. All key principles about intensifying screens, as well as film-screen combinations, can be illustrated in this way.

Artifacts

If students fully grasp all the principles involved in film exposure, development, and handling along with the use of intensifying screens, they will already have encountered most of the causes of artifacts. These can be briefly reviewed using the same diagrams used earlier. At this point you can widen the discussion to include the specific steps of the development process and what events may occur there that can also result in artifacts.

Silver Recovery

This final topic does not necessarily require much discussion. Make sure students understand why it is so important to recycle the silver from both the developer chemicals and old films. The type of silver recovery unit used in their clinical setting can be discussed in a little more detail, particularly if radiologic technologists in that department have any practical role in the recovery process. Otherwise, there may not be any need to discuss in depth the physical processes by which such units function.

Workbook Posttest Answers and Rationales

1. The silver halide crystals in the film emulsion are suspended in a gelatin that allows which of the following?
   a. Exposed crystals to remain on the film
   b. Unexposed crystals to wash away during development
   c. The film base to remain clear
   d. All of the above—As the gelatin washes away during development, the exposed crystals remain and the unexposed ones wash away; the film base remains clear.
   e. None of the above

2. What is needed to convert a latent image into a manifest image?
   a. Expose the film
   b. Develop the film—The latent image before development consists of atomic silver, which during development is converted into black metallic silver, which creates the manifest image.
   c. Place the film in a viewbox
   d. All of the above
   e. None of the above

3. What happens when photons interact with silver halide crystals in the film emulsion?
   a. Electrons are freed in the crystal.
   b. Electrons move to sensitivity specks.
   c. Sensitivity specks gain a negative charge.
   d. All of the above—These are the first key steps in forming the latent image, as the x-ray photon frees electrons that give the sensitivity specks a negative charge, thereby attracting the positive silver ions to them.
   e. None of the above

4. Atomic silver results from the joining of which of the following.
   a. Silver halide crystals with sensitivity specks
   b. Silver ions with the film developer
   c. Free elections at the sensitivity speck with silver ions—The silver ions are positively-charged and therefore attracted to the sensitivity speck, which is negatively-charged because of the free electrons that have migrated there.
   d. None of the above

5. With most modern films, which affects sharpness more?
   a. The size of the film crystals
   b. The size of the intensifying screen crystals—The phosphor crystals of the intensifying screen are larger than the silver halide crystals of the film and therefore have a greater effect on sharpness.
   c. The composition of the film/screen cassette
   d. All affect sharpness equally

6. Film storage temperatures that are too high could cause which of the following?
   a. **Fogging**—Fogging is a result of heat; film speed and the film base would be unaffected by anything but extremely hot conditions unlikely in any department.
   b. Slowing of film speed
   c. Breakdown of the film base
   d. All of the above
   e. None of the above

7. Light photons given off by the phosphors in an intensifying screen travel in what direction?
   a. **In all directions**—The direction of a light photon from a crystal is random, but since the film is immediately next to the screen and the reflective layer immediately next to it on the other side, it must strike one or the other.
   b. Toward the reflective layer, then toward the film
   c. Directly toward the film
   d. Direction depends on whether a grid is used

8. An intensifying screen may produce a poor image if it is which of the following?
   a. Dirty
   b. Scratched
   c. Warped
   d. **All of the above**—Any of these factors could affect how light photons from the screen reach or do not reach the film.
   e. None of the above

9. How long does it take modern automatic processes to develop the film to a final stage?
   a. 5-10 minutes
   b. 3-5 minutes
   c. 1-3 minutes
   d. **About 1 minute or less**—Although some take as long as 90 seconds, most now are under a minute.

10. Rollers inside an automatic film processor are used to do which of the following?
    a. **Move the film through different chemical baths**—The baths of chemicals remain constant, while the rollers move the film into and out of them.
    b. Transport the chemicals to the film in stages
    c. Evenly spread each chemical over the surface of the film
    d. Fix the image in the emulsion by applying pressure

11. What is the first chemical bath in the automatic processor?
    a. Fixer
    b. **Developer**—The film is first developed, then fixed, and finally washed and dried.
    c. Wash
    d. None of the above

12. The fixer does what in the development process?
    a. **Removes unexposed silver halide crystals from the emulsion**—This is called "fixing" not because crystals are fixed in place but because the image is fixed, because washing away the unexposed crystals prevents them from gradually becoming exposed later on and darkening the image.
    b. "Glues" the metallic silver to the film base
    c. Turns the atomic silver into black silver
    d. Turns the film base clear

13. What is the third step in the development process?
    a. Developer
    b. Fixer
    c. **Wash**—The film is first developed, then fixed, and finally washed and dried.
    d. Drying

14. Which variables should be controlled in the darkroom?
    a. **Temperature, humidity, light**—These factors can affect development just the same as they can affect unexposed film while being stored.
    b. Light
    c. Temperature, light, and sound
    d. Light and temperature

15. Which of the following is a type of silver recovery system?
    a. Metallic replacement unit
    b. Electrolytic unit
    c. Chemical precipitation unit
    d. **All of the above**—These are the three basic types of silver recovery units.
    e. None of the above

Testbank Questions

1. Putting emulsion on both sides of the film allows for which of the following?
    a. Reducing patient dose
    b. Eliminating the need for a grid
    c. Eliminating the need for an intensifying screen
    d. All of the above
    e. None of the above

2. The supercoat layer on the film serves to do which of the following?
    a. Hold silver halide crystals
    b. Bind the emulsion to the base
    c. Protect the emulsion
    d. All of the above
    e. None of the above

3. Film emulsion is composed of which of the following?
   a. Silver halide crystals
   b. Sensitivity specks
   c. A gelatin medium
   d. All of the above
   e. None of the above

4. Why do silver ions migrate to the sensitivity specks in film crystals after exposure?
   a. The silver ions with negative charges are attracted to the positively-charged sensitivity specks.
   b. The silver ions with positive charges are attracted to the negatively-charged sensitivity specks.
   c. The x-ray photon's kinetic energy "knocks" the ions to the sensitivity specks.
   d. The positively-charged ions are repelled by other positively-charged ions.

5. Intensifying screens are *not* used with which of the following?
   a. Grids
   b. Direct-exposure film
   c. Fast film
   d. High-contrast film

6. Mammography film is produced especially for which of the following?
   a. Imaging low-density differences in breast tissue
   b. Reducing exposure time
   c. Using fine grain crystals for better recorded detail
   d. All of the above
   e. None of the above

7. Cine radiographic film is used for which of the following?
   a. Mammography
   b. Dental radiography
   c. Magnification radiography
   d. Dynamic fluoroscopy

8. Larger silver crystals in a film emulsion result in which of the following?
   a. Larger film grain
   b. Faster film speed
   c. Less recorded detail when the film image is magnified
   d. All of the above
   e. None of the above

9. High-contrast films generally have which of the following?
   a. Silver halide crystals of even grain size
   b. Silver halide crystals of varying grain size
   c. Varying numbers of sensitivity specks intermixed in the film crystals
   d. Three or more sensitivity specks per silver halide crystal

10. Which of the following is true of recorded detail and film speed?
    a. They are inversely related.
    b. They are directly correlated.
    c. They are independent of each other.
    d. None of the above is true.

11. What condition(s) of humidity should be avoided for film storage?
    a. High humidity
    b. Very low humidity
    c. Both high humidity and very low humidity
    d. Any humidity at all

12. Accidentally exposing a radiographic film to light could cause which of the following?
    a. Artifacts in the image
    b. Generalized fogging
    c. Either artifacts or fogging
    d. None of the above

13. When removing film from the box, handle it carefully to prevent which of the following?
    a. Static electricity, which can cause artifacts
    b. Exposure to chemicals where fumes may be present
    c. Getting any hand cream or lotion on the film
    d. All of the above
    e. None of the above

14. Which is *not* a desired occurrence inside an intensifying screen?
    a. Luminescence
    b. Fluorescence
    c. Phosphorescence
    d. All of the above

15. An intensifying screen is positioned where?
    a. In direct, continuous contact with the film
    b. At a consistent buffered distance from the film
    c. In a holder immediately on the other side of the patient from the film
    d. Along the outside of the film cassette

16. The faster the intensifying screen,
    a. The fewer light photons it gives off per x-ray photon
    b. The fewer x-ray photons it is able to absorb
    c. The more light photons it gives off per x-ray photon
    d. The more x-ray photons it is able to absorb

17. What is the development process in which positively-charged silver ions are neutralized called?
    a. Fixation
    b. Reduction
    c. Hardening
    d. Ionization

18. A darkroom may be used to do which of the following?
    a. Load film into cassettes
    b. Remove film from cassettes
    c. Insert film into an automatic processor
    d. All of the above
    e. None of the above

19. Which of the following is true of a safelight?
    a. It protects film from being exposed while in storage.
    b. It is used to reveal specially encoded numbers on the film.
    c. It allows personnel to see inside the darkroom without exposing unprotected film.
    d. It prevents skin exposure to scatter radiation from the film.

20. An artifact is which of the following?
    a. Something a patient has swallowed that shows up on a radiograph
    b. An image on the radiograph of a button, zipper, jewelry, or other object inside the patient's body
    c. A result of the film being "burned" by a kVp that is too high
    d. Marks or images on a radiograph not resulting from attenuation of the x-ray beam in the examination

Answers to Testbank Questions

1. a	6. d	11. c	16. c
2. c	7. d	12. c	17. b
3. d	8. d	13. d	18. d
4. b	9. a	14. c	19. c
5. b	10. a	15. a	20. d

Audiovisual Script

SLIDE 8-1/CD 8-i Welcome
Welcome to Mosby's Radiographic Instructional Series.

SLIDE 8-2/CD 8-ii Film processing
The module you are about to experience is the last of eight in the Radiographic Imaging program: Film Processing.

This module will help you understand how film is processed in a modern, automatic processor. You will learn enough about how it works to be able to determine how the quality of the radiographs may be affected by your equipment and how to modify variables under your control.

SLIDE 8-3/CD 8-1 19th century photography

In 1895, Wilhelm Conrad Roentgen was the first scientist to recognize that x-rays could be produced. But long before he did, many had observed that some silver compounds reacted to light. At the beginning of the 1800s, a few people observed that reaction, put two and two together, and witnessed the birth of photography. Sensitivity to light is a characteristic of both photographic and radiographic film.

In those early days, it became clear that images of people or nature or anything you could see could not only be reproduced, but they could also be saved if they were treated with certain chemicals. Glass was the favorite substance to save the images on, although paper and other materials were used, too.

SLIDE 8-4/CD 8-2 Dr. Roentgen

By the time Roentgen was making his discoveries at the end of the nineteenth century, photography was a well established art. Like photographs, the first x-ray images were recorded on glass. The glass was coated on one side with an emulsion that was sensitive to light and to x-rays. After it was processed, it became the image you could see.

Because the use of glass plates had inherent problems such as their fragility, scientists developed a cellulose nitrate film base. This film could be coated with an emulsion (that is a mixture of gelatin and silver bromide crystals) on both sides. That reduced the radiation dose to the patient by half. The principle of applying the emulsion to both sides of the film is normal practice today.

Cellulose nitrate was highly flammable and contributed to the severity of several large hospital fires in the 1920s. Cellulose triacetate replaced it, which in turn was replaced by polyester, which is still used for the film base today.

SLIDE 8-5/CD 8-3 Modern radiographic film

Modern radiographic film has reached a high level of sophistication compared with early films. Different types of films provide a range of different film characteristics. Understanding the composition and types of film along with their different properties will help you understand why various films are used for specific procedures.

SLIDE 8-6/CD 8-4 Film cross section

Modern radiographic film is composed of a number of layers. All film starts with the base, now usually made of polyester. The base is strong, flexible, and clear.

A layer of adhesive binds the film emulsion to the base. Most film has an emulsion layer on both sides of the base; this is called double-emulsion film.

The emulsion contains the silver halide crystals that react to light and x-ray photons to form the latent image of the radiograph. We'll look at that process in a moment.

The final layer outside the emulsion is called the supercoat. This is a hard, clear layer that protects the emulsion from damage and gives strength to the film.

MORE INFO LEADS TO THIS AUDIO RESPONSE: The base and supercoat layers of film provide strength and protect the finished radiograph for years to come. This strength keeps radiographs from tearing or wearing out even with much handling, filing, and so on.

8-4A Silver halide crystals

The emulsion is made of a gelatin spread over the film base. The gelatin holds the silver halide crystals in suspension. This medium allows the unexposed crystals to be washed away in the development process and the exposed crystals, which are converted to dark grains, to remain. Shown here is a microphotograph of the crystals in the emulsion before exposure.

SLIDE 8-7/CD 8-5 Silver halide crystal matrix

You will remember that we talked about the latent image in an earlier unit. The latent image is an invisible change in the silver halide crystals of the film's emulsion resulting from their interaction with light or x-ray photons. After the film goes through chemical processing, the latent image becomes visible and is called the manifest image.

The latent image is formed from literally trillions of silver halide crystals in the emulsion. Each crystal is a lattice, something like the model shown here, made of silver, bromide, and iodine atoms. Tiny amounts of impurities, usually made of silver sulfide, are mixed into the crystals. These tiny impurities are called sensitivity specks.

MORE INFO LEADS TO THIS AUDIO RESPONSE: The exact composition of the crystals varies somewhat among different films and different manufacturers, as does the size of the crystals. What is important about silver halide crystals is that the silver atoms, after being converted into ions by x-ray or light photons, are free to move in the crystal.

SLIDE 8-8/CD 8-6 First steps in exposure

When x-ray or light photons interact with atoms in the crystals of the emulsion, electrons are freed. These electrons are attracted to and "caught" by the sensitivity specks, which then have a negative charge. These are the first steps in the process of latent image formation.

SLIDE 8-9/CD 8-7 Final steps in exposure

In the next step of the process, positively-charged silver ions are attracted to the negatively-charged sensitivity speck and migrate to it.

As this process is repeated over and over, more and more silver ions mass together at the sensitivity speck. The free electrons at the speck join with the positive silver ions to make atomic silver.

With the chemical processing of the film, described in more detail later on, this buildup of silver atoms is further developed into a silver grain that now becomes visible in the film as a tiny black spot. The latent image becomes a manifest image.

In crystals that do not interact with light or x-ray photons, such as in areas of the film where the x-ray beam was attenuated or absorbed by radiopaque body parts, atomic silver has not formed at the sensitivity specks. With the chemical processing, these areas do not turn into black silver grains but are removed from the film during processing, thus appearing as the "white" areas of a radiograph.

MORE INFO LEADS TO THIS AUDIO RESPONSE: Every x-ray photon can free thousands of electrons in the silver halide crystals, which migrate to the sensitivity specks. From 3 to 10 silver ions clump together at the speck, not enough to make a visible image, but enough to later develop into a visible silver grain during the chemical processing. Remember that trillions of crystals are present in even a small area of radiographic film, such that the film can show remarkable detailed differences in the amount of density at different areas of the image.

SLIDE 8-10/CD 8-8 Film speed

Because the size and concentration of silver halide crystals in the emulsion can be controlled during the manufacturing of radiographic film, films with different properties can be made for different imaging applications. These film properties are also called film characteristics.

Different types of film thus have different characteristics.

SLIDE 8-11/CD 8-9 Film characteristics

The two general types of radiographic film are films intended to be used with intensifying screens and those used without screens. As you recall from an earlier module, intensifying screens are used to decrease the radiation dose to the patient; the screen gives off light photons when struck by x-ray photons, and these light photons result in most of the latent image formation.

With direct-exposure films an intensifying screen is not used, and the x-ray photons are responsible for forming the latent image with the film's silver halide crystals.

The size and concentration of the crystals in the emulsion determine the four general characteristics of a film: speed, contrast, latitude, and recorded detail. We'll look at each of these separately.

MORE INFO LEADS TO THIS AUDIO RESPONSE: Most radiographic examinations now use screen film because of the reduced radiation exposure for the patient. Even though we can talk separately about different types of film and intensifying screens, as if they were chosen separately for an examination, remember that usually it is a film-screen combination that is standardized for most examinations.

CD 8-9A Mammogram

In addition to the two general types of film, screen film and nonscreen film, there is a number of specialty films for special applications.

Mammography film is a special single-emulsion, fine-grain film used to reduce the longer exposure time that in the past was necessary for imaging the low density differences in breast tissue, as shown here.

Other specialty films include the nonscreen films used in dentistry, duplicating films used to make copies of radiographs, and cine film used in dynamic fluoroscopy, such as in cardiac catheterization.

SLIDE 8-12/CD 8-10 Film crystal size and speed

Film speed refers to the amount of film blackening that occurs as a result of a set exposure. The faster the film, the shorter the exposure can be, and this has an obvious benefit. There are disadvantages to faster speeds, however, as we will see in a moment.

The primary factor in determining film speed is the size of the silver crystals in the film. The larger the crystals, the faster the film, because each crystal will produce a larger black area on the radiograph. Therefore fewer crystals need to interact with x-ray or light photons.

Film speed for radiographic film means the same thing as film speed for your own camera. Faster speed films can use shorter exposure times but may produce pictures that are more grainy than slower speed films.

CD 8-10A Film grain
When we talk of grain or film graininess, we are referring to the tiny black spots that make up the visible image, one grain from each silver halide crystal exposed. With modern films, usually the grain is not visible to the human eye.

But as shown here, when the film image is magnified many times, the grain does become apparent. The bigger the grain, the less sharp the image is.

SLIDE 8-13/CD 8-11 Contrast differences
Contrast is the differences in optical density on a radiographic image. Extremes of black and white are high contrast, while many different shades of gray are lower contrast. You can see the difference in the levels of contrast in the two radiographs shown here.

As discussed in an earlier module in this program, radiographic contrast results from subject contrast as well as film contrast. The primary factor in the film is the uniformity of the silver halide crystals. High-contrast films have a relatively even grain size, while low-contrast films have a range of grain sizes.

The choice of a high-contrast film or a low-contrast film depends in part on the body area being imaged. If body tissues have relatively small variations in density, such as in mammography, a high-contrast film is better at showing subtle differences. A lower-contrast film would be more appropriate in other cases, such as in obtaining some skeletal images.

MORE INFO LEADS TO THIS AUDIO RESPONSE: Radiographic contrast is partly a property of the film, but good contrast in the resulting image also depends on using the correct exposure factors. A film has a set exposure range that will produce an image within the diagnostically useful range of optical density. An exposure above or below this range will have poor contrast.

SLIDE 8-14/CD 8-12 Contrast in photographs
Film latitude refers to the range of exposure that can be used with a film to produce diagnostically useful densities. A film with a wide latitude can be adequately exposed over a wider range of mAs values than a film with narrow latitude and will show many shades of gray. However, a film with narrow latitude will differentiate more strikingly between subtle differences in tissue densities because it has a higher contrast than a wide latitude film. The photograph on the left here shows more shades of gray than the one on the right and is said to have a wider latitude.

You can see that latitude and contrast are inversely related. The wider the latitude, the lower the contrast. The narrower the latitude, the higher the contrast.

MORE INFO LEADS TO THIS AUDIO RESPONSE: Another way to consider latitude is in terms of exposure factors. Latitude is a measure of the width of the range of exposures that result in a diagnostic image.

SLIDE 8-15/CD 8-13 Differences in recorded detail

Recorded detail refers to the extent to which very small anatomical differences can be recorded on the film. An image with good recorded detail is said to have sharpness or high resolution.

In general, the size of the silver halide crystals in the film affects sharpness: the smaller the crystals and therefore the smaller the image's grain, the more detail it can show. Recorded detail is therefore inversely related to film speed, since faster films have larger grain.

Most modern films have such small grain, however, that the human eye cannot detect differences in recorded detail caused by film differences. The crystals in the intensifying screen are larger than in the film, on the other hand, and affect recorded detail both because of their size and because the light photons given off move in all directions and thus strike the film in a manner that blurs some detail. As discussed in an earlier module, this is part of the trade-off of using screens: you get slightly less detail but the patient receives a significantly lower exposure dose.

SLIDE 8-16/CD 8-14 Film-screen combination

In most modern imaging departments, there is a standardized approach to using certain film-screen combinations for standard imaging applications. Yet it is important to understand the different film characteristics in order to understand the rationales for the standardized approach and make decisions when appropriate about film selection and processing.

SLIDE 8-17/CD 8-15 Film storage

Because radiographic film is sensitive and is affected by many factors in addition to the x-ray exposure, proper storage and careful handling of film is essential.

SLIDE 8-18/CD 8-16 Film storage considerations

Film that is improperly stored or handled can produce poor quality images because of fogging or artifacts that might appear on the image. Storage considerations include temperature, humidity, light, radiation, shelf life, storage position, and handling.

Film is sensitive to temperature because heat photons can interact with the silver halide crystals in the emulsion and over time produce a gradual darkening or fog on the film. Film should be stored at a temperature under 68 degrees Fahrenheit, or 20 degrees Celsius. The longer the film is stored before use, the cooler the storage area should be; some radiographic units refrigerate or freeze films that will not be used within a set period. As a general rule, film should be used within about 45 days of arrival in the department.

MORE INFO LEADS TO THIS AUDIO RESPONSE: Refrigerated film should be in a moisture-proof package. The film should be brought to room temperature before use.

SLIDE 8-19/CD 8-17 Severely fogged radiograph
Humidity must also be controlled in the storage area. Film is delivered in moisture-proof packaging, but once a package of film is opened, it is susceptible to the effects of high humidity. Humidity over about 60% can produce fogging, the same way high temperatures can. The radiograph shown here is severely fogged. Low humidity also can cause damage, because tiny static electricity sparks are more likely with low humidity, and such sparks leave artifacts on the film.

SLIDE 8-20/CD 8-18 Lightproof cassettes
Radiographic film can be damaged by exposure to light, just as regular photographic film can. Exposure to bright light may cause artifacts on the film, and low-level exposure may cause generalized fogging. Film packages that have been opened must therefore be kept in a dark storage area.

Film is loaded into lightproof cassettes for use, as shown here. The cassette can then be handled in regular lighted areas without fear of exposing it to light.

Film outside of lightproof packaging or cassettes must be handled only in a darkroom. This protects it from light exposure before and after the radiographic exposure, until the film is put through the film processor. Darkrooms have a special light called a safelight that lets you see well enough to handle the film but that does not damage the film.

MORE INFO LEADS TO THIS AUDIO RESPONSE: Many imaging departments now use daylight processing systems. As we'll discuss in a few minutes, daylight processing systems eliminate the need for darkrooms or to handle film directly.

SLIDE 8-21/CD 8-19 Film storage area
Radiographic film, obviously, is very sensitive to radiation. Film therefore must be stored in areas protected from any possibility of radiation leakage from x-ray equipment. Typically the film storage area and darkroom are lead-lined for this protection. Film should be protected from the time of its arrival in the department until it is sent through the film processor.

MORE INFO LEADS TO THIS AUDIO RESPONSE: Remember that there is always the possibility of some radiation leakage during radiographic examinations. The housing around the tube and the collimator help prevent x-rays escaping except those in the primary beam, but scattering can occur from x-rays striking atoms in the patient, the examination table, even the air. Film should be protected from any possible exposure in the radiographic department.

SLIDE 8-22/CD 8-20 Film expiration date
The shelf life of radiographic film is another important consideration. Film should always be used before its expiration date. Usually film is ordered in small enough quantities that any given shipment of film is used up well before the expiration date. Still, it's a good idea to check the date on the package before opening it. Old film may not have good contrast and may have fog.

Finally, another film storage consideration is that film should be stored on end on shelves, not flat. This puts less pressure on the film, avoids stacking film boxes, and minimizes the risk of film warping and pressure marks on the film.

MORE INFO LEADS TO THIS AUDIO RESPONSE: Every imaging department has a standard system for monitoring expiration.

SLIDE 8-23/CD 8-21 Handling film

The careful handling of film includes all the factors we've just discussed: temperature, humidity, light, radiation, shelf life, and storage position.

Safe handling also involves the physical handling of film. Film boxes should be opened and closed carefully and slowly, and film sheets removed slowly to prevent artifacts caused by static electricity or abrasion. Take care to prevent creasing or bending the film. Make sure your hands are clean and dry before handling film, and avoid any hand creams or lotions that could leave fingerprint artifacts on the film. Keep film away from any chemicals that may produce fumes, including cleaning solutions and developing chemicals.

This completes the section on film characteristics and film handling.

MORE INFO LEADS TO THIS AUDIO RESPONSE: Film is most sensitive after exposure and before being developed, but the developed film with the image also should be handled carefully to prevent damage. Scratches or marks from careless handling could make diagnosis difficult or require a repeat examination with additional exposure to the patient.

SLIDE 8-24/CD 8-22 Intensifying screen

You have begun the topic of intensifying screens and film holders. This subject builds on information covered in the preceding topic on film characteristics and handling. If you have not yet worked through that topic, you may want to quit this section now and return later after going through the earlier topic.

You have already learned about the purpose of intensifying screens in an earlier module. Now we will review the structure and purpose of screens and then discuss their use in the context of this module: that is their use and handling with radiographic film.

SLIDE 8-25/CD 8-23 Cross section of screen

The purpose of intensifying screens, you'll recall, is to lower the radiation dose to the patient. X-ray photons that penetrate the patient strike the screen, which gives off a larger number of light photons that create the latent image in the film emulsion. Fewer x-ray photons are needed to create the image because each x-ray photon produces many light photons from the screens.

A screen is composed of several layers. The base is strong, flexible, and radiolucent. It serves as a support for the phosphor layer. The phosphor layer contains the phosphors, which give off light photons when struck by x-ray photons. These light photons are emitted in all directions. The reflective layer is on the side of the phosphor layer away from the film; its function is to reflect back to the film the light photons that were emitted in the opposite direction, thereby doubling the intensity of the light reaching the film and allowing a lower radiation exposure to the patient.

The protective coating is a thin layer of plastic that protects the phosphor layer from scratches and artifacts caused by handling. If this coating wears off over time or is scratched by fingernails or other items touching it, some of the phosphors may also be removed, which could cause artifacts to appear in films exposed using the screen.

SLIDE 8-26/CD 8-24 Functioning of screen

The term luminescence refers to the process by which a material gives off light photons from an interaction with other radiated photons. Fluorescence is a type of luminescence that happens instantaneously upon exposure to x-rays and stops immediately when the exposure is terminated. Phosphorescence is a type that continues to emit light after the initial interaction with the x-ray photon has been terminated. Phosphorescence is not desirable in an intensifying screen because the light photons do not all reach the film immediately to form the latent image. Yet phosphorescence can occur when a screen grows old and the phosphors are exhausted. For this reason screens must be replaced after a number of years.

CD 8-24A Phosphor crystals

The light photons generated in the intensifying screen are emitted by phosphor crystals. These crystals are significantly larger than the silver halide crystals in the film. Therefore, use of a screen reduces image sharpness somewhat. Some examinations requiring extremely fine detail, therefore, require the use of screens with small size crystals.

SLIDE 8-27/CD 8-25 Separation of screen and film

For best results, it is important that the intensifying screen be in direct, continuous contact with the film. Remember that the light photons are emitted from the crystals in the phosphor layer of the screen. From this point the photons may move in any direction as they spread out from the phosphors. The closer to the film the phosphor layer is, the less the photons can spread out, thus striking the film in a smaller area. This means the resolution of the image will be greater.

This illustration compares the effects of striking two phosphor crystals at different distances from the film. The light photons at the left do not spread out as far as those at the right, which originate farther away from the film. Therefore the x-ray photon on the right may produce a more dispersed area of darkening on the film, making the image less sharp.

As we'll see in a minute, cassettes include foam pressure pads to press the film and screen together to help ensure the good contact between the screen and the film.

SLIDE 8-28/CD 8-26 Fine detail screen

Intensifying screens are classified according to their speed and resolution.

The variables that influence the speed of a screen are similar to those that influence the speed of a radiographic film. The larger the phosphor crystals and the thicker the layer of phosphor, the faster the screen. The faster the screen, the more light photons it gives off per x-ray photon, and therefore the more it intensifies the formation of the latent image. This is sometimes called the intensification factor of a screen, which measures how much a screen amplifies the latent image by converting x-ray photons to light photons.

The greater the intensification factor of a screen, therefore, the lower can be the x-ray dose to the patient. There is a trade-off, however, because the same factors that increase screen speed decrease resolution. As with the film emulsion, larger crystals or a thicker layer of them will decrease resolution.

Screens are generally described as high-speed screens, medium (or par) speed screens, or fine-detail screens.

The two radiographs shown here compare a fine-detail and a high-speed screen; the difference in resolution can be seen.

SLIDE 8-29/CD 8-27 Cassette

Intensifying screens must be handled carefully. As mentioned earlier, if the protective coating is scratched or worn through, the phosphor layer can be damaged, producing artifacts on the radiograph.

In addition to preventing scratches and wear, screens must be cleaned periodically. Special cleaning materials and preparations should be used, following the manufacturer's directions.

Part of good screen care includes ensuring that the film and screen are held in close contact within the film holder or cassette. Uneven contact will produce an uneven image with blurring in areas of poor contact. Any warping in the screen or cassette, foreign material between the screen and film, or bends or breaks in the hinges, latches, or other parts of the cassette may cause poor contact and result in a poor image.

CD 8-27A Artifact

Can you guess what caused the problem in the radiograph shown here?

The blurry area on the image was caused by the film having poor contact with the intensifying screen because of a warped cassette.

SLIDE 8-30/CD 8-28 Cross sections

Intensifying screens and film are held together in film holders or cassettes. These are lightproof and allow for ease of handling and processing the film.

Many different types of holders and cassettes are commercially available. Most share certain characteristics. The cassette, usually made of a plastic, has a rigid back for strength and a simple system for opening and latching closed. One or more pads made of felt or foam rubber inside provide pressure to keep the film in contact with the screen. Typically there is a layer of lead in the backing to absorb any backscatter radiation that would otherwise reexpose the film.

Like intensifying screens, cassettes must be handled carefully and kept clean. Special materials are used for cleaning.

SLIDE 8-31/CD 8-29 Daylight film processing unit

Many radiology departments now use daylight film processing units, which eliminate the need for a darkroom. The unit automatically inserts the film into the cassette, so handling the film itself is no longer a factor. The unit removes the exposed film from the cassette and transfers it into the developing part of the processor.

With these contemporary units, film handling has become simpler and much less likely to cause handling artifacts on radiographs.

This completes the section on intensifying screens and film holders.

SLIDE 8-32/CD 8-30 Historic darkroom

You have begun the topic of film processing. This subject builds on information covered in the preceding topics. If you have not yet worked through those topics, you may want to quit this section now and return later after going through the earlier topics.

In the past, exposed radiographic films were processed by hand. It took about an hour for a darkroom technician to develop and dry the film, transforming the latent image into the fixed visible image that could be used for diagnosis.

That changed in 1956, when the first automatic processor was introduced. It could process film in 15 minutes. Refinements since then have reduced the processing time to between 45 and 120 seconds. With continuing improvements, the standard is moving toward a total processing time of between 20 and 45 seconds.

Because of the advantages of time and the quality of automatic processors, virtually no radiographic processing is done by hand anymore. In this module, we'll be talking only about automatic processing.

MORE INFO LEADS TO THIS AUDIO RESPONSE: Developing film in the old manual method involved moving the film from one tray of chemicals to another. Timing and solution temperature were critical. Often the results were less than ideal. Automated processes eliminated these difficulties.

SLIDE 8-33/CD 8-31 Development process

As we discussed earlier, an exposed radiographic film has a latent image composed of silver ions attracted to the sensitivity specks in the crystals of the emulsion. The chemical development process converts the clumps of silver ions into metallic silver that is deposited and fixed in place on the film, thereby making the visible, permanent image. Several different chemical solutions are required in this process.

SLIDE 8-34/CD 8-32 Developing unit

In the days of manual processing, films were developed using several tanks that held the different chemicals needed for the various steps. Automatic processors now use a roller transport system that move the film through the process automatically. The rollers grip the film as it enters the processor and move it through the processing stages, exposing it to the correct chemistry for just the right length of time, drying it, and delivering it as a final permanent image: all in 90 seconds.

SLIDE 8-35/CD 8-33 Automatic processor

You should have enough understanding of how automatic processing works to know when it might be causing problems that affect the quality of images. You might also need to remove film that gets stuck, or you may be responsible for cleaning the processor, so you need to be familiar with it.

This illustration shows how automatic processing works. The film enters the roller system at the feed tray. Rollers and racks take it through the tanks of wet chemicals and then to the drying chamber. It ends up at the receiving bin.

The 90-second transport time is carefully controlled by the transport system. The film spends precise amounts of time in each tank and is exposed to precise amounts of chemistry as it moves along.

SLIDE 8-36/CD 8-34 Transport rollers

The movement of the film through the automatic processor is controlled by the transport system. The transport system includes rollers, transport racks, and a drive system.

The transport system has two kinds of rollers: the transport roller and the master roller. The first, the transport rollers, are small (about an inch in diameter). They provide the tension that keeps the film moving along and can move films traveling in a downward or upward path at the same time. As you can see here, they're positioned either back to back in pairs, or staggered down from each other.

SLIDE 8-37/CD 8-35 Master roller

At the bottom of the transport rack is a turnaround assembly. It consists of a larger roller, or the master roller, which is about 3 inches in diameter, planetary rollers, and guide shoes. Together, they turn the leading edge of the film from its downward path to an upward path so it can progress to the top of the tank. At the top of the tank a crossover assembly transports the film into the next tank.

SLIDE 8-38/CD 8-36 Replenisher tanks

These two kinds of rollers move the film through at least three chemical wet tanks and then through the dryer.

The temperature of each of the chemical wet tanks is precisely maintained by heating elements controlled by thermostats.

Because some of the chemicals are absorbed by the film and carried into the next tank or used up in the processing itself, the tanks through which the film is transported are continually replenished with fresh chemicals from replenisher reservoirs as shown here. The water in the wash tank is not recirculated but is replaced with a continual flow of fresh water.

MORE INFO LEADS TO THIS AUDIO RESPONSE: Radiologic technologists seldom are responsible for checking the solutions in the replenisher reservoirs or adding solution. Still, it's important to understand these processes; for example, if the image in the developed film is not as diagnostically useful as expected, you may be able to determine which step in the process from exposure to final image is not functioning properly.

SLIDE 8-39/CD 8-37 Developer tank

Let's look in a little more detail at each of the stages in the automatic processor as the film moves through the whole process.

First, the film is fed into the unit through a feed tray in a conventional unit or directly from the cassette in daylight systems. The film first enters the developer tank.

The developer solution gives up electrons that neutralize the positively-charged silver ions in the film in a process called reduction. The chemical in the developer solution responsible for this is called the reducing agent. Metallic silver builds up in visible black specks at the sensitivity specks.

Other chemicals in the developer help control this process precisely and prevent overexposure. A hardener also prevents the film emulsion from becoming too soft or swollen during the processing.

To obtain the best visible image, the development process depends on precise control of the concentration and temperature of the developer, and the length of time the film is in the developer. All these are controlled automatically by the film processor.

SLIDE 8-40/CD 8-38 Radiograph without fixing
The rollers transport the film from the developer into the next tank, the fixer.

After development of the exposed silver halide crystals in the emulsion into metallic silver, some unexposed silver halide crystals remain on the film. Once the film is exposed to the light, these crystals would gradually become metallic silver, thereby darkening the film, as shown here on the unfixed film on the right. The use of a clearing agent in the fixer prevents this by bonding to unexposed silver halide crystals and removing them from the emulsion. (Clearing agent is also sometimes called hypo.) The film is now clear except for the desirable image resulting from the exposed crystals that were developed into metallic silver.

Other chemicals in the fixer include a preservative and a hardener.

SLIDE 8-41/CD 8-39 Washing stage
From the fixer the film is transported next to the wash tank, where a continual flow of fresh water dissolves any residual chemicals on the film. If any hypo in the fixer were allowed to remain on the film, the image would gradually turn brown or yellow over time.

After the wash the film moves through the drying chamber where hot air is blown over it. This hardens the emulsion and seals the film's supercoat.

This entire process takes only 90 seconds!

SLIDE 8-42/CD 8-40 Darkroom
Daylight processing systems make radiographic darkrooms unnecessary, although they still exist in most settings.

Darkrooms are used to load film into cassettes, remove film from cassettes, and insert film into automatic processors.

The radiography department may have one large centralized darkroom or several smaller ones spread out among the examining rooms. The centralized approach is generally more cost-effective and offers more uniform quality control, although multiple small darkrooms may offer convenience in a large department.

SLIDE 8-43/CD 8-41 Inside the darkroom
Darkrooms are protected at all times from outside light entering the room. Various entrances have been devised to allow personnel to enter without letting in the outside light. Such entrances include double interlocking doors, lightproof entrance mazes, and revolving doors.

Darkrooms can be designed in different ways, but all designs should be based on ease of operations. Lightproof pass boxes in the wall allow films to be brought into the darkroom without having to be carried in through the entrance. The automatic processor is centrally located, and countertops provide convenient work areas. Storage cabinets on the wall and under counters hold supplies.

Floor drains should also be present in case of a spill.

SLIDE 8-44/CD 8-42 Darkroom safelight

A darkroom is not completely dark, of course. The room is illuminated by a special red lamp, called a safelight. Radiographic film does not react to light at this wavelength, so it does not affect the film but provides enough light for personnel to perform their darkroom functions. The safelight produces the correct wavelength either with the special bulb or by using a special red filter. Tests are performed periodically to ensure that safelights will not produce fogging of film.

At times the darkroom must be illuminated by regular light, such as for cleaning or maintenance. Therefore regular lighting is present too, usually with switches that are positioned where they will not be accidentally turned on.

If the darkroom has a single door entrance that is not lightproof, there must be a warning light outside the room to indicate when the room should not be entered so as to prevent someone from accidentally entering and letting light in that may affect films inside.

SLIDE 8-45/CD 8-43 Processor feed tray

Finally, the film processing environment must be controlled in the same manner as film handling and storage. Processing can be affected adversely by temperature or humidity extremes, the presence of light or radiation, or careless handling of equipment or supplies.

Since film processing equipment varies considerably among different facilities, the best approach is to follow the protocols within the particular imaging department for how these various factors are controlled.

This completes the section on film processing.

SLIDE 8-46/CD 8-44 Radiograph with artifacts

You have begun the section on other processing factors: artifacts and silver recovery. This subject builds on information covered in the preceding topics on films and processing. If you have not yet worked through those topics, you may want to quit this section now and return later after going through the earlier topics.

Now let's look at two other processing factors: artifacts and silver recovery. Artifacts is the term for markings or images that appear on the finished film that did not result from the attenuation of the x-ray beam passing through the patient. The presence of artifacts, therefore, is undesirable. They may appear because of poor conditions related to the film, mishandling, or processing problems. Artifacts can cause an image to be misinterpreted, can make interpretation difficult or impossible (as in the image shown here on the right), and may require a repeat procedure resulting in unnecessary additional patient exposure.

SLIDE 8-47/CD 8-45 More artifacts

Different kinds of artifacts can occur, but virtually all can be prevented. Fog artifacts can be caused by high temperatures, bright light, high humidity, or ionizing radiation. Scratches or pressure on the film can cause white or dark areas. Poor contact between the screen and film can cause localized blurring or darker areas. Dirt on the screen or film can cause white spots. Damaged cassettes or screens can cause a range of artifacts, as can improperly functioning automatic processors. Shown here are films marred by a variety of artifacts.

Only by following accepted and safe procedures for handling and storing film and for processing exposed film, as described in earlier sections of this module, can artifacts be prevented.

SLIDE 8-48/CD 8-46 Silver recovery unit

Our final consideration when discussing film processing is silver recovery. This term refers to the process by which silver in the processing chemicals is reclaimed and recycled. This recycling is important for two reasons. Silver has economic value in its recycled form and helps recover some of the cost of the unexposed film, which is expensive in part because of the silver in it. Secondly, federal regulations require that heavy metals like silver be reclaimed from waste solutions before they are disposed of, to prevent pollution of the environment.

Roughly half the silver in the film ends up dissolved in the fixer in the automatic processor. Different kinds of silver recovery units are used to process the used fixer to recover the silver.

SLIDE 8-49/CD 8-47 Electrolytic unit

There are three types of silver recovery systems. They are metallic replacement units, electrolytic units, and the chemical precipitation units.

With metallic replacement units, the used fixer circulates through a tank in which iron molecules in steel screens break down and are replaced by metallic silver precipitates. This method is less efficient than other methods and less commonly used now.

With electrolytic units, such as the one shown here, an electric current is passed through the fixer and ionized silver molecules in the fixer are attracted to and form a plating on the negatively-charged cathode in the circuit.

Other units use a process of chemical precipitation in which other chemicals react with the silver in the fixer solution. Silver molecules are freed and precipitate out of the solution, falling to the bottom of the tank where they can be recovered from the silver sludge that forms.

SLIDE 8-50/CD 8-48 Waste film recycling area

The final form of silver recovery is from film itself. Any scrap film should not be discarded but kept in a special area for recycling, such as is shown here. This applies also to any original films removed from patient records for disposal. The recycling and processing of these films is usually handled by an outside company that specializes in this. Every imaging department has its own protocol for storing and recycling waste films.

This concludes this section.

SLIDE 8-51/CD 8-49 Quiz instructions

THIS AUDIO FOR SLIDE/TAPE ONLY: This concludes the presentation section of this module. If you are not going to work through the self-assessment quiz that now follows, you may stop the program at this point and turn off the equipment.

If your instructor has asked you to take this self-assessment quiz on the material you have learned in this module, you should have a piece of paper ready. There will be 10 questions with multiple-choice or short answers. After this self-assessment we will go back through these questions and briefly talk about the reasons for the correct answers. Ready?

THIS AUDIO IN CD ROM LECTURE MODE ONLY: You have reached the self-assessment quiz for this module. Here you will be asked 10 questions to help you assess how well you understand what you have learned in this module. The questions are multiple-choice or have short answers. After this self-assessment we'll go back through these questions and briefly talk about your answers and the reasons for the correct answers. Ready?

THIS AUDIO IN CD ROM STUDENT MODE ONLY: You have reached the self-assessment quiz for this module. Here you will be asked 10 questions to help you assess how well you understand what you have learned in this module. The questions are multiple-choice or have short answers. For multiple-choice questions, click on the box next to your answer choice. For those questions that require a short answer, type in your answer at the keyboard and press Enter. After this self-assessment we'll go back through these questions and briefly talk about your answers and the reasons for the correct answers.

SLIDE 8-52/CD 8-50 Quiz question 1

1. What part of the film contains silver halide crystals?
   a. Emulsion
   b. Supercoat
   c. Base

SLIDE 8-53/CD 8-51 Quiz question 2

2. The latent image forms when the film is exposed by movement of electrons to which of the following?
   a. Silver halide crystals
   b. Supercoat
   c. Sensitivity specks

SLIDE 8-54/CD 8-52 Quiz question 3

3. Which of the following refers to film speed?
   a. How fast the film package must be used up once opened
   b. How much film blackening occurs following an exposure
   c. The kVp of the exposure

SLIDE 8-55/CD 8-53 Quiz question 4

4. A film with a wide latitude generally has which of the following?
   a. The ability to show many shades of gray
   b. The ability to show few shades of gray
   c. A high contrast

SLIDE 8-56/CD 8-54 Quiz question 5

5. Which is the best storage condition for unexposed film?
   a. Warm temperature, high humidity
   b. Warm temperature, medium humidity
   c. Cool temperature, high humidity
   d. Cool temperature, medium humidity

SLIDE 8-57/CD 8-55 Quiz question 6

6. Intensifying screens function because of what process?
   a. The number of x-ray photons is doubled by the screen.
   b. X-ray photons striking the screen produce light photons.
   c. The screen produces free electrons that migrate to the sensitivity speck.

SLIDE 8-58/CD 8-56 Quiz question 7

7. It is important that the intensifying screen be which of the following?
   a. In direct contact with the film
   b. Spaced the proper distance away from the film

SLIDE 8-59/CD 8-57 Quiz question 8

8. What does the developer solution in an automatic film processor contain?
   a. The hypo
   b. The phosphor layer
   c. The reducing agent

SLIDE 8-60/CD 8-58 Quiz question 9

9. Film processing requires careful control of which of the following?
   a. Temperature and solution strengths
   b. Film size and speed
   c. Film and intensifying screen construction

SLIDE 8-61/CD 8-59 Quiz question 10

10. What is the term for markings or images on the final film not resulting from the attenuation of the x-ray beam passing though the patient?

SLIDE 8-62/CD 8-60 Quiz review

That concludes the self-assessment quiz for Module 8: Film Processing. Let's quickly go back through the questions and see how you did.

SLIDE 8-63/CD 8-61 Review question 1

Question 1 asked you which part of radiographic film contains silver halide crystals.

The correct answer is a, the emulsion. Congratulate yourself if you got it right! The emulsion contains all the silver halide crystals and is the part of the film that changes during exposure and development. The base is the strong clear part of the film to which the emulsion adheres, and the supercoat is the outside protective coating.

CD 8-61A Review question 1

Question 1 asked you which part of radiographic film contains silver halide crystals.

PRESENT THIS AUDIO IF ANSWER WAS a: Yes, you're right. The correct answer is a, the emulsion. The emulsion contains all the silver halide crystals and is the part of the film that changes during exposure and development. The base is the strong clear part of the film to which the emulsion adheres, and the supercoat is the outside protective coating.

PRESENT THIS AUDIO IF ANSWER WAS b or c: No, sorry, your answer is incorrect. The correct answer is a, the emulsion. The emulsion contains all the silver halide crystals and is the part of the film that changes during exposure and development. The base is the strong clear part of the film to which the emulsion adheres, and the supercoat is the outside protective coating.

SLIDE 8-64/CD 8-62 Review question 2
Question 2 asked about the formation of the latent image when the film is exposed, caused by movement of electrons to one of these: a, the silver halide crystals; b, the supercoat; or c, the sensitivity specks.

The correct answer is c, the sensitivity specks. The electrons are already in the silver halide crystals, and they are freed by the interaction of photons with the crystals. Then they migrate to the sensitivity specks, which then have a negative charge and attract the silver ions. The supercoat is the protective coating of the film and has nothing to do with the image.

CD 8-62A Review question 2
Question 2 asked about the formation of the latent image when the film is exposed, caused by movement of electrons to one of these: a, the silver halide crystals; b, the supercoat; or c, the sensitivity specks.

PRESENT THIS AUDIO IF ANSWER WAS c: Yes, you correctly answered c, the sensitivity specks. The electrons are already in the silver halide crystals, and they are freed by the interaction of photons with the crystals. They then migrate to the sensitivity specks, which then have a negative charge and attract the silver ions. The supercoat is the protective coating of the film and has nothing to do with the image.

PRESENT THIS AUDIO IF ANSWER WAS a or b: No, you incorrectly answered this one. The right answer is c, the sensitivity specks. The electrons are already in the silver halide crystals, and they are freed by the interaction of photons with the crystals. They then migrate to the sensitivity specks, which then have a negative charge and attract the silver ions. The supercoat is the protective coating of the film and has nothing to do with the image.

SLIDE 8-65/CD 8-63 Review question 3
Question 3 asked what the term film speed refers to.

The correct answer is b, how much film blackening occurs following an exposure. A fast film has more blackening, a slow film less. This means that with a fast film, the patient exposure can be decreased.

Answer choice a, how fast the film package must be used up once opened, has nothing to do with film speed. But it is true, nonetheless, that film does not last forever but has an expiration date.

Answer choice c, the kVp of the exposure, also is incorrect. Every film is manufactured with a set film speed, and this speed exists independently of the settings for the exposure.

CD 8-63A Review question 3
Question 3 asked what the term film speed refers to.

PRESENT THIS AUDIO IF ANSWER WAS b: Yes, you're correct in answering b, how much film blackening occurs following an exposure. A fast film has more blackening, a slow film less. This means that with a fast film, the patient exposure can be decreased.

PRESENT THIS AUDIO IF ANSWER WAS a: You incorrectly answered a. The correct answer is b, how much film blackening occurs following an exposure. A fast film has more blackening, a slow film less. This means that with a fast film, the patient exposure can be decreased. Answer choice a, how fast the film package must be used up once opened, has nothing to do with film speed. But it is true, nonetheless, that film does not last forever but has an expiration date.

PRESENT THIS AUDIO IF ANSWER WAS c: You incorrectly answered c. The correct answer is b, how much film blackening occurs following an exposure. A fast film has more blackening, a slow film less. This means that with a fast film, the patient exposure can be decreased. Answer choice c, the kVp of the exposure, is incorrect. Every film is manufactured with a set film speed, and this speed exists independent of the settings for the exposure.

SLIDE 8-66/CD 8-64 Review question 4
Question 4 asked about the characteristics of a film with a wide latitude.

The correct answer is a, the ability to show many shades of gray. That's basically the definition of wide latitude. Answer b, the ability to show few shades of gray, is incorrect because showing few shades of gray would be a narrow latitude. Answer c, a high contrast, means the same thing as narrow latitude.

CD 8-64A Review question 4
Question 4 asked about the characteristics of a film with a wide latitude.

PRESENT THIS AUDIO IF ANSWER WAS a: You're right! The correct answer is a, the ability to show many shades of gray. That's basically the definition of wide latitude.

PRESENT THIS AUDIO IF ANSWER WAS b: Sorry, your answer is wrong. Answer b, the ability to show few shades of gray, is a narrow latitude. The correct answer is a, the ability to show many shades of gray. That's basically the definition of wide latitude.

PRESENT THIS AUDIO IF ANSWER WAS c: Sorry, your answer is wrong. Answer c, a high contrast, means the film has a narrow latitude. The correct answer is a, the ability to show many shades of gray. That's basically the definition of wide latitude.

SLIDE 8-67/CD 8-65 Review question 5
Question 5 asked about the best storage conditions for unexposed film.

The correct answer is d, cool temperature and medium humidity. High temperatures can cause film fog. Colder temperatures are sometimes used for long periods of storage. Humidity should be in the medium range. Low humidity increases the risk of static electricity, which can cause film artifacts. High humidity can cause fogging.

CD 8-65A Review question 5
Question 5 asked about the best storage conditions for unexposed film.

PRESENT THIS AUDIO IF ANSWER WAS d: You're right! The correct answer is d, cool temperature and medium humidity. High temperatures can cause film fog. Colder temperatures are sometimes used for long periods of storage. Humidity should be in the medium range. Low humidity increases the risk of static electricity, which can cause film artifacts. High humidity can cause fogging.

PRESENT THIS AUDIO IF ANSWER WAS a, b, or c: Sorry, you missed this one. The answer is d, cool temperature and medium humidity. High temperatures can cause film fog. Colder temperatures are sometimes used for long periods of storage. Humidity should be in the medium range. Low humidity increases the risk of static electricity, which can cause film artifacts. High humidity can cause fogging.

SLIDE 8-68/CD 8-66 Review question 6
Question 6 asked what process accounts for the functioning of intensifying screens.

The correct answer is b, x-ray photons striking the screen produce light photons. The greater number of light photons interact with the film more quickly, thereby allowing the exposure to be shorter.

Answer a was that the number of x-ray photons is doubled by the screen. This is not true, the number of x-ray photons depends on the x-ray beam, and the intensifying screen does not produce any new x-ray photons.

Answer c, that the screen produces free electrons that migrate to the sensitivity speck, confuses what is happening in the screen and in the film. The migration of electrons to sensitivity specks occurs in the film, not in the screen.

CD 8-66A Review question 6
Question 6 asked what process accounts for the functioning of intensifying screens.

PRESENT THIS AUDIO IF ANSWER WAS b: You correctly answered b, x-ray photons striking the screen produce light photons. The greater number of light photons interact with the film more quickly, thereby allowing the exposure to be shorter.

PRESENT THIS AUDIO IF ANSWER WAS a: No, you missed it by answering a, that the number of x-ray photons is doubled by the screen. This is not true, the number of x-ray photons depends on the x-ray beam, and the intensifying screen does not produce any new x-ray photons. The correct answer is b, x-ray photons striking the screen produce light photons. The greater number of light photons interact with the film more quickly, thereby allowing the exposure to be shorter.

PRESENT THIS AUDIO IF ANSWER WAS c: Oops, you missed it by answering c, that the screen produces free electrons that migrate to the sensitivity speck, confusing what is happening in the screen and in the film. The migration of electrons to sensitivity specks occurs in the film, not in the screen. The correct answer is b, x-ray photons striking the screen produce light photons. The greater number of light photons interact with the film more quickly, thereby allowing the exposure to be shorter.

SLIDE 8-69/CD 8-67 Review question 7
Question 7 asked whether the intensifying screen should, a, be in direct contact with the film, or b, be spaced a proper distance away from the film.

The correct answer is a, the intensifying screen should be in direct contact. The farther it is away from the film, the more the light photons generated in the screen can spread out before they reach the film, thereby reducing sharpness.

CD 8-67A Review question 7

Question 7 asked whether the intensifying screen should, a, be in direct contact with the film, or b, be spaced a proper distance away from the film.

PRESENT THIS AUDIO IF ANSWER WAS a: Yes, you were right, the answer is a, the intensifying screen should be in direct contact. The farther it is away from the film, the more the light photons generated in the screen can spread out before they reach the film, thereby reducing sharpness.

PRESENT THIS AUDIO IF ANSWER WAS b: You missed it. The correct answer is a, the intensifying screen should be in direct contact. The farther it is away from the film, the more the light photons generated in the screen can spread out before they reach the film, thereby reducing sharpness.

SLIDE 8-70/CD 8-68 Review question 8

Question 8 asked what the developer solution in an automatic film processor contains.

The answer is c, the reducing agent, sometimes just called the developer. Hypo is another word for the fixer. The phosphor layer has nothing to do with developing, that is the layer in the intensifying screen where x-ray photons cause the development of light photons.

CD 8-68A Review question 8

Question 8 asked what the developer solution in an automatic film processor contains.

PRESENT THIS AUDIO IF ANSWER WAS c: Yes, of course you're correct. The answer is c, the reducing agent, sometimes just called the developer.

PRESENT THIS AUDIO IF ANSWER WAS a: No, you missed this one. You answered a, hypo, which is just another word for the fixer. The correct answer is c, the reducing agent, sometimes just called the developer.

PRESENT THIS AUDIO IF ANSWER WAS b: No, you missed this one. You answered b, the phosphor layer. Remember that the phosphor layer is the layer in the intensifying screen where x-ray photons cause the development of light photons. This has nothing to do with the developer. The correct answer is c, the reducing agent, sometimes just called the developer.

SLIDE 8-71/CD 8-69 Review question 9

Question 9 asked which factors in film processing must be carefully controlled.

The correct answer is a, temperature and strength of the solutions. A film can be over- or underdeveloped if the temperature is either too high or too low or the solution strength is too strong or too weak.

Answer b, film size and speed, involves factors to select before making the exposure, not during the film processing.

Answer c, film and intensifying screen construction, is not correct because these are not processing factors.

CD 8-69A Review question 9
Question 9 asked which factors in film processing must be carefully controlled.

PRESENT THIS AUDIO IF ANSWER WAS a: Yes, you're right. The correct answer is a, temperature and strength of the solutions. A film can be over- or underdeveloped if the temperature is either too high or too low or the solution strength is too strong or too weak.

PRESENT THIS AUDIO IF ANSWER WAS b: Sorry, but you missed it. Answer b, film size and speed, involves factors to select before making the exposure, not during the film processing. The correct answer is a, temperature and strength of the solutions. A film can be over- or underdeveloped if the temperature is either too high or too low or the solution strength is too strong or too weak.

PRESENT THIS AUDIO IF ANSWER WAS c: Sorry, but you missed it. You answered, c, about the construction of the film and screen; these are important, but these are not processing factors. The correct answer is a, temperature and strength of the solutions. A film can be over- or underdeveloped if the temperature is either too high or too low or the solution strength is too strong or too weak.

SLIDE 8-72/CD 8-70 Review question 10
Question 10 asked you for the term for markings or images on the final film not resulting from the attenuation of the x-ray beam passing though the patient.

The correct answer is artifact. Artifacts can be caused by mishandling the film or by many environmental factors such as temperature, humidity, radiation, and so on.

CD 8-70A Review question 10
Question 10 asked you for the term for markings or images on the final film not resulting from the attenuation of the x ray beam passing though the patient.

PRESENT THIS AUDIO IF ANSWER WAS artifact or artifacts: Yes, you're right. The correct answer is artifact. Artifacts can be caused by mishandling the film or by many environmental factors such as temperature, humidity, radiation, and so on.

PRESENT THIS AUDIO IF ANSWER WAS anything else: Sorry, you missed it. The correct answer is artifact. Artifacts can be caused by mishandling the film or by many environmental factors such as temperature, humidity, radiation, and so on.

SLIDE 8-73/CD 8-71 Quiz conclusion
This concludes the self-assessment quiz. This was not intended as a test, so don't feel bad if you missed some. All that means is that you probably need to review this module or study your textbook more carefully.

CD 8-71A Quiz feedback
FOR SCORE OF 10, THIS AUDIO: You've done an excellent job here with a difficult subject. Clearly you are studying well, and you seem to have worked through the tutorial carefully.

FOR SCORE OF 9, THIS AUDIO: You've done well with a difficult subject. Clearly you are studying and paying attention to the subject. Maybe next time you'll get the perfect score!

FOR SCORE OF 7-8, THIS AUDIO: Your score is about average. I'd suggest you review this material in your textbook. You may also find it helpful, next time, to read the material in your book before coming to the computer to take the tutorial. And don't hesitate to talk to your instructor if you have trouble after both reading the textbook and working through the multimedia tutorial.

FOR SCORE OF 5-6, THIS AUDIO: Your score is below average. You need to review this material in your textbook, and perhaps you should come back and take this tutorial again afterwards. You may have just been unprepared this time, or if you are having trouble after both reading the textbook and working through the multimedia tutorial, be sure to talk to your instructor.

FOR SCORE OF 0-4, THIS AUDIO: Your score is rather low. Don't feel too bad; these are, after all, difficult concepts to grasp. If you tried your best here but are having this much difficulty with the material, you should first go to your textbook and see if you can understand the material there. If it still seems difficult, please ask your instructor for additional study aids.

SLIDE 8-74/CD 8-72 Exam instructions

In the next 7 or 8 minutes you will be presented with 15 multiple-choice questions. Select the one best answer choice. Get ready a blank sheet of paper, numbered 1 to 15 down the left side. As you take the examination, write the letter corresponding to your answer choice next to the number for each question. Ready? You will not be asked to perform any complicated calculations.

CD 8-72A More exam instructions

In the next 7 or 8 minutes you will be presented with 15 multiple-choice questions. Select the one best answer choice. This examination covers the material you've been learning about in this tutorial over the last hour or so. It is designed to help you and your instructor determine how well you now grasp this material. You can use scratch paper during the exam if you want, but it shouldn't be necessary for any complicated calculations.

SLIDE 8-75/CD 8-73 Exam question 1

1. When does the latent image occur in the film?
   a. When the reducing agent is applied
   b. When the film is exposed
   c. When the film is loaded into the automatic processor
   d. When the film is manufactured

SLIDE 8-76/CD 8-74 Exam question 2

2. Why do silver ions move to the sensitivity specks?
   a. They are attracted by the negative charge.
   b. They are pushed by the x-ray photons' energy.
   c. The intensifying screen directs them toward the specks.
   d. All of the above are true.

SLIDE 8-77/CD 8-75 Exam question 3

3. Film speed relates to which of the following?
   a. The number of x-rays striking the film
   b. The use of silver or gold in the emulsion
   c. The thickness of the film's supercoat
   d. The size of the crystals in the film

SLIDE 8-78/CD 8-76 Exam question 4

4. High-contrast film is usually used for which type of body area?
   a. Ones that are very thick
   b. Ones that are very thin
   c. Ones that have much variation in density
   d. Ones that have little variation in density

SLIDE 8-79/CD 8-77 Exam question 5

5. A film with a wide latitude has which of the following?
   a. Low contrast
   b. High contrast
   c. Any degree of contrast

SLIDE 8-80/CD 8-78 Exam question 6

6. Which has the most effect on recorded detail?
   a. The thickness of the emulsion
   b. The size of the crystals in the film
   c. The size of the crystals in the screen
   d. All have the same effect.

SLIDE 8-81/CD 8-79 Exam question 7

7. For any particular application, which is true?
   a. The film and screen are selected in combination.
   b. The film is selected, and any screen available can be used.
   c. The screen is selected, and any film available can be used.

SLIDE 8-82/CD 8-80 Exam question 8

8. What may happen to unexposed film that has been left too long in a hot place?
   a. It may be underdeveloped after an exposure.
   b. It may require increasing the exposure to the patient.
   c. It may produce fog in the final image.
   d. All of the above are true.

SLIDE 8-83/CD 8-81 Exam question 9

9. Light photons are produced in which layer of an intensifying screen?
   a. The base layer
   b. The reflective layer
   c. The coating layer
   d. The phosphor layer

SLIDE 8-84/CD 8-82 Exam question 10

10. Where does fluorescence occur?
    a. Inside the x-ray tube
    b. Inside the patient during an exposure
    c. Inside the intensifying screen
    d. Inside the automatic processor

SLIDE 8-85/CD 8-83 Exam question 11

11. True or false: Using a fine-detail screen requires more patient exposure than a high-speed screen.
    a. True
    b. False

SLIDE 8-86/CD 8-84 Exam question 12

12. A damaged film cassette could cause which of the following?
    a. Radiation leakage
    b. Artifacts
    c. Fogging
    d. All of the above

SLIDE 8-87/CD 8-85 Exam question 13

13. Which of the following is an advantage of daylight processing units?
    a. No one handles the film directly.
    b. They are the only kind of unit that controls temperature.
    c. They are smaller and more affordable.
    d. They produce less radiation leakage.

SLIDE 8-88/CD 8-86 Exam question 14

14. What is the primary function of the fixer?
    a. To allow the film to dry flat
    b. To harden the film so it can be handled later on
    c. To remove unexposed silver halide crystals from the film
    d. To speed the developing action of the reducing agent

SLIDE 8-89/CD 8-87 Exam question 15

15. Why is the silver recovery process used?
    a. Because reclaiming the silver reduces pollution
    b. Because radiographic departments can then make their own film
    c. Because film inventory taxes are reduced
    d. All of the above

SLIDE 8-90/CD 8-88 Exam conclusion

INSTRUCTOR CD/SLIDE AUDIO: This concludes the examination section of Module 8 of Radiographic Imaging. Please follow your instructor's directions for your answer sheet to the questions.

STUDENT CD AUDIO: This concludes the examination section of Module 8 of Radiographic Imaging. Your score has been saved on the computer. Your instructor will report it to you later.

Answers to the Multimedia Examination

1. b	6. c	11. a
2. a	7. a	12. d
3. d	8. c	13. a
4. d	9. d	14. c
5. a	10. c	15. a